Practical Diagnostic Imaging

For The Veterinary Technician

PRACTICAL DIAGNOSTIC IMAGING

For The VETERINARY TECHNICIAN

CONNIE M. HAN, RVT
CH2 Veterinary Imaging Consultants, Inc.
West Lafayette, Indiana

CHERYL D. HURD, RVT
CH2 Veterinary Imaging Consultants, Inc.
West Lafayette, Indiana

THIRD EDITION

with **464** *illustrations*

ELSEVIER
MOSBY

ELSEVIER
MOSBY

11830 Westline Industrial Drive
St. Louis, Missouri 63146

PRACTICAL DIAGNOSTIC IMAGING FOR THE
VETERINARY TECHNICIAN

NOTICE

Radiography is an ever-changing field. Standard safety precautions must be followed, but as new research and clinical experience broaden our knowledge, changes in treatment and drug therapy may become necessary or appropriate. Readers are advised to check the most current product information provided by the manufacturer of each drug to be administered to verify the recommended dose, the method and duration of administration, and contraindications. It is the responsibility of the licensed prescriber, relying on experience and knowledge of the patient, to determine dosages and the best treatment for each individual patient. Neither the publisher nor the author assumes any liability for any injury and/or damage to persons, animals, or property arising from this publication.

The Publisher

First Edition 1994. Second Edition 2000.

ISBN-13: 978-0-323-02575-1
ISBN-10: 0-323-02575-7

Publishing Director: Linda L. Duncan
Managing Editor: Teri Merchant
Editorial Assistant: John N. Dedeke
Publishing Services Manager: Patricia Tannian
Project Manager: Sarah Wunderly
Design Manager: Gail Morey Hudson

Transferred to digital print 2013

Last digit is the print number: 9 8

Contributors

JEFFREY SIEMS, MS, DVM, Dipl ACVR
Inland Empire Veterinary Imaging
Spokane, Washington

KIMBERLY K. ZODY, RVT
Purdue University Diagnostic Imaging Department
West Lafayette, Indiana

GAIL ORZECHOWSKI, RT
Summit Industries, Inc.
2901 West Lawrence Avenue
Chicago, Illinois

Preface

The third edition of *Practical Diagnostic Imaging for the Veterinary Technician* captures many of the advances in technology, techniques, procedures, and products to come about in the last 4 years. Each chapter has been refined, and updated illustrations have been added throughout.

As in earlier editions, Chapters 1 through 7 contain the fundamentals of radiology. Chapter 5 on x-ray equipment has been expanded to keep pace with the latest technological advances. Chapter 15 on diagnostic ultrasound has also been expanded to include a section on basic cardiac ultrasound.

We believe that we have covered many of the topics, techniques, and species that we come across in our travels to veterinary clinics throughout the Midwest. This opportunity gives us valuable perspective in recommending only those techniques that we find flexible enough to work in a variety of settings. As with all procedures, repetition leads to innovation, and we have tried to add to this edition any "time-saving" practices that we use daily.

It is our hope that this latest edition will fulfill the need for a text that includes all the diagnostic imaging modalities seen in a veterinary practice, as well as techniques to ensure radiographs of diagnostic quality every time.

Acknowledgments

We gratefully acknowledge the assistance of all the people involved with the publication of this book. To both Dr. Jeffrey Siems and Kimberly Zody for their valuable input and updates relating to Chapter 15, Diagnostic Ultrasound, and Chapter 13, Exotic Animal Radiography. To Gail Orzechowski from Summit Industries for her valuable input relating to Chapter 5, X-Ray Equipment. To all the wonderful people at Elsevier, who were patient and helpful in publishing this edition. To our families for all their encouragement and assistance.

Connie M. Han
Cheryl D. Hurd

Contents

PART ONE

Radiographic Technique and Equipment

1

X-Ray Generation

CHERYL HURD

CHAPTER OBJECTIVES

- List the effects of changing the focal spot size on the resolution of the image.
- Explain how focal spot size affects heat dissipation.
- State the significance between a rotating anode and a stationary anode.
- Describe how rectifiers control the efficiency of an x-ray machine.
- Explain how to read a tube rating chart.
- Describe how to take advantage of the anode heel effect.

Definition of X-Rays

X-rays are a form of electromagnetic radiation. Other forms of electromagnetic radiation include gamma rays, radio waves, and visible light. X-rays are similar to visible light with shorter wavelengths. *Wavelength* is the distance a wave can move in the time it takes to complete one cycle. The wavelength of an x-ray is measured in nanometers (nm). A nanometer is equal to one millionth of a millimeter. Medical x-rays are typically 0.05 to 0.01 nm. A short wavelength such as this allows x-rays to penetrate objects where visible light is reflected or absorbed. X-rays can be thought of not only as having waveform, but also as representing small packets of energy called *quanta* or *photons*.

Fundamental Properties of X-Rays

X-rays have short wavelengths and demonstrate the following properties:

1. Are able to penetrate materials that absorb or reflect light, with the amount of absorption dependent on atomic number, density of the object, and energy of the x-rays.
2. Cause certain substances to emit radiation of longer wavelengths or to fluoresce.
3. Can produce a latent image on photographic film, which can then be made visible by the development process.
4. Have the ability to excite or ionize atoms and molecules of a substance.

5. Can ionize gases (remove electrons from atoms to form ions) that can be used for measuring and controlling exposure.

X-Ray Tube Anatomy

X-rays are generated when fast-moving electrons collide with any form of matter. The x-ray tube uses a stream of electrons directed toward a metal target. The energy of the electrons interacting with the atoms of the target is converted to heat (99%) and x-radiation (1%). Heat generation in the x-ray tube is a limiting factor in the production of x-rays. This is why higher-output x-ray machines have rotating anode x-ray tubes.

> **Of electron interaction with the target, 99% results in heat; only 1% is x-ray generation.**

The x-ray tube contains a heated filament in the cathode where the electrons are generated and an anode containing a tungsten target where x-rays are generated. Both are enclosed in a vacuumed glass envelope. A beryllium window in the glass envelope allows the x-rays to pass with minimal filtration. An aluminum filter is placed across the window to absorb the low-energy (soft) x-rays while allowing the more energetic and useful x-rays to form the x-ray beam. The entire tube is surrounded by oil, which acts as an electrical barrier while absorbing heat generated by the tube. The tube and oil are encased in a metal housing to prevent damage to the glass envelope and to absorb stray radiation (Fig. 1-1).

At the cathode is a filament consisting of a tightly coiled tungsten wire. The cathode is housed within a focusing cup to focus the beam of electrons on the focal spot of the anode. As current is applied to the filament, electrons are "boiled off" and become available to be accelerated toward the anode and to participate in the formation of x-rays. As the filament becomes hotter, more electrons become available and thus more x-radiation is produced. The *milliamperage* (mA) control on the machine affects the current to the cathode and thereby controls the amount of radiation that is produced.

The anode contains a tungsten metal plate on which the electrons are focused. This is the site of x-ray generation. The focal spot is oriented at an 11-degree to 20-degree angle so that a relatively large focal spot size is maintained while a relatively small effective focal spot size is used. The *effective* focal spot is the actual focal spot as it would be viewed from the position of the film. The stream of electrons is focused to the rectangular-shaped target, but because of the angle of the anode, the effective focal spot is smaller than that of the actual focal spot (Fig. 1-2). Small effective focal spots produce better resolution in the image but are less tolerant of heat. Remember that the majority of energy used in producing x-rays is converted into heat. Some equipment has the capability of using both small and large focal spots (100 mA for small and 300 mA for large focal spots).

> **Small effective focal spots produce better detail but lack the ability to dissipate heat.**

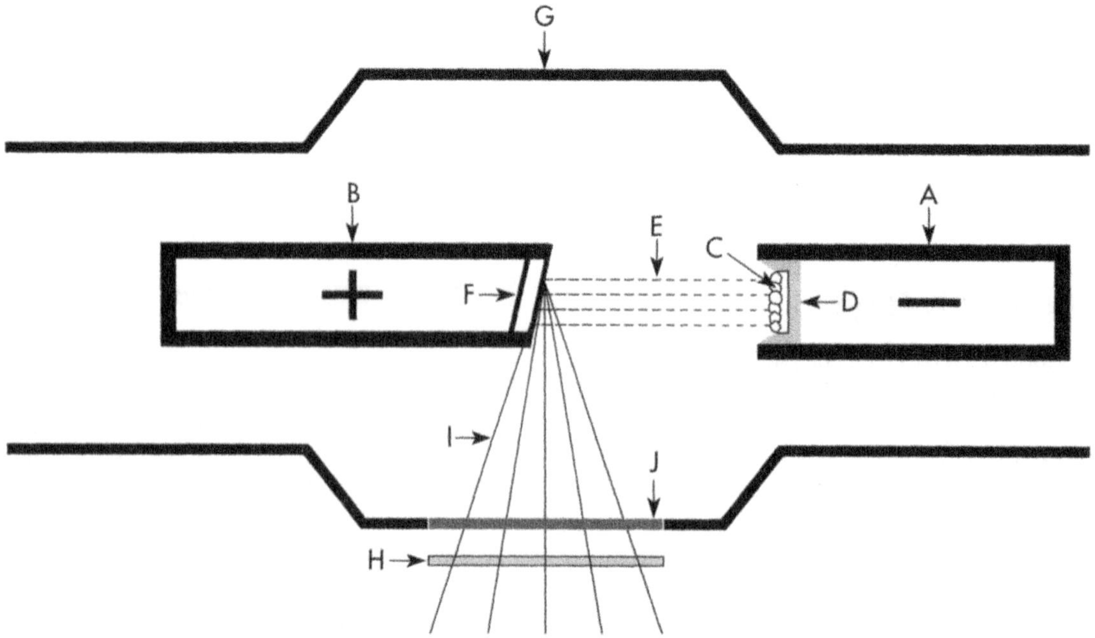

FIG. 1-1 Anatomy of an x-ray tube: *A*, cathode; *B*, anode; *C*, tungsten filament; *D*, focusing cup; *E*, accelerating electrons; *F*, tungsten target; *G*, glass envelope; *H*, aluminum filter; *I*, generated x-rays; *J*, beryllium window.

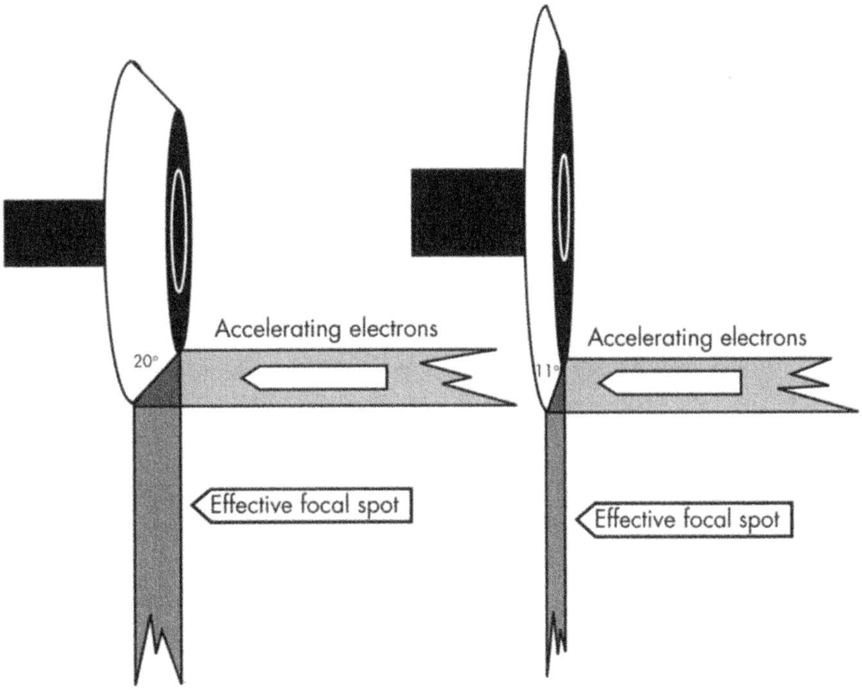

FIG. 1-2 The effective focal spot is the actual focal spot as it would be viewed from the position of the film. Because of the angle of the anode, the effective focal spot is smaller than the actual focal spot.

Manufacturers provide this dual capability by changing the size of the filament and focusing cup. A small focal spot will have a shorter filament and focusing cup compared with the large focal spot. Shortening the filament and focusing cup directs the electrons to a smaller section on the target, creating a smaller effective focal spot. A large focal spot allows the electrons to cover a larger area of the target by using a longer filament and focusing cup (Fig. 1-3).

The problem of heat production necessitated the development of two types of anodes: stationary and rotating. *Stationary* anodes are used in low-output machines with low-mA capabilities (e.g., 5 to 50 mA). A block of tungsten

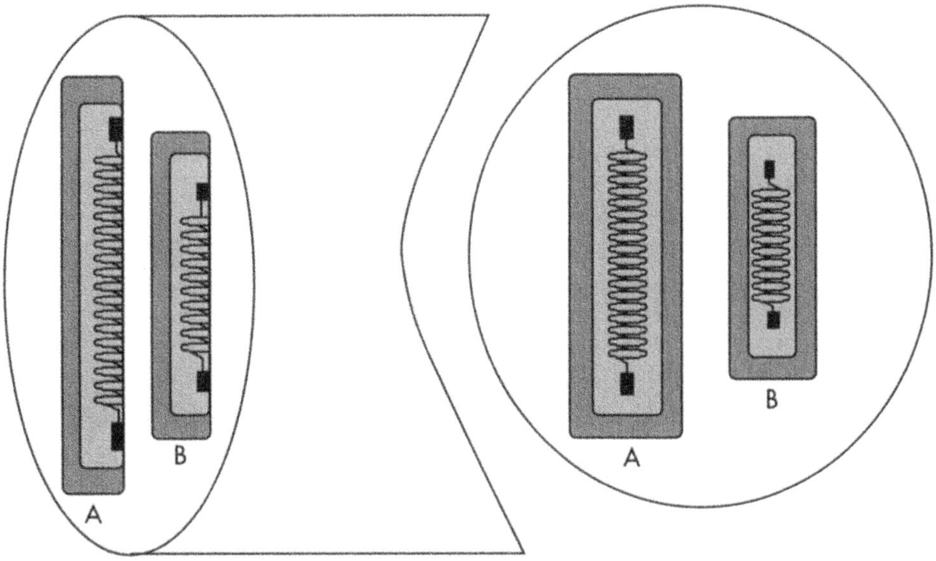

FIG. 1-3 A small focal spot has a shorter filament *(B)* and focusing cup compared with the large focal spot with a longer filament *(A)*. When using a small focal spot, the electrons are directed to a smaller section of the target, creating a smaller effective focal spot. This increases the detail on the finished radiograph.

is embedded into a block of copper on the anode side of the tube. The copper is a good conductor of electrical current, helping to conduct the heat away from the tungsten target. A *rotating* anode is a disc-shaped piece of metal (usually molybdenum alloy) containing a tungsten insert around its periphery. This type of anode is used in higher-output machines with capabilities of 100 to 1200 mA. The anode rotates at a high speed during exposure to dissipate the heat over a greater surface area while maintaining a relatively small effective focal spot.

To produce x-rays, the filament in the cathode is heated to supply a cloud of electrons. The focusing cup directs the electrons into the target in the focal spot area. Electrical potential is applied across the tube to accelerate electrons from the cathode and bombard the anode in the focal spot. The collision of electrons with the target causes heat and x-rays to be generated.

Transformers

High voltage potential is needed to accelerate the electrons from the cathode to the anode. The high voltage necessary on the anode side is produced by a step-up transformer. The *step-up* transformer increases the incoming volts (110 to 120 volts in some small portable machines and 440 to 880 volts in a large stationary machine) up to the required 40 to 150 kilovolts depending on the machine. Relatively low voltage is required by the filament on the cathode side. A *step-down* transformer is used to decrease the incoming voltage, while at the same time the amperage is increased to 5 to 1200 mA. Increasing the amperage in the filament circuit going to the cathode results in an increased number of electrons being produced by the filament, which increases the number of x-rays produced. Thus a direct relationship exists between mA and the total number of x-rays produced.

Rectifiers

The electrical current used in the United States alternates at 60 cycles per second. The electrical potential oscillates in a positive direction for 1/120 of a second and a negative direction for 1/120 of a second. The complete cycle requires 1/60 of a second. Available electrical current may also be single phase or three phase. *Single-phase* current has only one flow of current, cycling as described above. With *three-phase* current, three single-phase waves are superimposed over each other, but out of synchronization by 120 degrees. The second wave starts after the first has cycled 120 degrees, then the third starts after the first has cycled 240 degrees. This overlapping pattern allows a more nearly constant maximum positive and negative oscillation of electrical current.

Electrons only flow from the cathode to the anode when positive potential (voltage) is applied across the tube. During one half of the cycle, a negative potential is applied across the tube, resulting in no electron flow or x-rays being generated. Occasionally, rectifiers are placed in the high-voltage circuit to protect the anode from high negative voltages and the cathode from high positive voltages. Basically, the rectifiers limit the electron flow to one direction—from the cathode to the anode. With low-output portable equipment, the x-ray tube itself acts as a rectifier in a process called *self-rectification*.

X-ray machines are rectified in three different ways (Fig. 1-4). The first method is *half-wave* rectification using single-phase current. This method allows the electrons to flow from the cathode to the anode only on the positive phase of the incoming alternating current. The disadvantage is that only the positive half of the cycle is used for x-ray production. Half-wave rectified units provide 60 pulses of x-rays per second, with each pulse 1/120 of a second long. Longer exposure times are necessary to produce an image. These units are found in low-output portable equipment.

The second rectifier is the *full-wave* single-phase rectified unit. With this unit the positive phase is used, and the negative phase is converted to a positive phase so that it also can be used to produce x-rays. The full-wave rectified unit produces 120 pulses of x-rays per second. Faster exposure times can be used, since twice the number of x-rays is generated per unit time compared with the half-wave rectified machine.

The third rectification method is the *three-phase* rectified approach, which is the most efficient of the three methods. Using three-phase current, a more nearly constant potential can be applied to the x-ray tube. Each phase of the current can be rectified so that six pulses of positive potential per cycle are used to generate x-rays. The result is a more con-

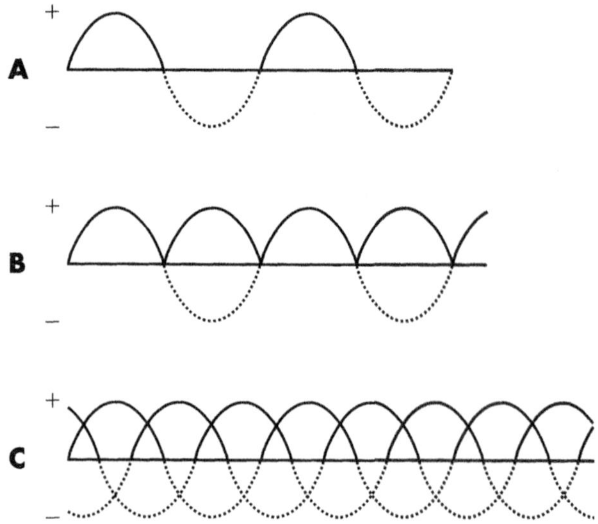

FIG. 1-4 Types of rectifiers. X-rays are generated only on the positive peak of the wave. **A,** Half-wave single-phase method: 60 pulses/second. **B,** Full-wave single-phase method: 120 pulses/second. **C,** Three-phase rectifier: almost continuous x-ray production.

tinuous potential across the terminals of the tube, resulting in a higher energy of electrons and a more constant energy x-ray beam.

Tube Rating Charts

Tube rating charts prolong the life of the x-ray tube by helping the operator determine the maximum exposure characteristics that provide safe operation of the machine. The exposure characteristics are *kilovoltage peak* (kVp), mA, exposure time, and focal spot size. Extremely high-exposure and low-exposure techniques should be checked on a chart provided by the x-ray tube manufacturer.

Fig. 1-5 and Fig. 1-6 are tube rating charts for a 2-mm focal spot x-ray machine. The manufacturer provides a tube rating chart in one of these two styles. In Fig. 1-5, plot the intersection of the kVp and the exposure time to be used. If that point falls below the mA value curve, then that exposure setting can safely be used with that machine. In Fig. 1-6, plot the intersection of the mA and exposure time to be used. The kVp curve directly above that point represents the maximum kVp setting for that mA and exposure time. Multiplying mA and exposure time results in mAs.

Two types of damage may occur from an improperly set exposure technique. *Tube overload* occurs when the combined kVp and mAs are too high for the machine. Too much heat is created, causing the anode to crack. *Tube saturation* occurs when the positive potential (voltage) between the cathode and anode is insufficient to pull all the electrons across the tube. The extra electrons build up on the glass envelope. This "electroplating" of the glass envelope may cause it to be almost as attractive to the electrons as the anode during a high-kVp exposure. If the electrons "short" to the glass envelope and tube housing, the tube will crack and be destroyed.

Tube overload: mAs and kVp too high

Tube saturation: kVp too low

Manufacturers of the larger x-ray generators usually build in circuits to protect the tube. These tube protection circuits usually only protect against tube overload and only at extreme tube saturation conditions. To protect against tube saturation, mA settings under 500 (with 60 kVp or less) should be used.

An excessive amount of time between starting the rotating anode and making the exposure also contributes to electroplating of the glass envelope. When the x-ray machine is on but no exposures are being made, a low current is applied to the filament in the cathode. When the rotating anode is started, the current is boosted up to the full mA selected. Electrons are boiled off from the filament and made available for the exposure. If an excessive filament boost is used and a low kilovoltage is selected, all the electrons produced are not attracted to the anode. The excess electrons contribute to the electroplating of the glass envelope.

Anode Heel Effect

Anode heel effect is the unequal distribution of the x-ray beam intensity emitted from the x-ray tube. Tubes with lower target angles (e.g., 11 degrees) have a distribution of x-ray beam intensity that decreases rapidly on the anode side of the tube (Fig. 1-7). This effect results from absorption of

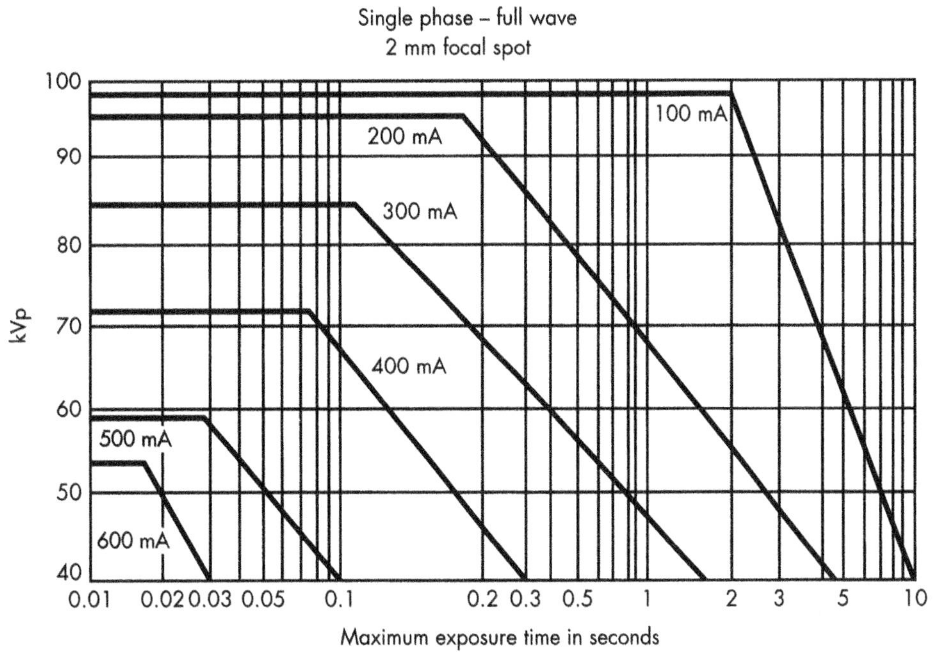

FIG. 1-5 Tube rating chart provided by the x-ray tube manufacturer to plot whether exposure setting is safe to use with the machine.

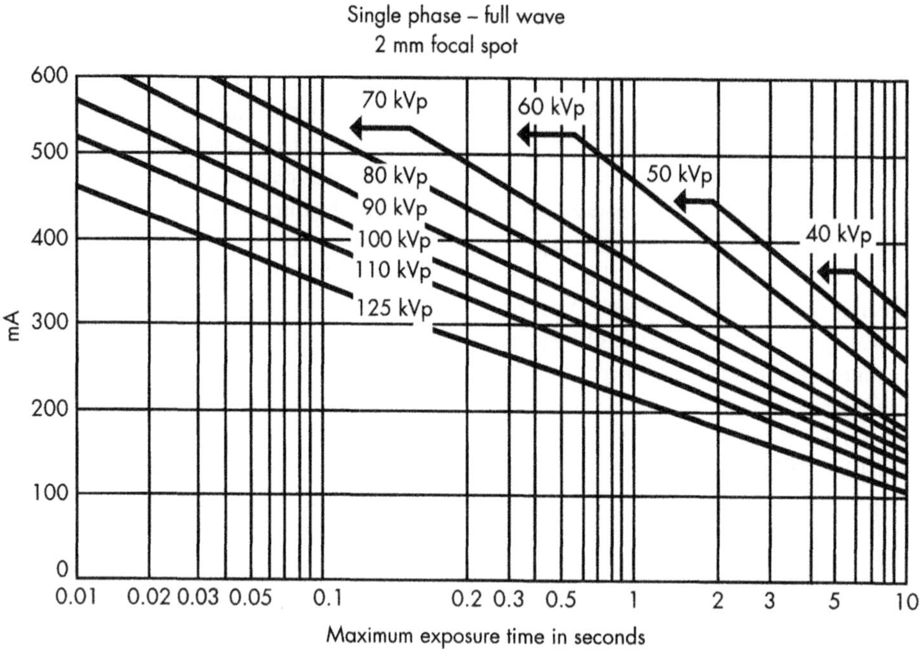

FIG. 1-6 Tube rating chart provided by the x-ray tube manufacturer to plot maximum kVp setting.

the x-ray beam by target and anode material. The anode heel effect is an advantage when radiographing areas of unequal thickness, such as the thorax or abdomen. By placing the patient's head toward the anode side, the part of the x-ray beam with the higher intensity (cathode side) is directed to the thickest area. This provides a more even film density. The heel effect is most noticeable when large films and short focal film distances are used.

Summary

By understanding how the x-ray machine works in general, it is much easier to understand how the x-ray machine controls may be used to produce quality radiographs. The kVp, mA, and exposure time are the three basic x-ray machine controls that a user must routinely adjust for proper exposure. The kVp mainly controls the quality of the x-ray

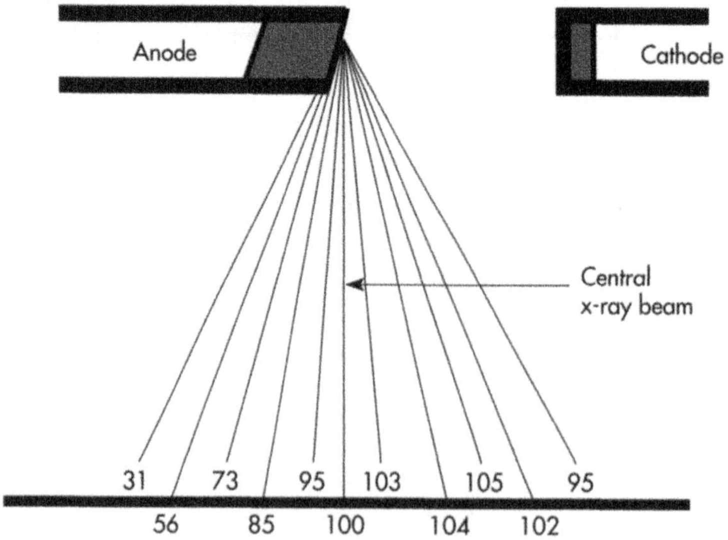

FIG. 1-7 Anode heel effect. X-ray beam intensity decreases toward the anode side because of absorption by the target and the anode material.

beam: the higher the kVp, the more potential is applied across the terminals of the x-ray tube. The electrons hit the target "harder" and produce a more energetic (more penetrating) x-ray. The mA and exposure time both affect the quantity of x-rays produced. If the mA is doubled, the amount of electrons boiled off at the filament and the number of x-rays produced are doubled as well. If the exposure time is doubled, the number of x-rays produced is also doubled because the electrons have more time to bombard the target and produce x-rays.

Both mA and exposure time (product = mAs) work together, as explained later in this text. These variables have a linear effect on film density. For example, if the mA or exposure time is doubled, the film density is also doubled. Conversely, if the mA or time is halved, the film density is also half as much.

Recommended Reading

Curry TS III et al: *Christensen's physics of diagnostic radiology*, ed 4, Philadelphia, 1990, Lea & Febiger.

Douglas SW et al: *Principles of veterinary radiography*, ed 2, London, 1987, Bailliere Tindall.

The fundamentals of radiology, ed 12, Rochester, NY, 1992, Eastman Kodak Company.

Lavin LM: *Radiography in veterinary technology*, ed 3, Philadelphia, 2003, Elsevier.

Morgan JP, Silverman S: *Techniques of veterinary radiography*, ed 5, Davis, Calif, 1993, Veterinary Radiology Associates.

Ticer JW: *Radiographic technique in veterinary practice*, ed 2, Philadelphia, 1984, Saunders.

2

Achieving Radiographic Quality

CONNIE HAN

CHAPTER OBJECTIVES

- Explain how changing the milliamperage (mA) and the kilovoltage peak (kVp) affects the radiographic density.
- List the factors that control the radiographic detail.
- List the types of distortion that can be created and how they affect the image quality.
- Describe the importance of using a grid to reduce scatter radiation.
- List the advantages and disadvantages of the different types of grids.

Radiographic Density

Radiographic density is the degree of blackness on a radiograph. The dark areas are made up of black metallic-silver deposits on the finished radiograph. These deposits occur in areas where x-rays have penetrated the patient and exposed the emulsion of the film (Fig. 2-1). Radiographic density can be increased by raising either the mA setting or the exposure time. Both methods increase the number of x-rays produced by increasing the number of electrons in the electron cloud or the amount of time the electrons are allowed to travel from the cathode to the anode. A higher kVp gives more radiographic density by increasing the penetrating power of the x-ray beam.

Radiographic Contrast

Radiographic contrast is defined as the differences in radiographic density between adjacent areas on a radiographic image. Radiographs that show a long scale of contrast have a few black and white shades with many shades of gray. On the other hand a short scale of contrast has black and white shades with only a few shades of gray in between. For most studies a long scale of contrast is desired. The amount of radiographic contrast depends on the following factors:

1. Subject density
2. kVp level
3. Film contrast
4. Film fogging

Subject density is the ability of the different tissue densities to absorb x-rays. X-rays penetrate the various tissues, depending on the differences in atomic number and thickness. These tissues are as follows from least dense to most dense (Fig. 2-2):

Subject densities: air, fat, water or muscle, bone, metal

1. Air
2. Fat
3. Water or muscle
4. Bone
5. Metal

Bone containing mainly calcium and phosphorus has a high average atomic number compared with muscle containing mainly hydrogen and nitrogen. Bone absorbs more x-rays than the muscle and appears whiter on the finished radiograph. The thickness of the area also affects the amount of x-rays absorbed. If you radiograph an area that is 3 to 15 cm in thickness, the area measuring 15 cm absorbs more x-rays than at 3 cm.

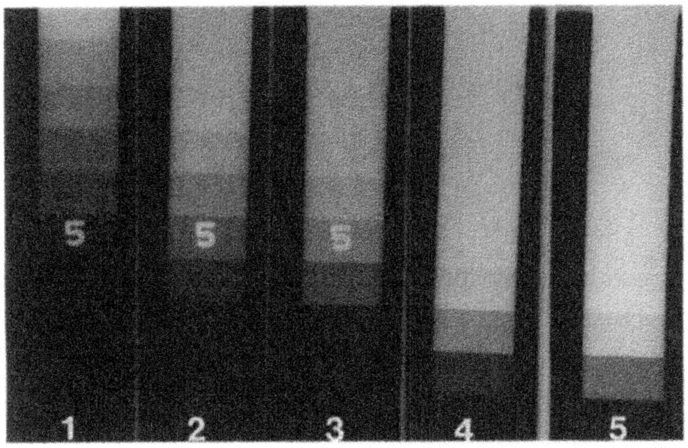

FIG. 2-1 The first image displays more radiographic density than the fifth one. This means the first image was exposed with higher mAs (mA × exposure time).

Radiographic contrast can be lengthened or shortened by increasing or decreasing the kVp. The higher the kVp, the longer is the scale of contrast (the more grays that can be visualized). Radiographs made with a high kVp have more exposure latitude. Minor errors in technique can still produce a diagnostic radiograph.

Film contrast is also a factor that affects the radiographic contrast. Some types of film have an inherent capability of producing a long scale of contrast or long latitude. Long-latitude film allows for more variation in technique while still producing a diagnostic radiograph. When using long-latitude film, changing the exposure technique can shorten the scale of contrast. However, the scale of contrast cannot be lengthened when using contrast film (film that produces a short scale of contrast).

Film fogging can greatly decrease the radiographic contrast by decreasing the differences in densities between two adjacent shadows (Fig. 2-3). Care must be taken in the storage and handling of the film to prevent fogging. Films can become fogged from low-grade light leaks in the darkroom, scatter radiation, heat, and improper processing.

Radiographic Detail

A diagnostic radiograph is one with good radiographic detail. Good radiographic detail is characterized by sharp tissue and organ interfaces. Many factors can affect the detail

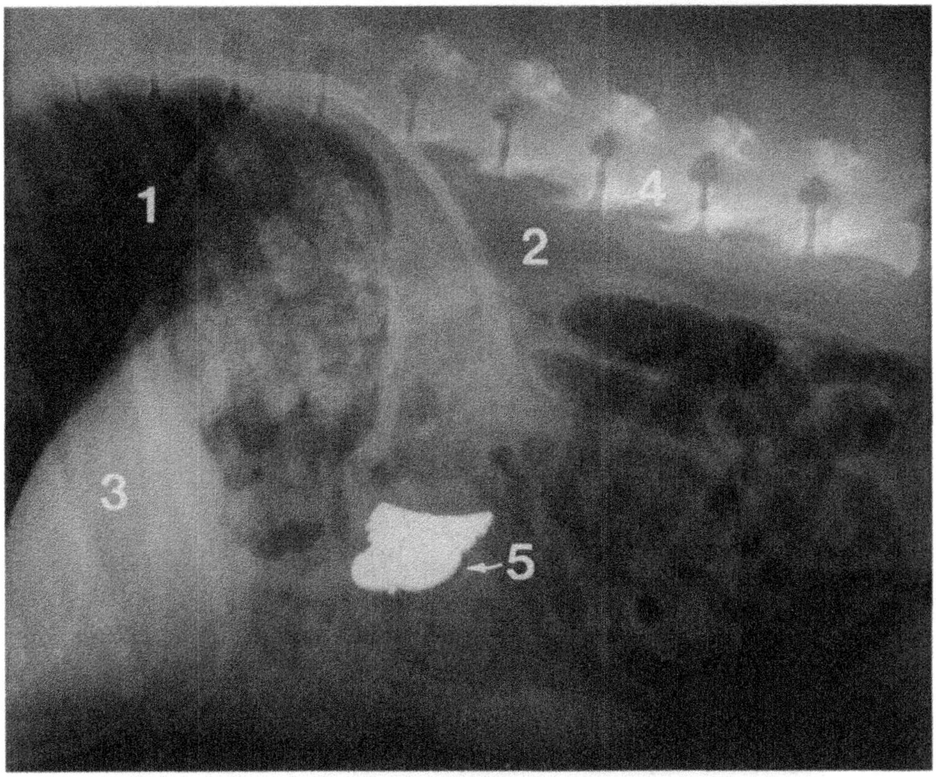

FIG. 2-2 Subject densities: *1*, air; *2*, fat; *3*, water or muscle; *4*, bone; *5*, metal. Air is the least dense, allowing the x-rays to penetrate and expose the film. Metal is the most dense, absorbing most of the x-rays and allowing only a few to penetrate, exposing the film.

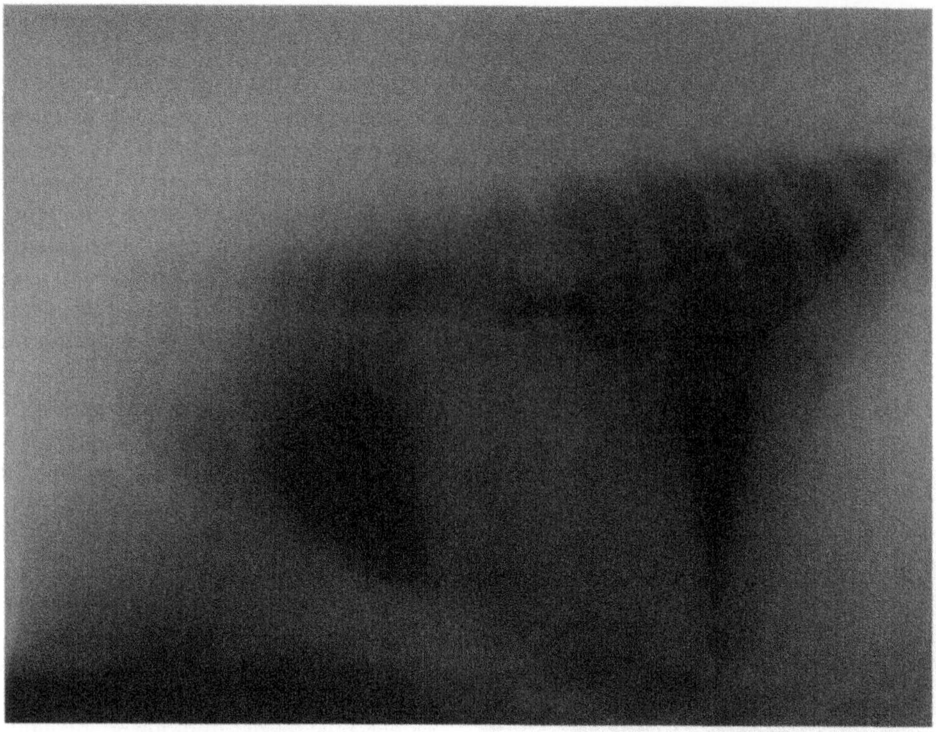

FIG. 2-3 Radiograph fogged from scatter radiation. Fogging decreases the differences in densities between two adjacent shadows.

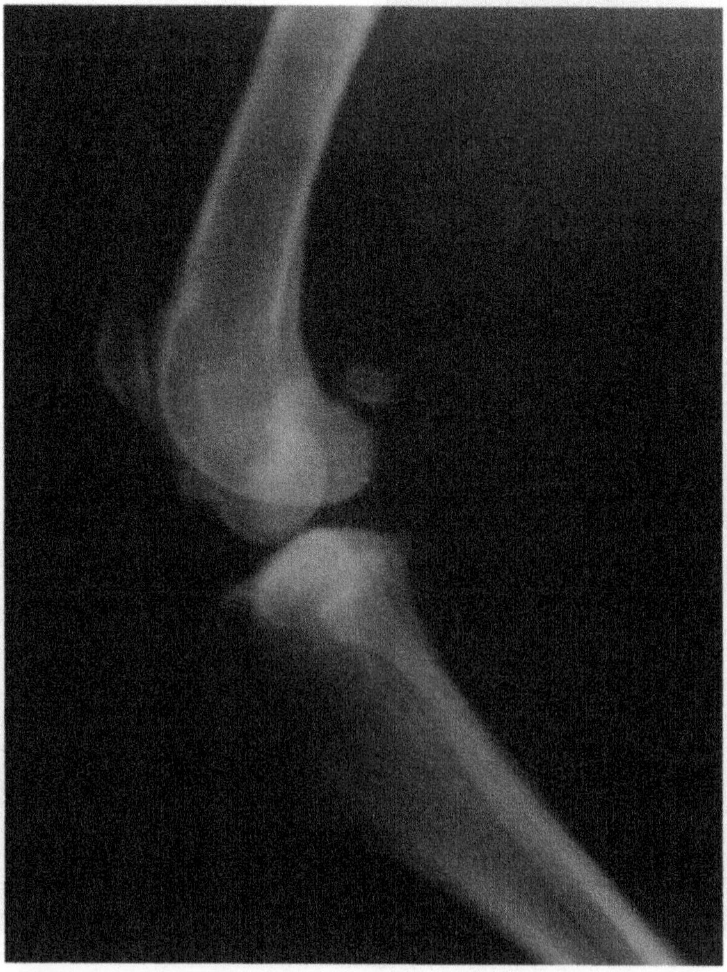

FIG. 2-4 A long exposure time with an animal that is panting causes a decrease in detail because of blurring from patient motion.

on a radiograph. The most common are patient motion and the penumbra effect.

Patient motion causes loss of detail because of blurred interfaces. It is generally a result of a long exposure time combined with patient motion (Figs. 2-4 and 2-5). Using the shortest possible exposure can control this factor. If this approach is not adequate, sedation of the patient is recommended.

A loss of detail is also caused by the *penumbra effect.* Excessive penumbra causes blurring at the edges of the shadows cast by the x-ray exposure. Changes to the following three main factors that affect the amount of penumbra on a radiograph can increase or decrease the radiographic detail:

1. *Size of the focal spot.* The larger the focal spot, the more pronounced is the penumbra effect (Fig. 2-6). Decreasing the focal spot size decreases the penumbra. Manufacturers design the focal spot size as small as possible without losing the ability to dissipate heat effectively.

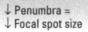

   ↓ Penumbra =
   ↓ Focal spot size

2. *Focal-film distance* (FFD). The distance from the target to the film is the FFD. Increasing the FFD can decrease the penumbra effect (Fig. 2-7). There is a limit to this effect because of the inverse square law, which states that the intensity decreases at a rate inverse to the square of the distance. In simpler terms, if the FFD is doubled, the mA must increase four times to maintain the radiographic density. In most cases this is not practical because the shortest possible exposure times are necessary to deal with the patient motion. An FFD of 36 to 40 inches is sufficient to minimize the penumbra effect.

   ↓ Penumbra =
   ↑ FFD

3. *Object-film distance* (OFD). The distance from the object that is being imaged to the film is the OFD. The penumbra is decreased by keeping OFD as short as possible (Fig. 2-8). By using a combination of these factors, the penumbra is minimized and good radiographic detail can be achieved.

   ↓ Penumbra =
   ↓ OFD

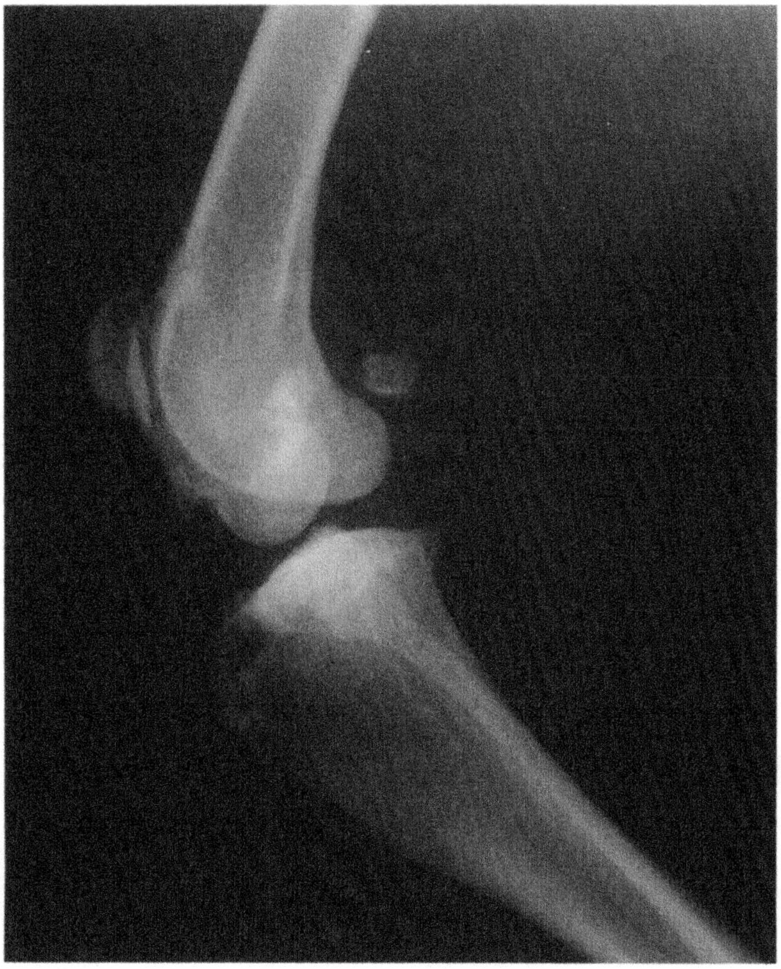

FIG. 2-5 Same animal as Fig. 2-4 but exposed without the animal panting. Notice the increase in detail.

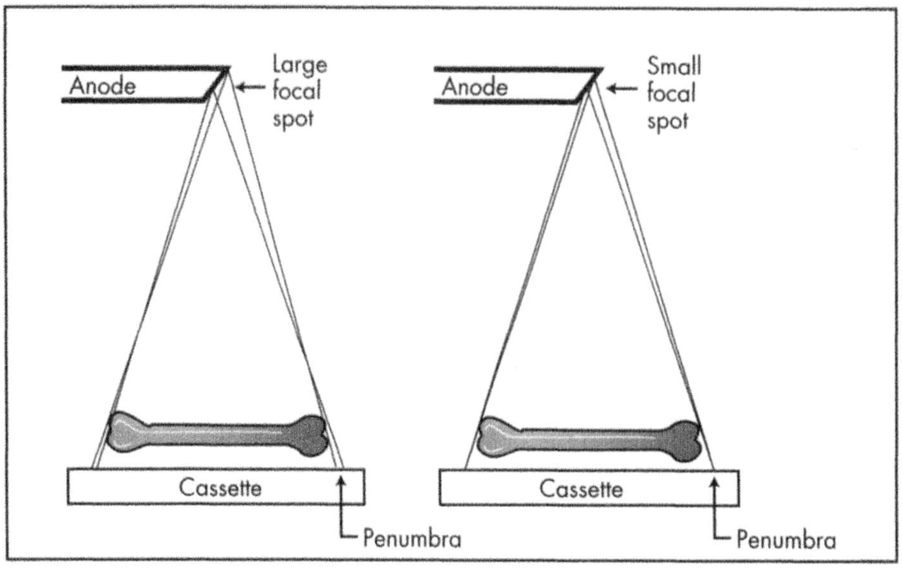

FIG. 2-6 Increasing the size of the focal spot increases the amount of penumbra, decreasing the radiographic detail.

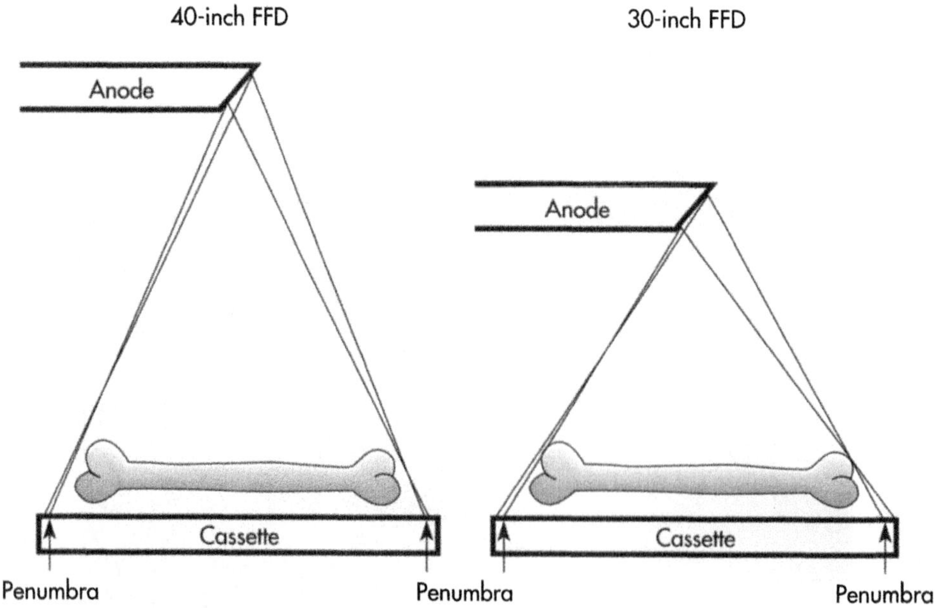

FIG. 2-7 Increasing the focal-film distance (FFD) decreases the amount of penumbra, increasing radiographic detail.

Quantum Mottle

Quantum mottle is a density variation seen on radiographs made using high-speed film-screen combinations. X-rays are produced in small packets of energy called *quanta,* and only small areas of the screens are struck by each quantum that exits the patient. Likewise, the light that is emitted by the intensifying screens strikes the film in discrete areas. If the product of mA and exposure time (mAs) is lower, fewer x-rays are generated, which means fewer quanta to expose the film. Quantum mottle is most evident on the edge of the exposure that did not penetrate the patient to expose the film. This area should be uniformly black; however, with quantum mottle, it appears as a dappled pattern. The increased x-ray–to–light conversion efficiency of the rare earth film-screen systems allows low-mAs techniques. When these efficient systems are used, quantum mottle is

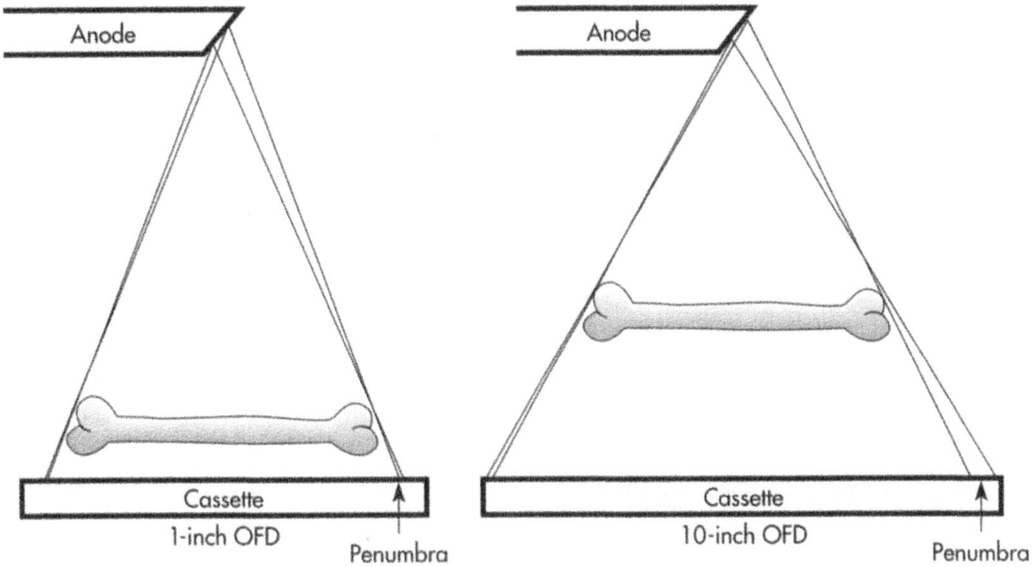

FIG. 2-8 Increasing the object-film distance (OFD) increases the amount of penumbra, decreasing the radiographic detail.

more noticeable because of the fewer number of x-rays needed to produce a given density.

Distortion

A diagnostic radiograph must accurately record the size, shape, and location of the anatomic structures of the patient. Distortion occurs when there is a misrepresentation of these factors. Therefore it is important to understand how the x-rays project the objects on the film.

Foreshortening occurs when the object is not parallel to the recording surface. This distorts the size of the object by shortening the length of the object (Fig. 2-9). Foreshortening occurs mainly when imaging the long bones, such as the humerus and femur. If one end of the bone is farther away from the recording surface than the other, the bone appears shorter.

↓ OFD = ↓ Magnification and penumbra

Not only does the object need to be parallel to the recording surface, but also the OFD needs to be as short as possible. Increasing the OFD increases the penumbra and greatly magnifies the size of the object (Fig. 2-10). The amount of magnification increases as the distance to the recording surface increases.

It is important to project areas accurately between a series of radiodense and radiolucent objects. The vertebral column is a good example. The vertebrae must be parallel to the recording surface. When radiographing the cervical vertebrae in lateral recumbency, if the patient is allowed to lie naturally, the midcervical vertebrae tend to sag. This produces a false narrowing of the intervertebral disk spaces

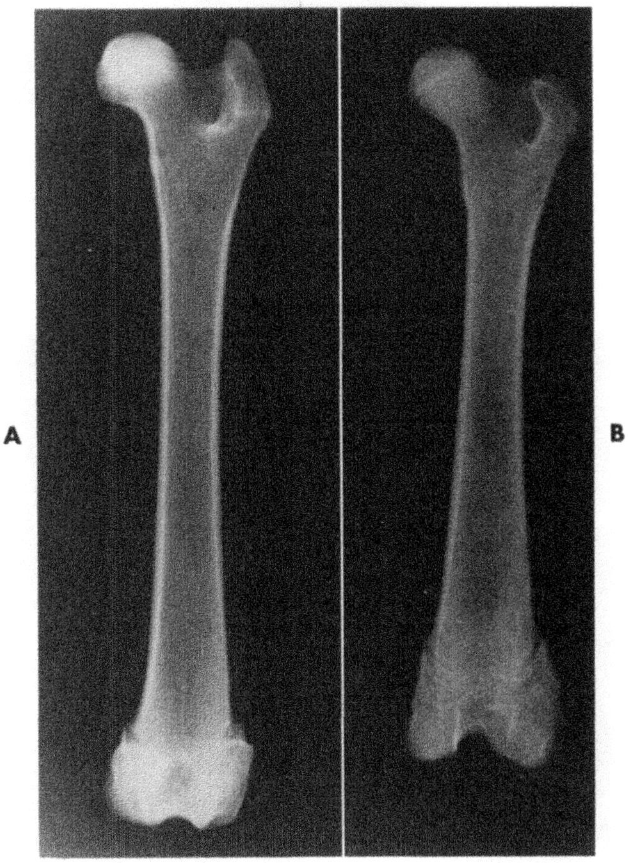

FIG. 2-9 Foreshortening. The same femur is used in both images. **A,** The femur is parallel to the cassette. **B,** The distal end of the femur is elevated 5 inches, placing the femur at a 45-degree angle to the cassette. Note that **B** appears shorter than **A.**

A

B

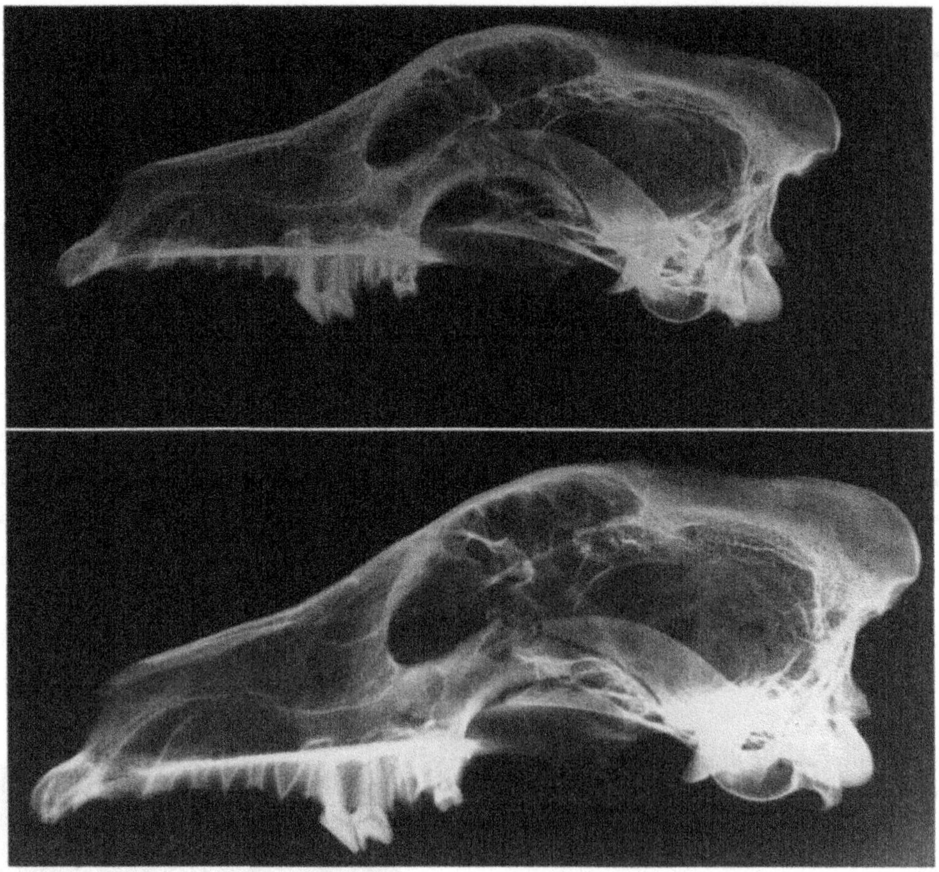

FIG. 2-10 Magnification. The same skull is used in both images. **A,** The skull is placed directly on the cassette (0 inches OFD). **B,** The skull is elevated 10 inches (10 inches OFD). Note that **B** is larger with decreased detail, especially around the tympanic bulla and carnassial tooth.

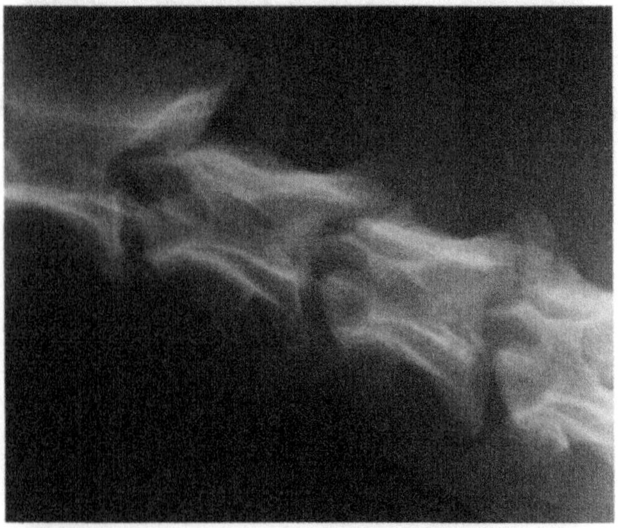

FIG. 2-11 A false narrowing of the intervertebral disk spaces occurs when the vertebrae are not parallel to the recording surface.

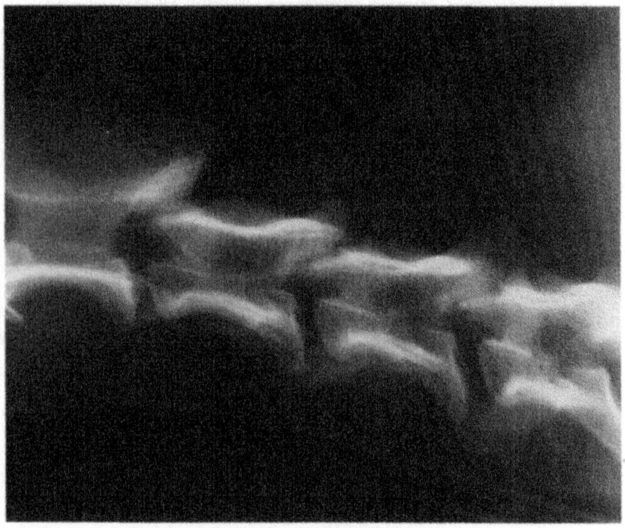

FIG. 2-12 The vertebrae are placed parallel to the recording surface by padding under the neck. Note the size of the intervertebral disk spaces compared with Fig. 2-11.

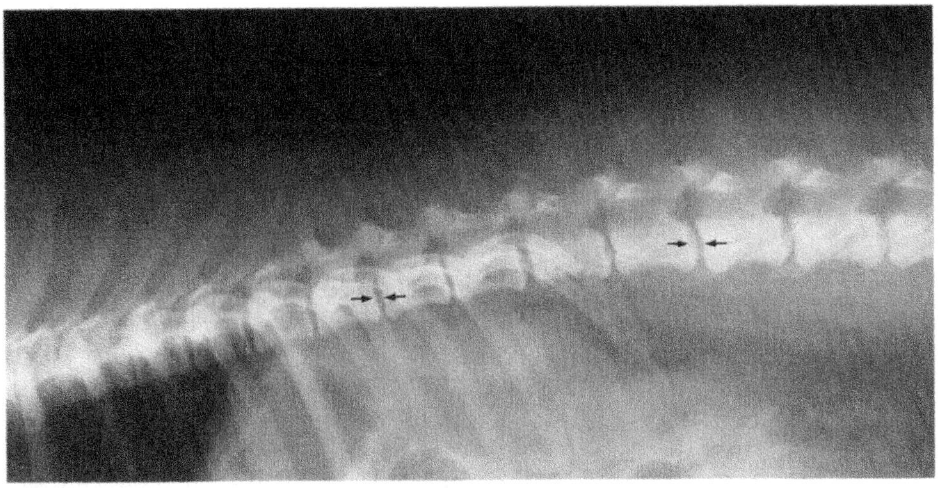

FIG. 2-13 The intervertebral disk spaces appear narrow toward the edges of the radiograph compared with the disk spaces in the center of the radiograph.

(Fig. 2-11). A small amount of padding brings the vertebral column parallel to the recording surface (Fig. 2-12). Care must be taken not to use too much padding because this elevates the column, also producing a false narrowing of the intervertebral disk spaces.

Distortion can occur when the x-ray beam is not perpendicular to the recording surface. The x-rays in the center of the primary beam penetrate perpendicular to the intervertebral disk spaces. As the distance from the center of the primary beam increases, the x-rays strike the intervertebral disk spaces at an increasing angle. A false narrowing of the intervertebral disk space results from this increase in distance from the center of the primary beam (Fig. 2-13). Sometimes it is necessary to make multiple images of the vertebral column, centering the primary beam over multiple areas. This type of distortion is also apparent when radiographing complex joints such as the stifle and elbow. When imaging these areas, it is best to center the primary beam directly over the joint.

Scatter Radiation

When an x-ray photon strikes an object, it does one of three things; the photon penetrates the object, is absorbed by the object, or produces scatter radiation (Fig. 2-14). Scatter radiation does not contribute to the formation of the useful image. It fogs the film, greatly decreasing the contrast, and is also a safety hazard to the patient and personnel. Scatter radiation has a longer wavelength than the primary beam and is projected in all directions. Because it has a long wavelength and is less energetic, scatter radiation is likely to be absorbed by the next object it strikes, whether the patient, staff, or film cassette.

↑ kVp =
↑ Scatter radiation

Exposure techniques that have a high kVp produce more scatter radiation. The thickness of the area being imaged

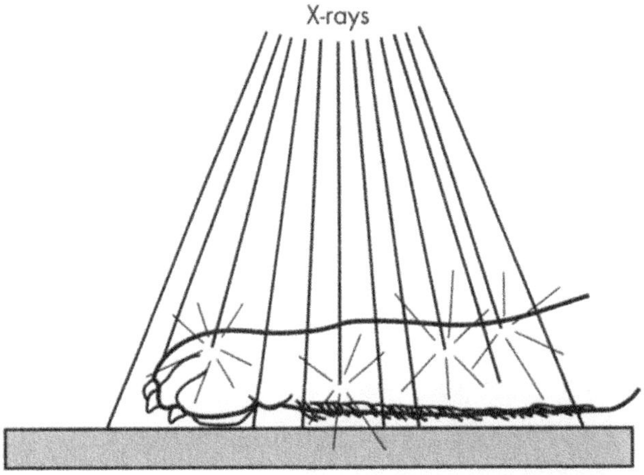

FIG. 2-14 X-ray photons penetrate the object, are absorbed by the object, and produce scatter.

dictates the amount of kVp needed. Areas measuring greater than 9 cm produce enough scatter radiation to decrease significantly the detail on the radiograph.

Beam-limiting devices are often used to decrease scatter radiation. These devices confine the primary beam to the area being examined. Available types of beam limitation devices are as follows:

- *Cones* are lead cylinders of fixed size and are placed over the collimator on the x-ray tube head. This restricts the primary beam to the size of the cone being used.
- *Diaphragms* are sheets of lead with rectangular, square, or circular openings. The sheets are a fixed size and fit on the tube head near the tube window. Diaphragms limit the size of the primary beam to the size of the diaphragm being used.
- *Collimators* consist of lead shutters installed in the tube head of the x-ray machine. The shutters are

adjustable and have a light that allows visualization of the actual size of the primary beam field.

- *Filters* are made of a thin sheet of aluminum and are placed over the tube window. Filters are used to absorb the less penetrating (soft) x-rays as they leave the tube head.

Grids

Grids are used to decrease scatter radiation and increase the contrast on the radiograph. As the thickness of the area being imaged increases, the amount of kVp needed also increases. If the kVp is higher, more scatter radiation is produced. To eliminate the increase of scatter radiation, grids are necessary with areas measuring greater than 9 cm (Fig. 2-15).

≤9 cm: tabletop technique; >9 cm: grid technique

A *grid* is a series of thin, linear strips made of alternating radiodense and radiolucent material. The radiodense strips are made of lead, whereas the radiolucent interspacers are plastic, aluminum, or fiber. The grid is placed between the patient and the cassette. X-rays that penetrate the patient and pass in perfect alignment between the lead strips expose the film. Scatter radiation diverges in all directions and is more likely to be absorbed by one of the lead strips.

The grid also absorbs a portion of the usable x-rays. To compensate for this loss, the number of x-rays generated must be increased by increasing the mAs. Depending on the type of grid used, the increase may be up to 6.6 times the mAs required for the tabletop exposure.

Grid Ratio

Grid efficiency is dependent on grid ratio. The grid ratio is the relationship of the height of the lead strips to the width between them. For example, a grid with lead strips 2.5 mm high and 0.5 mm apart would have a 5:1 grid ratio. If the grid ratio is higher, the grid is more efficient at absorbing the scatter radiation. Therefore a grid with a 5:1 ratio is less efficient than a 10:1 ratio grid. However, grids with high ratios absorb more scatter and available x-rays, so a greater increase in mAs is necessary with the more efficient high-ratio grids. mA must be increased as the grid ratio increases to maintain radiographic density (Table 2-1).

Types of Grids

Grids are manufactured with either parallel or focused lead strips, and these two types are made with either crossed or linear configuration (Fig. 2-16).

A

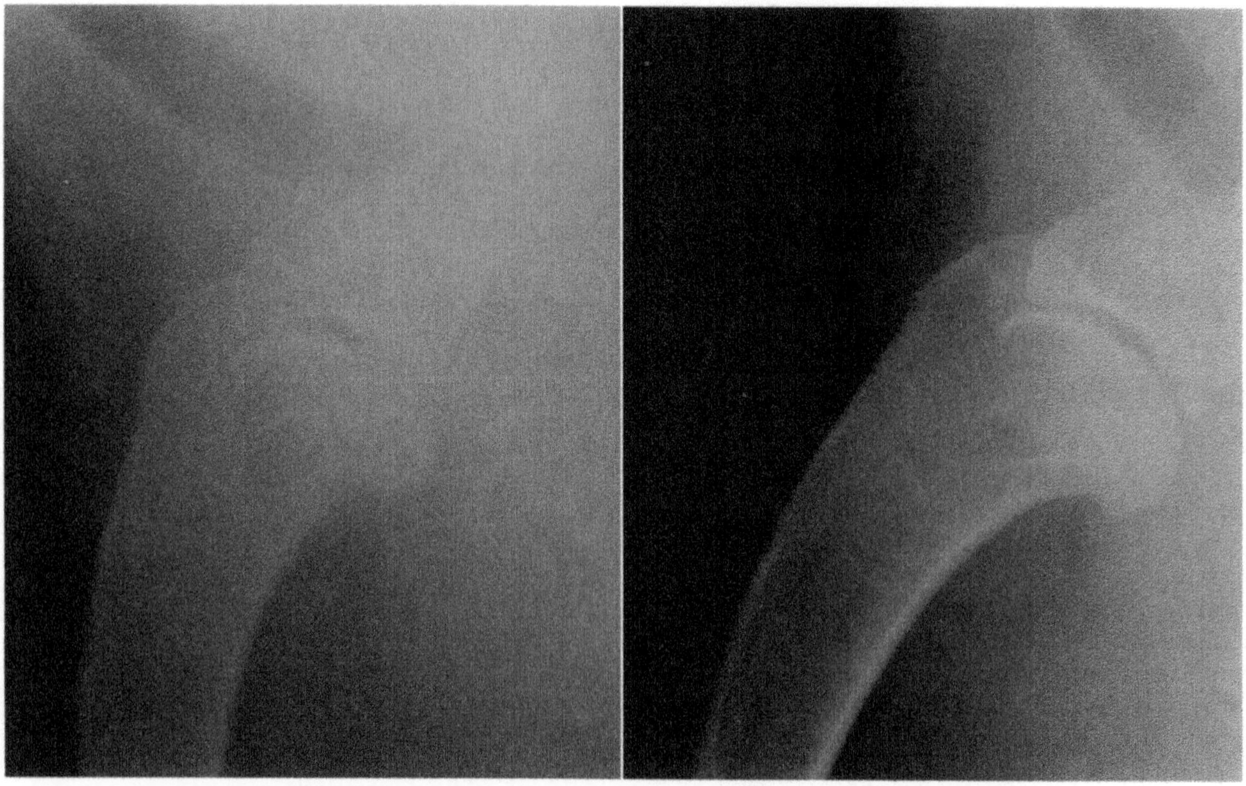

B

FIG. 2-15 Nongrid vs. grid technique. Both images are of the same subject, measuring 12 cm. **A,** Exposed image using a tabletop technique. **B,** Exposed image using a grid. Note the increase in contrast and a decrease in scatter with the second image.

With *parallel* grids, the lead strips are placed perpendicular to the grid surface. The x-rays and scatter radiation that interact with the lead strips are absorbed, whereas the ones that interact with the interspaces pass through to expose the film. A disadvantage of a parallel grid is that the x-ray beam diverges at increasing angles and is absorbed at the periphery of the grid. This decreases the amount of x-rays reaching the film near the grid edges, called *grid cutoff*. If the grid ratio is higher, the grid cutoff is more pronounced.

With *focused* grids, the lead strips are placed with progressively increasing angles to match the divergence of the x-ray beam (Fig. 2-17). By angling the lead strips, the cutoff of the primary beam is eliminated, and the density of the radiograph is uniform. For the focused grid to be effective, a distance or "window" of distances is set up by the manufacturer, called *grid focal distance*. Setting the FFD out of the grid focal distance results in primary beam cutoff on the periphery of the radiograph. Cutoff of the primary beam also occurs if the grid is not perpendicular to or centered with the x-ray tube (Fig. 2-18).

With *linear* grids, the lead strips are parallel to one other. The grid is placed so that the lead strips are parallel to the length of the table. With linear grids, the primary x-ray beam can be angled along the length of the grid without absorption of x-rays by the lead strips.

Crossed grids have two linear grids placed on top of one another. The lead strips on the top grid cross those on the bottom grid. This type of grid removes more scatter radiation than the linear grid. However, the tube cannot be tilted without producing cutoff. Because crossed grids contain more lead, an increased number of x-rays are absorbed. As a result, higher mAs is needed compared with a linear grid.

TABLE 2-1

INCREASE IN GRID RATIO AND mAs TO MAINTAIN RADIOGRAPHIC DENSITY

GRID RATIO	mAs ADJUSTMENT
No grid	1
5:1 grid	3 times
8:1 grid	4 times
12:1 grid	5 times
15:1 grid	6 times

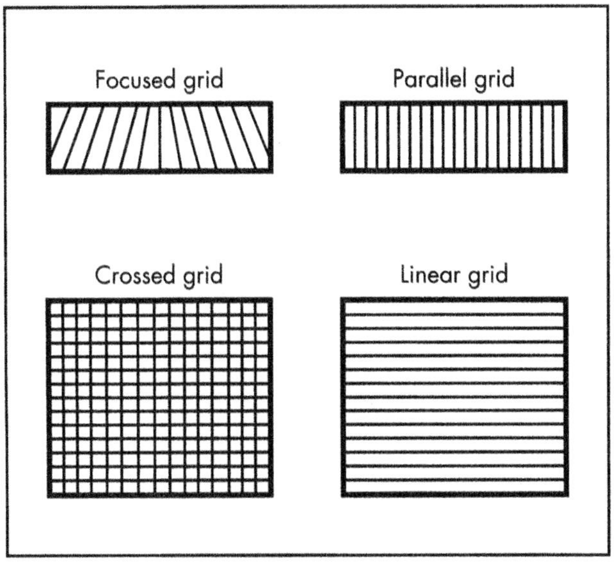

FIG. 2-16 Grids are manufactured with parallel or focused lead strips. These two types are made with linear or crossed configurations.

Eliminating Grid Lines

Grids produce thin white lines on the finished radiograph. The visibility of the grid lines can be decreased three ways. First, the lead strips can be made as thin as possible while retaining the ability to absorb scatter radiation effectively. If the lead is thinner, the white line produced on the radiograph is also thinner. Second, increasing the number of lines per inch make the individual lines less visible. To increase the lines per inch and keep the thickness of the lead the same, the width of the radiolucent strips must be decreased. This produces a grid with more lead in it, which can absorb more of the primary beam and may require higher mAs. A grid with 80 to 100 lines per inch is sufficient to make the grid lines less visible.

The third way to decrease grid lines is to use a *Potter-Bucky diaphragm*, also called a "Bucky." This device sets the grid in motion, blurring the white grid lines on the radiograph. The distance and speed of travel are sufficient so that the lines cannot be seen. The Bucky is placed in a cabinet beneath the x-ray table with a tray to hold the cassette. When using a grid in combination with a Bucky, fewer lines

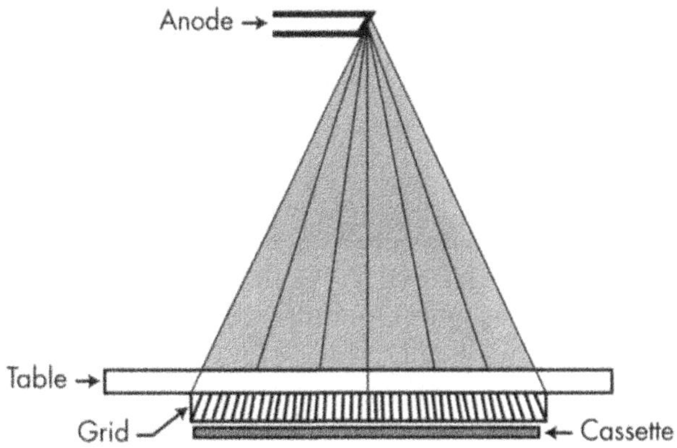

FIG. 2-17 Focused grids contain lead strips placed with progressively increasing angles to match the divergence of the x-ray beam.

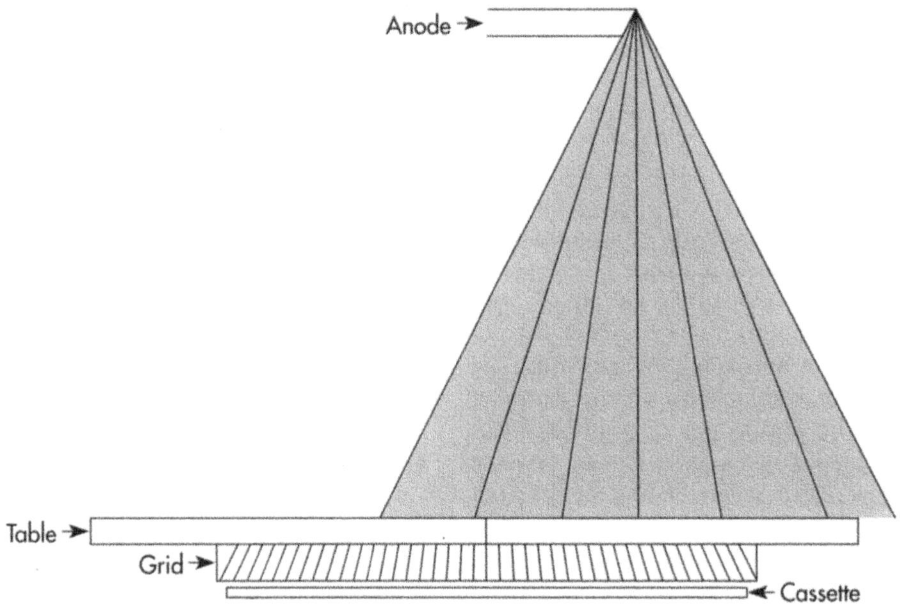

FIG. 2-18 When the grid is not centered with the x-ray tube, grid cutoff occurs. This produces visible grid lines more prominently on one end of the film and an overall decrease in radiographic density.

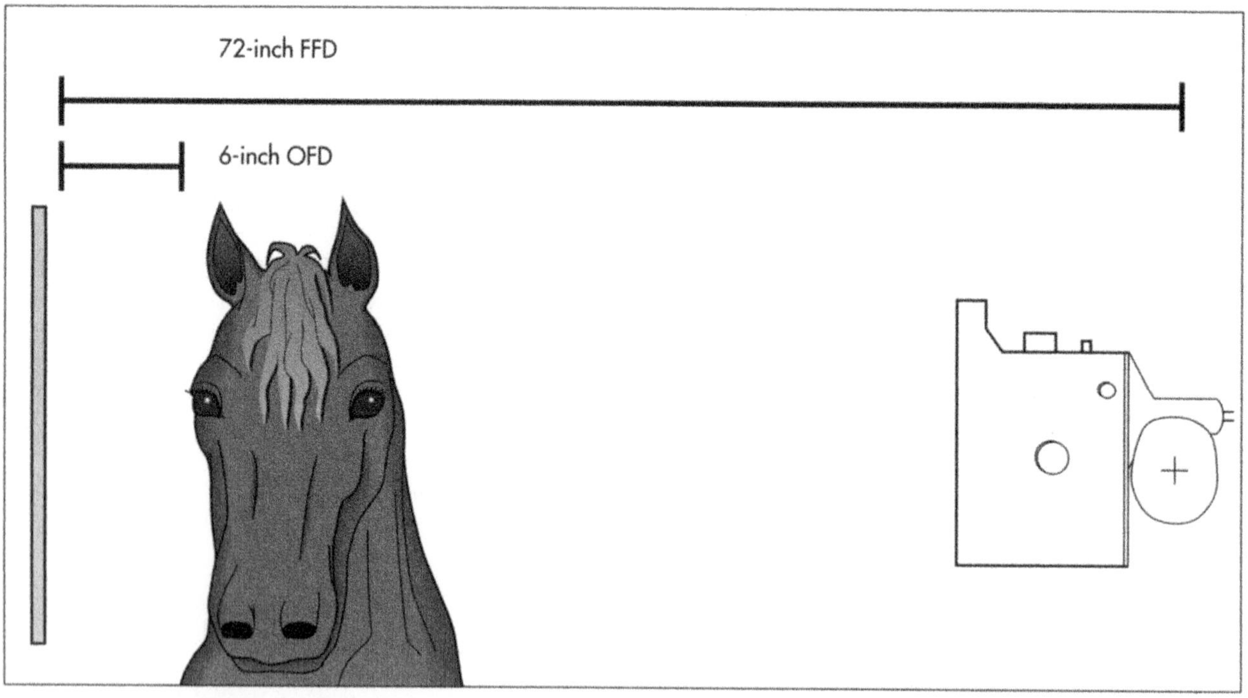

FIG. 2-19 Air gap technique. By increasing the OFD to 6 inches, the scatter is allowed to pass by the cassette without affecting the film. Next, increasing the focal-film distance to 72 inches decreases the magnification and penumbra that occurred from increasing the OFD.

per inch are necessary. This allows for lower mAs. One disadvantage of using a Bucky mechanism in veterinary medicine is the resultant noise and vibration, which may cause some animals to struggle or move during the x-ray exposure.

Air Gap Technique

Scatter radiation can also be reduced with the use of the air gap technique. This method is most useful in large animal radiography, when the use of a grid cassette may not be possible. With this technique, the FFD is increased to 6 feet and the OFD is increased to 6 inches. By increasing the OFD, the amount of scatter that can reach the cassette is decreased. Increasing FFD decreases the penumbra and magnification that occur with a greater OFD. The air gap acts similar to a grid by allowing the scatter to pass by the cassette (Fig. 2-19).

Recommended Reading

Characteristics and applications of x-ray grids, Cincinnati, 1989, Liebel-Flarsheim.

Curry TS III et al: *Christensen's physics of diagnostic radiology*, ed 4, Philadelphia, 1990, Lea & Febiger.

Douglas SW et al: *Principles of veterinary radiography*, ed 4, London, 1987, Bailliere Tindall.

The fundamentals of radiology, ed 12, Rochester, NY, 1992, Eastman Kodak Company.

Lavin LM: *Radiography in veterinary technology*, ed 3, Philadelphia, 2003, Elsevier.

Morgan JP, Silverman S: *Techniques of veterinary radiography*, ed 5, Davis, Calif, 1993, Veterinary Radiology Associates.

Myer W: Radiography review: radiographic density, *J Am Vet Res Sci* 18(5):138, 1977.

Ticer JW: *Radiographic technique in veterinary practice*, ed 2, Philadelphia, 1984, Saunders.

Wrigley RH, Borak TB: The effect of kVp on the dose equivalent from scattered radiation by radiography personnel, *Vet Radiol* 24:181, 1983.

3

Exposure Variables

CONNIE HAN

CHAPTER OBJECTIVES

- Explain how changing the milliamperage (mA) affects the quantity of x-rays generated and the radiographic density.
- Describe how changing the kilovoltage peak (kVp) affects the quality of x-rays generated and the radiographic density.
- State the principles behind the inverse square law.
- Explain how to compensate for increasing or decreasing one of the exposure variables by increasing or decreasing another variable to maintain radiographic density.

Four exposure factors control the radiographic density contrast and detail: (1) mA, (2) kVp, (3) focal-film distance (FFD), and (4) object-film distance (OFD). Changing one of these factors usually requires adjustments in another factor to maintain the same radiographic density.

Milliamperage

The term *mAs* is a product of the milliamperage and the exposure time. Milliamperes control the number of electrons in the electron cloud generated at the filament of the cathode. This is done by controlling the temperature of the cathode filament. When mA is increased, the temperature of the filament is increased, producing more electrons to form the electron cloud. Therefore, increasing the mA increases the amount of radiographic density because an increased number of x-rays are generated. The other factor is the length of time the electron current is allowed to flow from the cathode to the anode. The total number of x-rays generated is controlled by varying the exposure time. Using a longer exposure time allows the electrons a longer period to cross from the cathode to the anode, generating more x-rays. The mA and exposure time are inversely related—the higher the mA, the shorter the exposure time required to maintain the desired number of x-rays generated. The following are some different combinations of mA and exposure time to achieve the same mAs:

- ◆ 300 mA at 1/60 sec = 5 mAs
- ◆ 200 mA at 1/40 sec = 5 mAs
- ◆ 100 mA at 1/20 sec = 5 mAs

> mAs controls the quantity of x-rays produced.

When faced with a choice of which combination of mAs to use, always choose the one with the highest mA and the fastest exposure time. The mAs can be used to adjust the radiographic density by following these rules (Figure 3-1):

- To double the radiographic density → double the mAs.
- To halve the radiographic density → halve the mAs.

Double the mAs → double the radiographic density
Halve the mAs → halve the radiographic density

Kilovoltage Peak

The kVp is the voltage applied between the cathode and the anode. It is used to accelerate the electrons toward the target. The negatively charged electron cloud waits on the cathode side. Increasing the kVp increases the positive charge on the anode. This causes the electrons to move across faster, increasing the force of the collision with the target. The result is an x-ray beam of shorter wavelength with more penetrating power. The correct kVp setting is determined by the thickness of the part being imaged—the thicker the part, the higher the kVp setting, because more penetration is needed. A higher kVp gives a longer scale of contrast and more exposure latitude. Greater exposure latitude allows for more variation in exposure factors in producing the most diagnostic radiograph. As with mAs, changing the radiographic density with kVp involves following these rules (Figure 3-2):

kVp controls the quality of the x-rays produced.

- To double the radiographic density → increase the kVp by 20%.
- To halve the radiographic density → decrease the kVp by 16%.

Increase the kVp 20% → double the radiographic density
Decrease the kVp 16% → halve the radiographic density

Focal-Film Distance

FFD is the distance from the target to the recording surface (film). For most radiographic procedures this distance is held constant at 36 to 40 inches. FFD may need to be changed in some situations. This requires changing one of

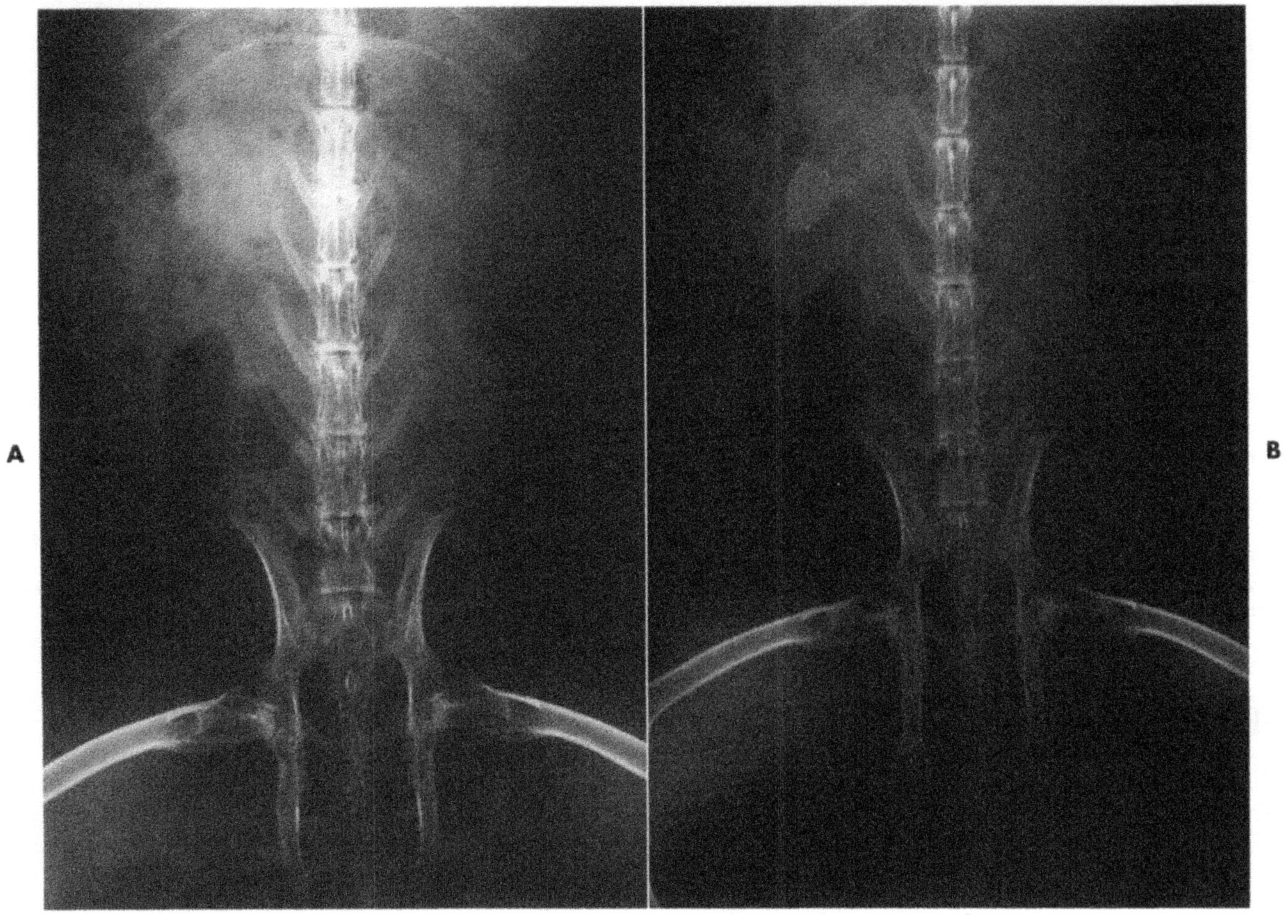

FIG. 3-1 Radiographic density can be doubled by doubling the mAs, or it can be halved by halving the mAs. **A,** Exposed at 8 mAs and 56 kVp. **B,** Exposed at 16 mAs and 56 kVp. Note that **B** has more radiographic density than **A** because the mAs was double that of **A.**

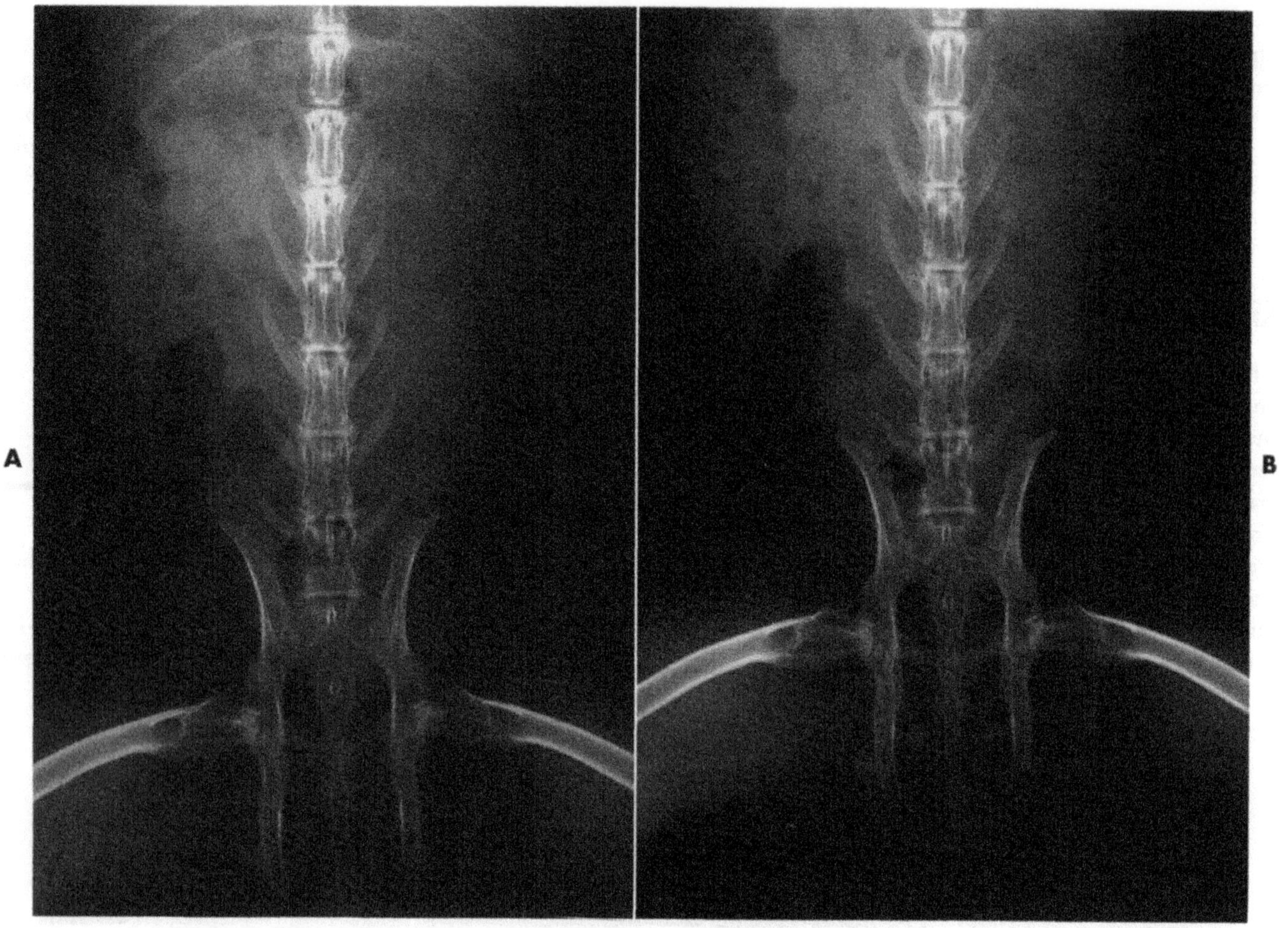

FIG. 3-2 Radiographic density can be doubled by increasing the kVp by 20%, or it can be halved by decreasing the kVp by 16%. **A,** Exposed at 8 mAs and 56 kVp. **B,** Exposed at 8 mAs and 64 kVp. The kVp was increased 20% from **A** to **B,** whereas the mAs remained constant. Note that **B** has double the radiographic density of **A.**

the other factors to maintain the radiographic density. The *inverse square law* states that the intensity of the x-ray beam is inversely proportional to the square of the distance from the source of the x-ray. This means if the FFD is doubled, the mAs must be increased four times to maintain radiographic density. The same number of x-rays must diverge, covering an area that is four times as large. Changing the FFD does not affect the penetrating power of the beam, so kVp remains constant.

Object-Film Distance

OFD is the distance from the object being imaged to the recording surface (film). This distance should be as short as possible to minimize the penumbra effect and the magnification that occurs with a large OFD.

Recommended Reading

Curry TS III et al: *Christensen's physics of diagnostic radiology*, ed 4, Philadelphia, 1990, Lea & Febiger.

The fundamentals of radiology, ed 12, Rochester, NY, 1992, Eastman Kodak Company.

Lavin LM: *Radiography in veterinary technology*, ed 3, Philadelphia, 2003, Elsevier.

Ticer JW: *Radiographic technique in veterinary practice*, ed 2, Philadelphia, 1984, Saunders.

4

Recording the Image

CONNIE HAN

CHAPTER OBJECTIVES

- Define the latent image and its relationship to exposure and development.
- List the different types of film.
- Explain how the speed of the film can be changed and how the detail is affected.
- Describe how the speed of the intensifying screens can be changed and how the detail is affected.
- Describe the proper procedures for the cleaning and care of intensifying screens.

When x-rays generated by an x-ray tube are directed toward an object, part of the x-ray interacts with the object and part is deflected or absorbed. Some of the x-rays pass through the object. Use of x-ray film and intensifying screens provides a method of recording an image created by varying degrees of x-ray penetration within the patient.

X-Ray Film

X-ray film consists of several layers: a thin protective layer, an emulsion that contains silver halide crystals, and a polyester film base (Figure 4-1).

The first layer is a thin, clear gelatin that acts as a protective coating on both sides of the x-ray film. This protective material helps decrease damage to the sensitive film emulsion.

The second layer is the *emulsion*, which contains finely precipitated silver halide crystals in a gelatin base. The emulsion coats both sides of the film base. This gives the film greater sensitivity, increasing the speed, density, and contrast. By increasing the speed of the film, the exposure required to produce an image can be decreased, thus decreasing exposure to the patient and staff. The silver halide emulsion is 90% to 99% silver bromide crystals and 1% to 10% silver iodide crystals. The gelatin that suspends the silver halide crystals is a colloid. It liquefies in high temperatures and remains solid in cool temperatures. When placed in the chemicals, the emulsion swells, allowing the chemicals to act on exposed or sensitized crystals without damaging or destroying the crystals. Once dry, the emulsion hardens again, trapping the black metallic silver.

The *film base* at the center of the film provides support for the x-ray film. The base does not produce a visible light pattern or absorb the light, although a blue tint has been added to ease eyestrain.

When exposed to electromagnetic radiation, the silver halide crystals become more sensitive to chemical change. These sensitized crystals make up the *latent image*. When the film is placed into the developer, the latent image is

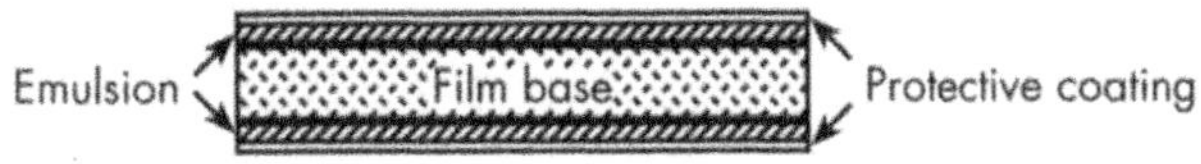

FIG. 4-1 Layers of the x-ray film.

reduced to black metallic silver. The removal of the remaining silver halide crystals occurs in the fixer. The results are varying shades of black metallic silver and the clear film base.

Film is sensitive to all types of electromagnetic radiation, including gamma rays, particulate radiation (alpha and beta), x-rays, heat, and light. Film is also sensitive to excessive pressure, so care must be taken when handling and storing the film.

Film Types

Screen-type film

Screen-type film is most sensitive to the light produced by intensifying screens. The two types of screen-type films are blue-sensitive film and green-sensitive film. *Blue-sensitive film* is most sensitive to the light emitted from screens containing blue light–emitting phosphors. Calcium tungstate and some rare-earth phosphors are the most common blue light–emitting phosphors. They emit light in the ultraviolet, violet, and blue light range. *Green-sensitive film* is most sensitive to the light from green light–emitting phosphors. Rare-earth phosphors are the most common green light–emitting phosphors. Use of screen-type film reduces radiation exposure and also shortens the exposure time, which decreases blurring motion on the finished radiograph.

Direct-exposure film

Direct-exposure film is more sensitive to direct x-rays than it is to light. Because it does not use the intensifying effect of the screens, direct-exposure film requires a higher mAs (product of mA and exposure time) than screen film. General anesthesia or heavy sedation may be necessary to prevent a motion artifact from appearing on the radiograph as a result of higher mAs. Direct-exposure film is mainly used for extremities or the rostral mandible or maxilla, where high detail is needed. It comes packaged in a paper folder enclosed in a stout, lightproof envelope. Care must be taken when handling this film because it is protected only by paper. Pressure artifacts can also easily occur. Some direct-exposure film can only be manually processed because of the thickness of the emulsion. However, direct-exposure film that can be automatically processed is available.

Film Speeds

Film speeds are rated as *high* (regular or fast), *average* (par), and *slow* (detail). If the film speed is faster, it is more sensitive and requires a lower mAs. High-speed film requires less exposure than slow-speed film to produce a given radiographic density.

Film speed is changed by increasing the size of the silver halide crystals. High-speed film has larger silver halide crystals than average-speed or slow-speed film. The drawback to using high-speed film is that with the larger crystal size, the image has a more granular appearance. This decreases the detail considerably. Average-speed (par) film is used for most veterinary radiography.

Par-speed film is used for most veterinary radiographic procedures.

Film Latitude

Film latitude is the film's inherent ability to produce shades of gray. Film with a long or an increased latitude can produce images with a long scale of contrast (many shades of gray). Longer-latitude film is desirable because it allows for greater exposure errors while still producing a diagnostic radiograph.

Film Storage and Handling

Proper storage and handling of the film ensure a good diagnostic radiograph. Unexposed film should be stored in a cool, dry place away from strong chemical fumes. A base fog can occur if film is kept under adverse conditions over a long period. Film is pressure sensitive, so it should be stored on end and not laid flat on its side.

Intensifying Screens

Intensifying screens contain fluorescent crystals bound to a cardboard or plastic base. When exposed to x-rays, these crystals emit foci of light. Placing the film in direct contact with the screens accurately records any x-rays that penetrate the patient and irradiate the screens. Approximately 95% of the film's radiographic density is caused by fluorescence of the intensifying screens, whereas only 5% is related to direct x-ray exposure. With each x-ray photon the screen absorbs, it emits 1000 light photons, amplifying the photographic effect of the x-rays. The film is sandwiched between two screens mounted inside a lightproof cassette. The cassettes hold the film in close uniform contact with the screens (Figure 4-2).

Ninety-five percent of film density is caused by the light from the intensifying screens.

The screens are supported by a plastic or cardboard base. Next to the base is a thin reflecting layer that reflects the light back toward the film side or front of the screen. The third component is the phosphor layer. The two most common phosphors used are calcium tungstate and compounds containing rare-earth elements. Calcium tungstate emits a blue light, as do some of the rare-earth phosphors. Lanthanum oxybromide and gadolinium oxysulfide are two rare-earth phosphors that emit green light. All rare-earth phosphors differ from calcium tungstate in that they have an increased ability to absorb x-rays and convert them into light energy. Rare-earth screens allow a reduction in exposure technique compared with a calcium tungstate screen of the same thickness. Over the phosphor layer is a thin, waterproof,

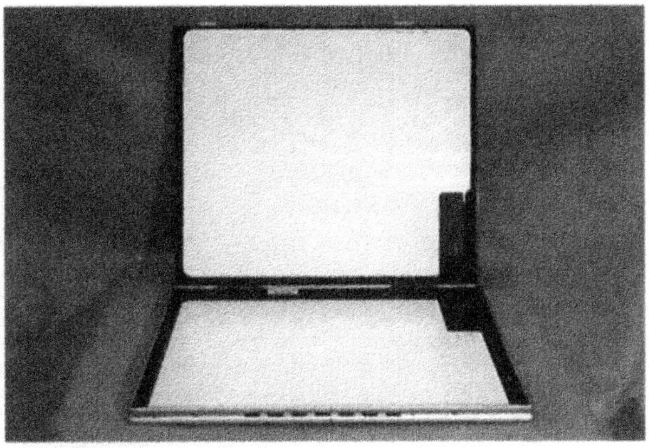

FIG. 4-2 Cassettes hold the film in close uniform contact with the screens.

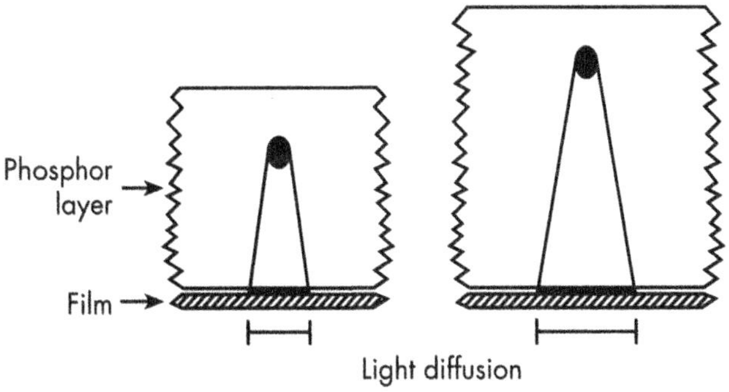

FIG. 4-3 As the phosphor layer becomes thicker, screen speed becomes faster. However, a thick phosphor layer allows for more light diffusion, giving the image a grainier appearance.

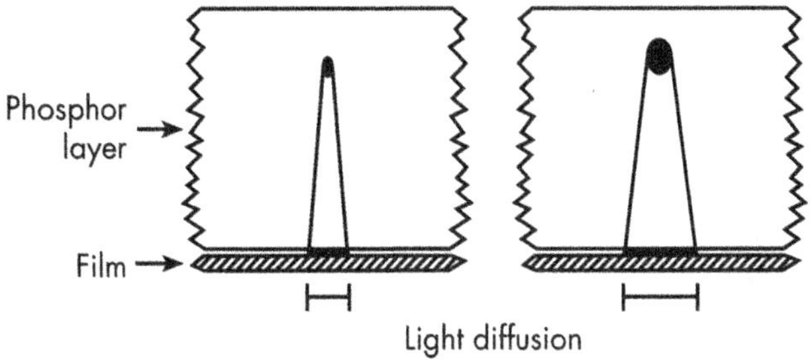

FIG. 4-4 Increasing the size of the phosphor crystals increases the speed of the screen; however, the image appears grainier.

protective coating. This coating serves to (1) prevent static when loading and unloading, (2) provide physical protection, and (3) provide a surface that can be cleaned.

Screen Speeds

Intensifying screens have three different speeds: (1) *high* (regular), (2) *par* (medium), and (3) *slow* (detail or fine). High-speed screens require less exposure compared with the par or slow speeds, but detail is decreased. With shorter exposure times, the high-speed screens are ideal for soft tissues with unavoidable movement, such as the thorax and abdomen. Better detail can be achieved with slow-speed screens requiring a longer exposure time. When changing from a high-speed to a par-speed screen, the mAs needs to be increased two times. When changing from a high-speed to a slow-speed screen, the mAs needs to be increased four times to maintain the radiographic density.

Three methods are available for changing the speed of screens, as follows:

1. Increase the thickness of the phosphor layer. A thicker layer absorbs more x-ray energies than a thin layer and emits more light. The disadvantage of increasing the thickness is that it allows the light to diffuse, causing the image to be blurred (Figure 4-3).
2. Increase or decrease the size of the phosphor crystals. Larger phosphor crystals can absorb more x-rays and emit a larger area of light (Figure 4-4). High-speed screens have larger crystals than par-speed or slow-speed screens. This means that high-speed screens require a lower mAs than the other screens, but the image has a grainier appearance.
3. Light-absorbing dyes are sometimes incorporated into the phosphor layer. These dyes absorb the lateral-spreading light that will blur the image. The amount of light that reaches the film is decreased, but the increase in detail is helpful.

By combining the factors of thickness, crystal size, and dyes, a good balance of speed and detail can be achieved.

Film-Screen Combinations

Fast-speed or slow-speed systems can be created by combining a different speed of film with the different screens. A slow-speed system produces an image with excellent detail that requires the highest exposure. As the speed of the system increases, the amount of exposure needed to produce the image decreases, as does the degree of detail. The image appears grainier at higher speeds.

> A 400-speed film-screen combination is used for most general veterinary radiography.

Most manufacturers classify their film screen systems as 100-, 200-, and 400-speed systems. The 100-speed system produces excellent detail; however, it is the slowest system, requiring the highest exposure. The 200-speed system produces good detail and is twice as fast as the 100-speed system. The 400-speed system is used for most veterinary applications, producing a good balance of speed and detail.

A par-speed film is used with these three systems. Faster systems can be created by using a high-speed film. High-speed film in a 400-speed screen increases the system to an 800-speed system. This means a radiograph can be taken at half the mAs, but the detail is decreased. Systems up to 1200 speed can be created by changing the speed of the screens and film. These fast speeds are most often used for special applications.

For most general veterinary radiography, a 400-speed system works well. A practice that does a substantial amount

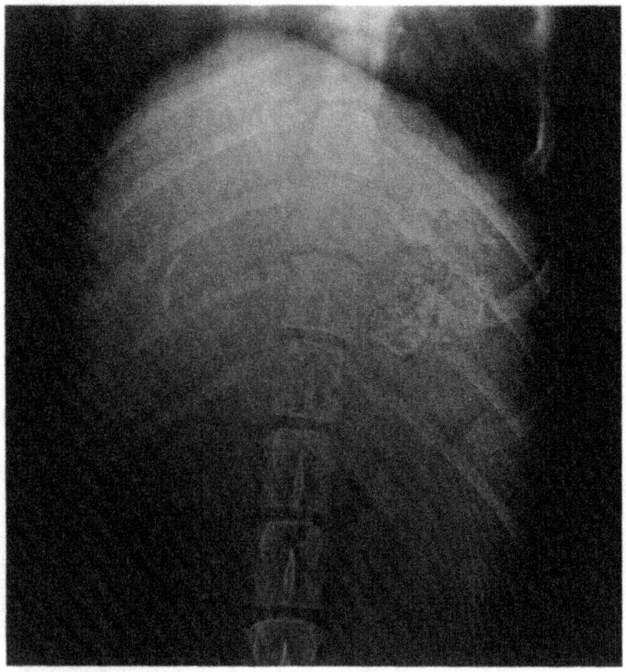

FIG. 4-5 Damaged cassettes can lead to poor film-screen contact. Note the blurry interfaces in the areas of the cranial abdomen and caudal thorax.

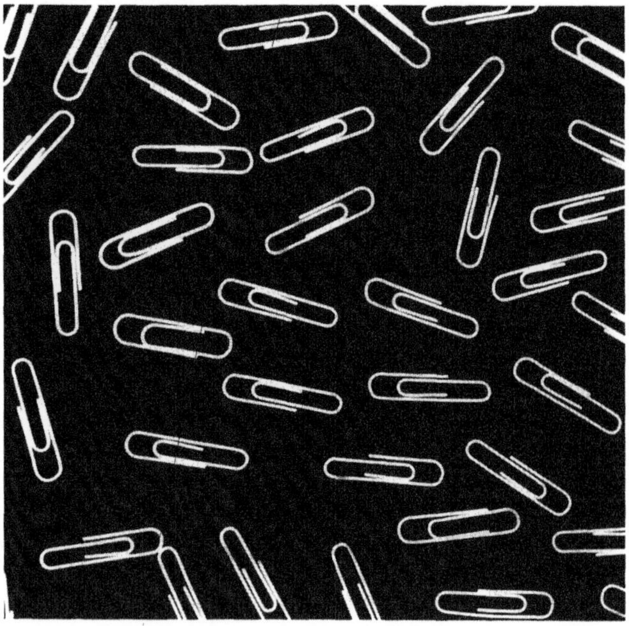

FIG. 4-6 Radiograph exposed to check the film-screen contact. Poor film-screen contact results in decreased detail on the finished radiograph.

of orthopedic radiography may have a 200-speed system for the bone radiographs and a 400-speed system for the thoracic and abdominal radiographs. Low-output equipment may require a system faster than 400 speed to produce radiographs without motion.

Care of Screens

Proper care of intensifying screens is important in veterinary radiography. Regular cleaning is necessary to ensure that the screens are free from dirt and foreign material. Such material can block the light emitted from the screens from reaching the film, leaving it unexposed. The result is a white area on the film in the likeness of the foreign material. Identifying the cassettes on the screens and outside the cassette enables the dirty cassette to be retrieved and cleaned.

Processing chemicals can permanently damage the screen's surface if not promptly cleaned. The screens should be cleaned with a soft, lint-free cloth and an intensifying screen cleaning solution. If a commercial cleaner is not available, warm water is the next best choice. Do not use denatured alcohol or abrasive products because they can damage the protective coating and phosphor layer. Be sure to allow the screen to dry completely before reloading.

The cassettes are precision instruments and should be handled that way. Do not drop them or set heavy objects on them. This can lead to poor film-screen contact and an area of the image that is blurred (Figure 4-5).

To check the film-screen contact of your screens, place paper clips over the surface of the cassette. Use enough clips to cover every area completely. Expose the cassette using 50 to 60 kVp and half the mAs that you would use for a nongrid extremity. Process the film and view it dry. If there are any areas with poor film-screen contact, the image of the paper clips will be blurred (Figure 4-6).

Recommended Reading

Curry TS III et al: *Christensen's physics of diagnostic radiology,* ed 4, Philadelphia, 1990, Lea & Febiger.

Douglas SW et al: *Principles of veterinary radiography,* ed 4, London, 1987, Bailliere Tindall.

The fundamentals of radiology, ed 12, Rochester, NY, 1992, Eastman Kodak Company.

Koblik PD et al: Rare-earth intensifying screens for veterinary radiography: an evaluation of two systems, *Vet Radiol* 21(5):224, 1980.

Morgan JP, Silverman S: *Techniques of veterinary radiography,* ed 5, Davis, Calif, 1993, Veterinary Radiology Associates.

Skucas J, Gorski J: Application of modern intensifying screens in diagnostic radiology, *Med Radiol Photogr* 56(2):25, 1980.

Ticer JW: *Radiographic technique in veterinary practice,* ed 2, Philadelphia, 1984, Saunders.

5

X-Ray Equipment

CONNIE HAN

CHAPTER OBJECTIVES

- Explain the differences among portable, mobile, and stationary x-ray equipment.
- Define the variables used in choosing x-ray equipment.
- Describe the basics of fluoroscopy and how it differs from conventional radiography.

There are many factors to consider when choosing x-ray equipment. The needs of an individual practice vary depending on the species majority, caseload, and degree of technology desired.

Types of Equipment

The three basic types of x-ray equipment are portable, mobile, and stationary units. The *portable* unit is one that can be carried to the animal. These machines generally have a fixed milliamperage (mA) that is set by the manufacturer at 15 to 30 mAs (product of mA and exposure time) with a variable kilovoltage peak (kVp) ranging from 40 to 90. The exposure times range from 1/20 of a second to 6 seconds. The portable unit is ideal for extremities of large animals and can be used to radiograph some small animals (Figure 5-1). Most portable x-ray machines use a fixed mA, meaning that only the exposure time can be changed to increase the radiographic density. For this reason, motion can be a problem for some exposures because of the prolonged exposure times.

The *mobile* x-ray machine is one that can travel to the patient; however, its size limits it to hospital use, such as in the treatment room or driveway (Figure 5-2). These units generally produce a maximum 300-mA, 125-kVp, and 1/120-second techniques. The tube head on a mobile unit can be either lowered to the ground for large animal radiography or suspended above a table for small animal radiography.

Stationary units are those that are installed in a room with proper shielding for radiography (Figure 5-3). These units come with many different exposure capabilities, depending on the quality desired. A general, small-animal practice that does mainly routine radiographic examinations may be well served by a 300-mA, 125-kVp, and at least 1/60-second machine. However, practices that provide specialty services, such as internal medicine or surgery referrals, may require higher-output equipment.

Caseload is one factor taken into account when choosing x-ray equipment. *Caseload,* or the number of radiographs that are made in a week's time, is classified as low, medium, and high volume. A *low-volume* caseload averages one or

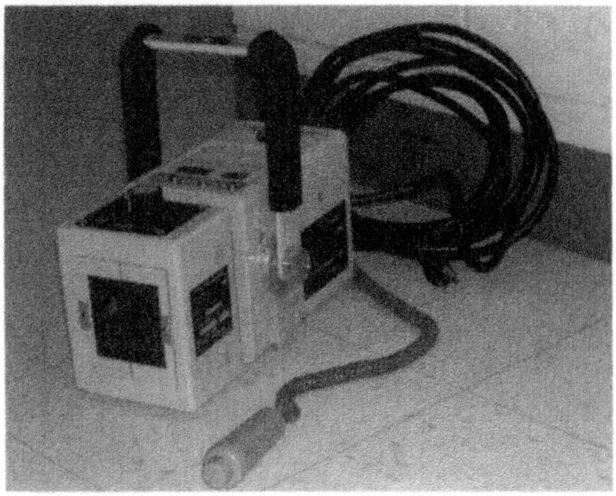

FIG. 5-1 XTec 90P Laseray portable x-ray unit.

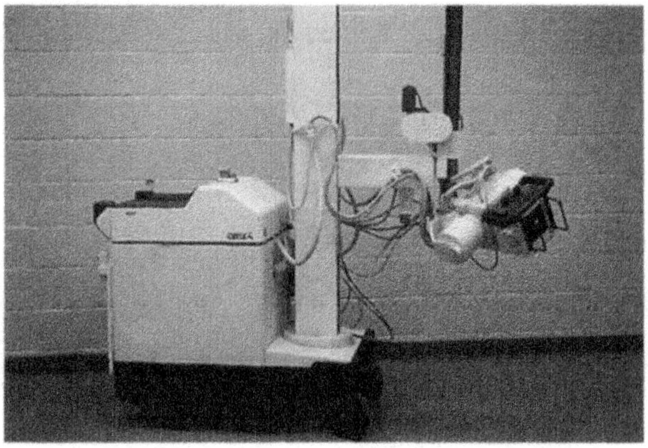

FIG. 5-2 AMX-4 mobile x-ray unit. This unit has been modified to allow the tube head to be lowered to the ground.

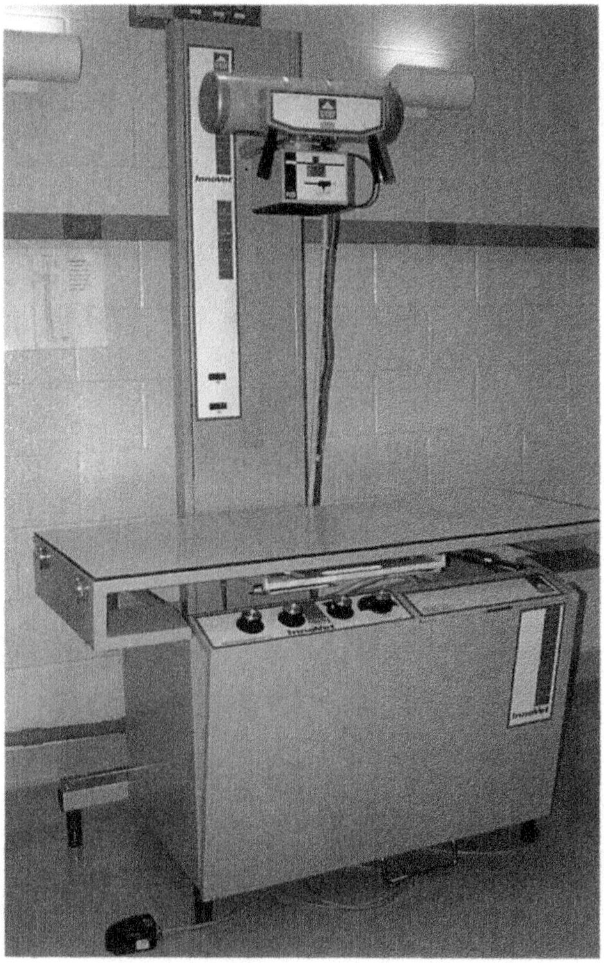

FIG. 5-3 InnoVet stationary x-ray unit.

two cases per week, with the majority involving the extremities of large animals; small animals are occasionally seen. For a low-volume practice a portable unit might be considered. A *medium-volume* practice averages 3 to 15 cases per week. These cases can be a mixture of both large and small animals. For a medium-volume practice a mobile unit might be considered. A *high-volume* practice averages 16 or more cases per week. The high-volume practice would benefit from the use of a stationary unit.

Accessory equipment needs vary depending on the type of x-ray machine used. Basic equipment requirements for a fixed x-ray machine include the x-ray generating system, collimator, grid, table, tube stand, and positioning aids. Since most large animal extremity radiographs are made with portable or low-output x-ray machines, tube stands and cassette holders should be used. These pieces of accessory equipment allow examiners to be positioned farther from the primary beam, thus decreasing personnel exposure. The cassettes or x-ray tubes should never be handheld.

Fluoroscopy

With fluoroscopy, an image intensifier converts and transfers the image on the intensifying screen to a photoelectric surface. Fluoroscopy differs from conventional radiography in several ways. With fluoroscopy, the x-ray tube is beneath the table, with constant x-ray production directed up toward a fluoroscopic screen. The image is then transferred to a monitor and can be stored on spot film or videotape. Conventional radiography produces a single exposure from an x-ray tube suspended above a table. The image is captured on radiographic film. In addition to the stationary fluoroscopic unit, mobile C-arms and handheld units are also available. The mobile C-arm can be used during surgery, and handheld units are often used as a screening method for equine extremities.

Fluoroscopy should never be used in place of radiography. Radiation risks greatly increase with the constant x-ray production that is used in fluoroscopy. One method for decreasing the risk to staff while using fluoroscopy is to depress the x-ray button intermittently instead of holding it down continuously.

High Frequency Technology

Although a good-quality radiography depends on correct exposure factors, optimal processing conditions, and the skill of the operator, a high-quality radiograph is attainable with minimal exposure to the patient and operator by using a high-frequency generator. High-frequency technology has become widely used in human medicine over the past 15 years. In the past 5 years veterinarians have begun to realize the benefits of this technology.

Since single-phase (60-Hz) generators allow output to fluctuate, or vary, and produce an inconsistent amount of radiation, usable x-ray is not being produced as often as with high-frequency technology. High-frequency generators use a series of current conversions and manipulations to produce a more constant radiation output. The result is that more usable radiation is produced using the same amount of time than with a 60-Hz generator.

High-frequency technology has provided some significant advantages over 60-Hz technology when producing a radiograph. Exposure times are decreased since more radiation can be produced in shorter times. In addition, with more usable radition being produced, there is less scatter radiation overlying the image. The inherent benefits of a reduction in patient and operator dose are derived from less scatter and shorter times. Lower exposure factors also help prolong the life of the x-ray tube. Additional benefits include the smaller size of the high-frequency generator that allows the veterinarian to free up valuable floor space and easier serviceability as a result of the greater use of printed circuit boards.

Recommended Reading

Douglas SW et al: *Principles of veterinary radiography,* ed 4, London, 1987, Bailliere Tindall.

The fundamentals of radiology, ed 12, Rochester, NY, 1992, Eastman Kodak Company.

Morgan JP, Silverman S: *Techniques of veterinary radiography,* ed 5, Davis, Calif, 1993, Veterinary Radiology Associates.

Ticer JW: *Radiographic technique in veterinary practice,* ed 2, Philadelphia, 1984, Saunders.

6

Darkroom Techniques

CHERYL HURD

CHAPTER OBJECTIVES

- Describe the proper layout of a darkroom.
- List the different methods of identifying x-ray film.
- Explain the importance of proper safelight illumination.
- Describe what the developer does to exposed x-ray film.
- Describe what the fixer does to the exposed x-ray film.
- Explain the different methods used to maintain the manual processing tanks.
- List the steps to manual process film.
- Describe the care of the manual processing tanks.
- Describe the care and use of an automatic processor.

Along with a good technique chart, proper darkroom techniques should also be followed to ensure consistent-quality radiographs. Improperly exposed radiographs can quickly become nondiagnostic with poor film-handling and darkroom techniques.

Darkroom Layout

Bench Areas

For most veterinary practices, whether using manual or automatic processing, the darkroom does not need to be large or elaborate as long as the layout is designed for efficiency. The room must be just large enough to provide a "dry bench" area away from the "wet bench" area (Figure 6-1). The dry bench area is for unloading and loading cassettes and film storage. The wet bench is for film processing and drying. These areas must be separated to prevent splashes of processing chemicals from damaging the dry films or the sensitive intensifying screens. This can be achieved in a small room by placing a partition between the two areas. An adequate number of electrical outlets should also be provided to supply the safelights, viewboxes, and labeling equipment.

Dry bench: loading and unloading the cassettes

Wet bench: film processing and drying

Light Proofing

A darkroom's most important feature is that it must be *light-proof.* White light that leaks from around the door, through a blackened window, or around ventilation fans can fog the film. Film is more sensitive after it has been exposed to x-rays, so even low-grade light leaks decrease the quality of the finished radiograph.

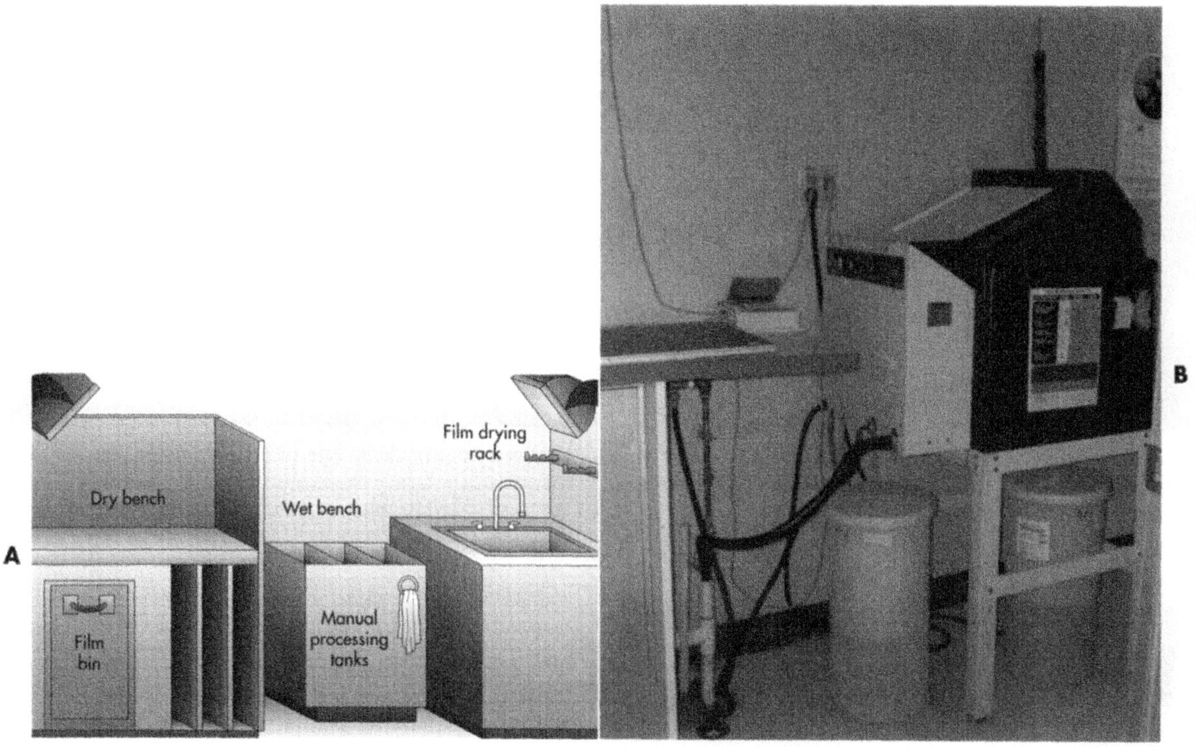

FIG. 6-1 **A**, Schematic drawing of a darkroom using manual processing. Note that the dry bench has been separated from the wet bench by a partition. **B**, Darkroom using an automatic processing system.

When checking for light leaks, staff should stand in the darkroom for at least 5 minutes to allow the eyes to adjust to the darkness. The door frame, ventilation fan, or blackened windows should be checked for any signs of white light. When performing this test, it is helpful to vary the intensity of light outside the door. Because the work done in the darkroom is with a limited amount of light, painting the walls and ceiling colors that reflect the available light helps greatly.

Ventilation

The darkroom should have adequate ventilation to prevent volatile chemical fumes from accumulating in the room. These fumes can cause fogging of the film, damage to electrical equipment, and even health problems for the staff. A lightproof ventilation fan installed in the ceiling helps remove the fumes and controls the temperature and humidity in the room. The exhaust from automatic processors and film dryers should also be vented away from the darkroom because they contain volatile chemical fumes.

Cleanliness

Cleanliness is important in the darkroom because intensifying screens and films are exposed to this area. Dirt and hair on countertops can fall into cassettes, causing white artifacts on subsequent radiographs from that cassette. Chemical spills also cause artifacts on the radiographs and damage the intensifying screens. Keeping both wet and dry areas of the darkroom clean prevents these problems. Film hangers for manual processing as well as rollers in automatic processing units should also be cleaned regularly. Residual chemicals cause artifacts on finished radiographs.

Film Identification

Permanent labeling is necessary for all radiographs. Each film must be identified before the film is processed for legal purposes and for certification organizations. The labeling can occur during the exposure or after the exposure but before the film is processed. The label should include the clinic's name and address, the clinic owner's name, the date, and the patient's name, species, gender, and age.

Methods for film identification include the following:

1. The photo labeler uses a cassette containing a leaded window that protects the area during exposure (Figure 6-2). During identification, the window slides back, exposing the information from a card

Films should be identified during or after exposure but before processing.

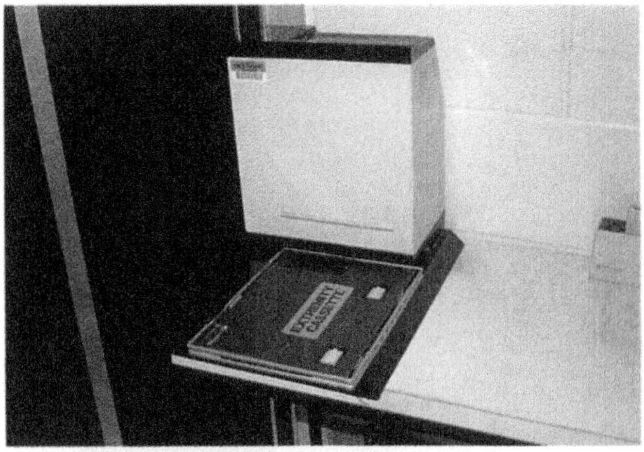

FIG. 6-2 Kodak X-Omatic Identification Labeler, Model II, a method of identifying the film outside the darkroom before processing.

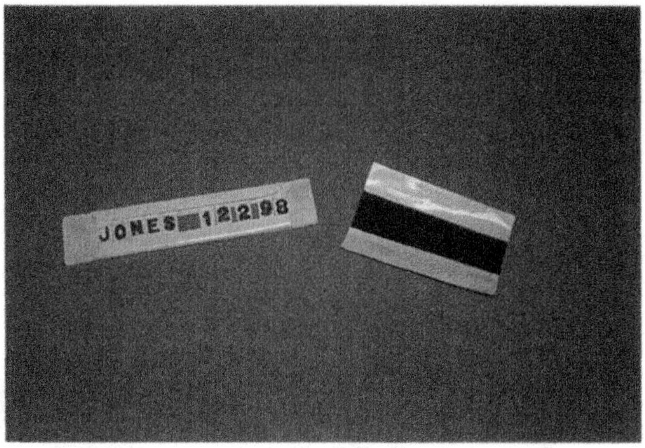

FIG. 6-4 Radiopaque tape or lead letters can be used to identify film during the exposure.

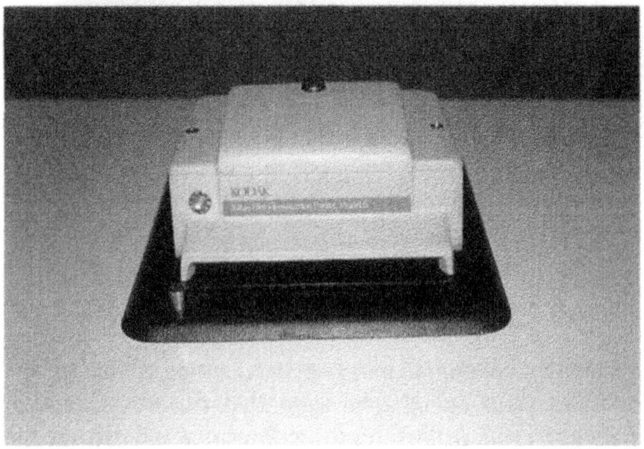

FIG. 6-3 Kodak X-Ray Film Identification, Model B manual film identification printer, a method of identifying the film inside the darkroom before processing.

onto the protected area. This forms a latent image of the information on the film.

2. Manual printers are similar to photo labelers except they use a flash of light through an information card to produce a latent image on the film (Figure 6-3). The manual printer is placed in the darkroom, and the film is taken out of the cassette to be identified.
3. Lead letters or radiopaque tape are placed on the cassette during exposure of the radiograph (Figure 6-4).

Safelights

Safelight illuminators are important for darkroom processing. The purpose of a safelight is to provide a sufficient amount of light to the room without fogging the film. Safelights can be mounted to provide light either directly or indirectly. With *direct* lighting, the safelight is mounted at least 48 inches above and directed toward the workbench. *Indirect* lighting has the safelight directed toward the ceiling and uses the reflecting light to illuminate the room. With indirect lighting, the safelight can be mounted closer to the bench but should be as high as possible (Figure 6-5).

Many types of safelight filters are available that filter out light in different areas of the light spectrum. The type of film used dictates which filter is necessary. Blue-sensitive film requires a safelight that filters out blue and ultraviolet light. This can be done with a Wratten series 6B filter. Green-sensitive film requires a safelight to filter both green and blue light. The Kodak GS-1 filter accomplishes this and can also be used with blue-sensitive film. A white-frosted 7- to 10-watt bulb is recommended for most safelight filters.

A periodic check of the safelight filter is recommended. This procedure is done by first making a moderate exposure on a film using approximately 1 to 2 mAs and 50 kVp. Film that has been exposed to x-rays is more sensitive to low-grade light, producing an overall fogged appearance. Two thirds of the film should be covered with black paper or cardboard, and one third is allowed to be exposed to the safelight for 30 seconds. This is longer than it should take to place the film in an automatic processor or on a hanger and into the manual tanks. After 30 seconds, another one third of the film is uncovered, waiting 30 more seconds. The process is repeated for the final one third, then the film should be developed. This test exposes portions of the film to the safelight for 30, 60, and 90 seconds. Once dry, the film should be examined for areas of increased film density. If an increase in density is detected, a close check of the darkroom is necessary. Improper safelight distance, a cracked safelight filter, or light leaking from around the safelight filter can all cause film fogging.

A red light bulb should never be used to replace a safelight filter. A red bulb does not filter the light; it only colors it.

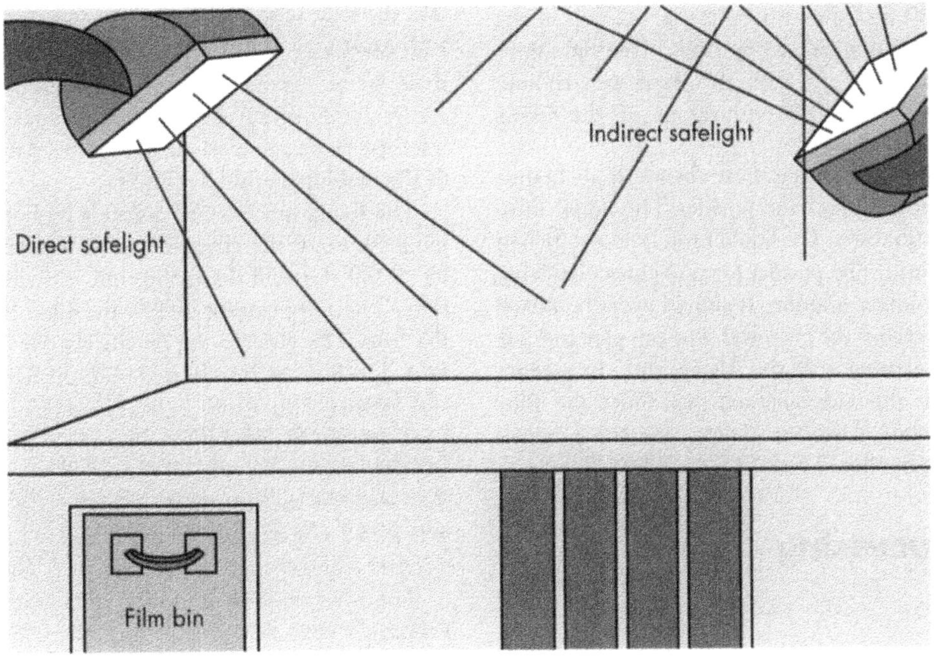

FIG. 6-5 Direct and indirect safelight illumination.

Processing Chemistry

Developer

The developer's main function is to convert the sensitized silver halide crystals into black metallic silver. Sensitized silver halide crystals are those that have been exposed to electromagnetic radiation, making them susceptible to chemical change. The developer contains five ingredients: a solvent, reducing agents, a restrainer, an activator, and a preservative.

> **Developer changes the sensitized silver halide crystals into black metallic silver.**

Water is used as the *solvent* to keep all the ingredients in solution. Water also causes the film emulsion to swell so that the reducing agents can penetrate the sensitized crystals. The *reducing agents* change the sensitized silver halide crystals into black metallic silver. The most common reducing agents are a combination of hydroquinone and *p*-methylaminophenol. The *restrainers* are used to protect the unexposed silver halide crystals by preventing the reducing agents from affecting the unsensitized silver halide crystals. Potassium bromide and potassium iodide are the most common restrainers. Bromide ions are produced during the exchange between the reducing agents and the sensitized crystals. In a fresh solution the bromide ions are not available. They are added as a starter solution but are not placed in replenishing solutions. Excessive bromide ions inhibit the reducing agents. The *activator* helps to soften and swell the film's emulsion so that the reducing agents can work effectively. Reducing agents cannot function in an acidic or neutral solution. The activators, usually a carbonate or hydroxide of sodium or potassium, provide an alkaline pH in the range of 9.8 to 11.4. The *preservative* prevents the solution from rapidly oxidizing. Sodium sulfite and potassium sulfite are the most common preservatives.

Developing chemicals are manufactured in two forms: liquid and powder. The liquid form is used most often and requires dilution with water. The powder form should never be mixed in the darkroom because the chemical dust contaminates unprotected film, causing artifacts. Always mix the powder in a bucket outside the darkroom and then finish the dilution in the darkroom.

Fixer

The fixer removes the unchanged silver halide crystals from the film emulsion, leaving the black metallic silver. It also hardens the film emulsion, decreasing the susceptibility to scratches. The fixer contains five ingredients: a solvent, a fixing agent, an acidifier, a hardener, and a preservative.

> **Fixer clears the remaining silver halide crystals from the film's emulsion.**

As with the developer, the *solvent* for the fixer is water. It keeps the ingredients in solution and causes the film emulsion to swell, allowing the fixing agents to reach the unexposed crystals. The *fixing agent* is sodium or ammonium thiosulfate. This clears the remaining silver halide crystals from the film emulsion. The *acidifier* is acetic or sulfuric acid and is used to neutralize any alkaline developer remaining on the film. Ammonium chloride is used as a *hardener*. It hardens and prevents excessive swelling of the film emulsion, shortening the drying time. The final ingredient is the *preservative*. As with the developer, sodium sulfite is used to prevent decomposition of the fixing agents.

As with developing chemicals, fixer chemicals are manufactured in two forms: liquid and powder. The liquid form requires dilution with water. The liquid form is more efficient than the powder form. The powder form requires dissolving and mixing to become a solution. It should never be mixed in the darkroom because the chemical dust can contaminate unprotected film, causing artifacts. Always mix the powder in a bucket outside the darkroom and then finish the dilution in the darkroom. Also, the powder requires a longer clearing time than the liquid form.

Manual Processing

Equipment

Manual processing tanks are usually made from stainless steel and are large enough to accept 14 × 17–inch film hangers. Tanks with 5-gallon capacity are sufficient. Plastic or wooden lids are needed to cover the developer and fixer tanks. This reduces the rate of evaporation and oxidation of the chemicals. Ideally, separate stirring rods for the developer and fixer are used to mix the chemicals before processing. One stirring rod can be used if rinsed in the wash tank thoroughly between tanks. Also, an accurate timer and a floating thermometer should be available.

Procedure

Developing x-ray film is a chemical process that depends on the duration of immersion in the chemicals and the temperature of the chemicals. The recommended time for development is 5 minutes. This allows just enough time for the reducing agents to convert the sensitized silver halide crystals. The temperature of the chemicals is also important. The warmer the temperature, the more the emulsion swells and the faster the chemicals work. Cold temperatures also affect the chemicals by decreasing their ability to penetrate the film emulsion. Most manufacturers recommend a temperature for the chemicals they produce, usually 68° F (20° C), with 5 minutes of developing time. For some cases this may not be possible, so the time can be adjusted to compensate for the increase or decrease in temperature. The time can be decreased by 30 seconds for every 2° F increase in developer temperature. Also, the time can be increased by 30 seconds for every 2° F decrease in developer temperature. This applies only between 65° F (18° C) and 74° F (23° C).

> Developing time is 5 minutes at 68° F (20° C) for most manufacturers' chemicals.

The rinse bath removes developer from the film, preventing carryover into the fixer tank. Agitating the film in the running water bath for 30 seconds adequately removes the developer. The rinse water should be continually exchanged to prevent accumulation of developer. The temperature of the incoming rinse water can often be used to regulate the temperature of the developer and fixer tanks.

The fixing process also depends on immersion time and temperature of the chemicals. The standard temperature is 68° F (20° C), and the fixing time is double the developing time. The temperature affects the time the film is left in the fixer. The warmer the chemicals, the shorter the fixing time. The film can be removed from the fixer after 30 seconds and viewed with white light. However, it must be placed back into the fixer for the remainder of the time. The clearing time increases as the thickness of the emulsion increases. Direct-exposure film has a thicker emulsion and requires a longer time in the fixer.

> Fixing time is double the developing time.

The final wash rinses away the processing chemicals. Failure to rinse the film completely results in a film that eventually becomes faded and brown. This results from oxidation of the chemicals remaining in the film emulsion. The wash tank should have fresh circulating water to decrease the time needed for the final wash. Generally, the wash time is at least 30 minutes.

Box 6-1 details the steps for manual processing.

Maintaining the Tanks

There are two methods for maintaining manual processing tanks. With the *exhausted method*, the chemicals are allowed to drain back into their respective tanks and not into the wash tank. This permits the exhausted chemicals to remain in the tank, maintaining the chemical levels. With the *replenishing method*, the chemicals are *not* allowed to drain back into their respective tanks, but instead are placed in the wash tank. The chemical levels are maintained with replenishing chemicals that are more concentrated than the initial solutions. In this way the potency and levels of the chemicals can be preserved. With either method, the chemicals should be changed every 3 months.

Automatic Processing

Use of an automatic processor has many advantages over manual processing. Automatic processors can develop film more quickly, processing and drying a film in 90 to 120 seconds. Also, automatic processors consistently provide high-quality radiographs. This eliminates the need for repeat radiographs because of processing errors.

Automatic processors move the film through the developer, fixer wash bath, and dryers at a uniform rate of speed (Figure 6-6). Chemicals and film are specially manufactured to withstand the high temperatures involved in automatic processing. The chemicals are kept at temperatures around

BOX 6-1

STEPS FOR MANUAL PROCESSING

DAILY CHECKLIST

1. Check chemical temperature. Optimal chemical temperature is 68° F (20° C).
2. Stir both chemicals.
3. Check chemical levels.
4. Clean countertops.
5. Turn on water to wash tank.

PROCESSING INDIVIDUAL FILMS

1. Locate the correct size of hanger(s).
2. Set timer.
3. Turn on safelight.
4. Turn off white lights.
5. Unload cassette and place film on hanger.
6. Immerse film in developer. Optimal time is 5 minutes at 68° F (20° C).
7. Gently agitate film to dislodge any air bubbles that may cling to surface of the film.
8. Reload empty cassette.
9. After 5 minutes of developing time, place film in wash tank and agitate for 30 seconds.
10. Lift film out of wash tank, allowing the excess water to drain back into wash tank.
11. Place film into fixer tank and agitate gently to dislodge any air bubbles that cling to surface of the film.
12. White lights can be turned on without causing problems after 30 seconds of clearing time in fixer.
13. Remove film from fixer tank after 10 minutes, or twice the developing time.
14. Place film in wash tank for 30 minutes or longer, depending on the amount of water replenishing.
15. After washing film, hang until dry.

THREE-MONTH CHECKLIST

1. Completely drain all three tanks.
2. Clean tanks with a 1:32 solution of bleach and water.
3. Rinse tanks well.
4. Refill tanks with fresh chemicals.

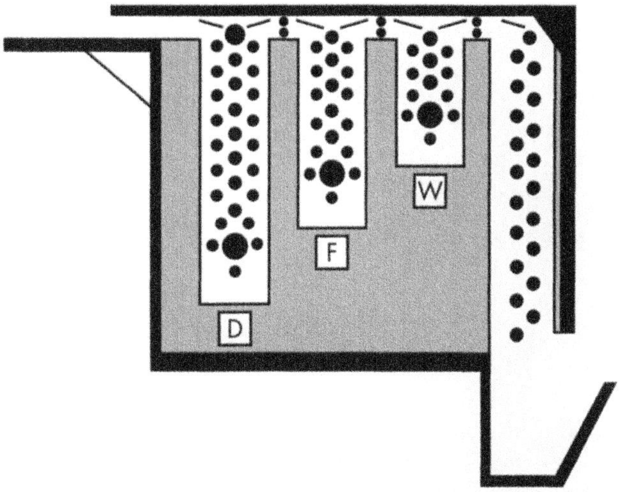

FIG. 6-6 Automatic processor. A series of rollers transports the film through the developer, fixer, washer, and dryer. From start to finish, this process varies from 90 to 120 seconds.

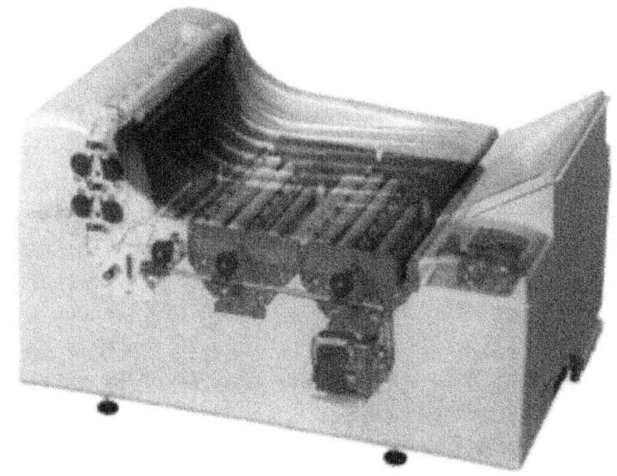

FIG. 6-7 Roller placement in an automatic processor. (Courtesy Summit Industries.)

95° F (35° C), depending on the type of film and equipment used (Figures 6-7 and 6-8). The emulsion on film designed for automatic processing is harder than on film designed for manual processing, preventing scratches from the roller. This film can also be manually processed in case of mechanical problems with the automatic processor.

Maintaining the Tanks

Small tabletop automatic processors are easily maintained in most veterinary practices. The equipment should be completely cleaned every 3 months. This includes draining and cleaning the tanks. A 1:32 solution of bleach (e.g., Clorox) helps to reduce algae and remove chemical buildup. The rollers can be cleaned with a mild detergent and soft sponge. When applying any cleaning solution to the tanks or rollers, rinse them thoroughly before replacing the chemicals. Also, check the springs and gears for signs of wear, and replace if necessary. Wipe the feed tray and top rollers with a clean, soft sponge every day. This helps to remove dirt, debris, and chemical residue between episodes of routine maintenance.

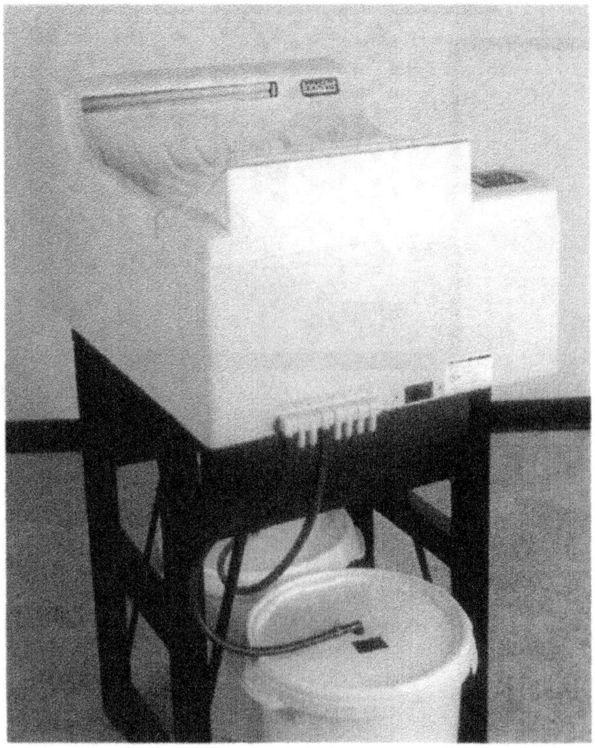

FIG. 6-8 InnoVet cold water automatic processor.

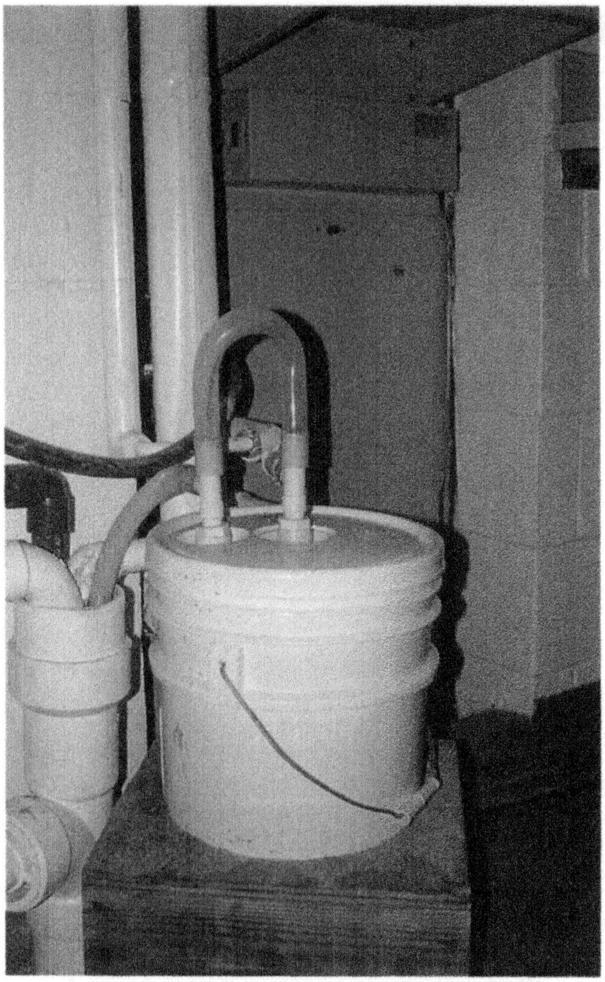

FIG. 6-9 Kodak Chemical Recovery Cartridge Type P-2 hooked to an automatic processor.

Silver Recovery

When an exposed film is placed in the developer, the exposed silver halide crystals are changed to black metallic silver. The remaining silver halide crystals are removed from the film in the fixer. Over time the fixer solution becomes rich with silver that can be reclaimed. Silver recovery systems can be attached to automatic processors to filter and store the silver that would normally be discarded down the drain (Figure 6-9). The black metallic silver found in the radiographs can also be recovered.

The manual processing fixer solution, silver recovery systems, and old radiographs can be sold to companies that reclaim the silver. These companies are usually listed in the telephone directory under the heading *Gold and Silver Refiners and Dealers.*

Recommended Reading

Douglas SW et al: *Principles of veterinary radiography,* ed 4, London, 1987, Bailliere Tindall.

The fundamentals of radiology, ed 12, Rochester, NY, 1992, Eastman Kodak Company.

Morgan JP, Silverman S: *Techniques of veterinary radiography,* ed 5, Davis, Calif, 1993, Veterinary Radiology Associates.

Ticer JW: *Radiographic technique in veterinary practice,* ed 2, Philadelphia, 1984, Saunders.

7

Radiation Safety

CHERYL HURD

CHAPTER OBJECTIVES

- Explain what radiation can do to living tissue.
- List the organ systems that are most sensitive to ionizing radiation and the features that these systems have in common.
- Describe how the developing fetus is affected by ionizing radiation.
- List and define the terminology used when describing doses of radiation.
- State the ways to minimize radiation exposure during general x-ray procedures.
- State the ways to minimize radiation exposure during fluoroscopic procedures.
- Describe the types of staff-monitoring devices.
- List the four sources of radiation exposure.
- Explain the care of protective apparel and how often it should be checked.

Ionizing radiation is a difficult concept to grasp, since at diagnostic levels it cannot be seen, felt, or heard by the patient or operators. Radiation safety is important because radiation ionizes intracellular water. This action releases toxic products that can damage critical components of the cell, such as deoxyribonucleic acid (DNA).

Radiation can have four effects when it comes in contact with the cells of living tissue:

1. Pass through with no effect.
2. Produce cell damage that is repairable.
3. Produce cell damage that is *not* repairable.
4. Kill the cell.

The cumulative effects of radiation damage the body in several ways and may have carcinogenic effects, which means that cancer can occur. The effects of radiation on the body may be *somatic*, occurring only within the lifetime of the individual, or may be *genetic*, occurring in future generations. Although these effects may result from one massive dose of radiation, they also may result from several small doses over many years.

> Doses of radiation are cumulative over a lifetime.

The organ systems that are most sensitive to ionizing radiation are systems that have rapidly growing or reproducing cells. The reproductive organs may experience temporary or permanent infertility, decreased hormone production, or mutations. The hematopoietic cells are relatively sensitive to ionizing radiation. Of these, the lymphocytic series is the most sensitive. Damage to these cells can cause lowered resistance to infection and clotting disorders.

The thyroid gland, intestinal epithelium, and the lens of the eye are also radiosensitive tissues. An increased incidence of squamous cell carcinoma may occur with chronic low-level skin exposure. Radiodermatitis (reddened, dry skin) can be an indicator of excessive, chronic low-level radiation exposure.

> Organ systems with rapidly reproducing cells are most sensitive to ionizing radiation.

The developing fetus is sensitive to the effects of ionizing radiation. The degree of sensitivity depends on the stage of pregnancy and the dose received. The preimplantation period (0 to 9 days) is the most critical time for the embryo regarding intrauterine lethality. Organogenesis (10 days to 6 weeks) carries the greatest risk of congenital malformation in the fetus, since this is the critical developmental period for fetal organs. The fetus may have skeletal or dental malformations. Other abnormalities include microphthalmia (microphthalmos) and overall growth retardation. A fetal dose of greater than 25 RADs (0.25 Gray) has been the advised threshold for significant damage to the fetus. The fetal period (6 weeks to term) is the least sensitive time for the fetus; however, growth and mental retardation may still occur. Irradiation after 30 weeks is less likely to cause abnormalities because the sensitivity of the fetus approaches that of the adult.

> The fetus is most sensitive to ionizing radiation during the first trimester of pregnancy.

Exposure Terminology

The following is a brief description of the terminology used when describing doses of radiation. *Roentgen equivalent man* (rem) is the amount used to express the dose equivalent that results from exposure to ionizing radiation. The rem takes into account the quality of the radiation so that doses from different types of radiation can be compared. *Sievert* (Sv) is used to define a rem: 1 Sv = 100 rem. A millirem (mrem) is equal to 0.001 rem (1/1000 rem). A rad is the *radiation absorbed dose. Gray* (Gy) is used to define rad: 1 Gy = 100 rad.

In dealing with x-rays only and not other types of radiation, rad is equivalent to rem. Other types of radiation must have a quality factor added to determine the dose. MPD is the *maximum permissible dose.* The National Council on Radiation Protection and Measurements (NCRP) recommends that the MPD (whole body) per year for occupational persons not exceed 5 rem or 0.05 Sv. Individual organs should not exceed 50 rem or 0.5 Sv, and the lenses of the eyes should not exceed 1.5 rem or 0.15 Sv per year. An occupationally exposed individual is one who normally performs his or her work in a restricted-access area and who has duties that involve exposure to radiation. ALARA stands for "as low as reasonably achievable." The MPD for nonoccupational persons is as low as 0.1 rem per year, depending on the state. This is known as the ALARA MPD.

> MPD for occupationally exposed persons should not exceed 5 rem per year.

In some states, regulations specify that a fetus cannot receive more than 0.5 rem for the entire gestational period. A pregnant staff member who chooses to continue working around radiation-producing devices should wear an additional badge at waist level underneath the lead gown to monitor the fetal dose. This second badge should not exceed 0.05 rem per month.

Sources of Exposure

Ionizing radiation can come from one or all of the following sources of exposure: primary beam, scatter radiation, x-ray tube head, and fluoroscopy.

The primary beam is one source of occupational exposure to ionizing radiation. Lead gloves are used to protect the hands and forearms from scatter radiation, but they cannot protect from primary beam exposure. The 0.5 mm of lead typically used in protective apparel only decreases the primary beam exposure by 25%. If an exposure were made using 10 mAs and 80 kVp with an ungloved hand in the primary beam, the hand would receive approximately 100 mrem of exposure. A gloved hand in the primary beam using the same exposure technique would still receive 75 mrem of exposure.

Scatter radiation is another source of exposure. *Scatter radiation* is defined as the x-rays degraded by collision with tissue molecules. Scatter radiation comes from the patient, floor, and sides of the table. Again, using 10 mAs and 80 kVp, the radiation exposure at the side of the table is 5 mrem without protective apparel.

When an exposure is made, a small amount of radiation can leak from the x-ray tube housing. This only becomes a problem when portable x-ray equipment is handheld or cradled in a lap for the exposure.

During *fluoroscopy,* a flow of x-rays is continuously produced and a real-time image is viewed on a monitor. Approximately 5000 mrem per minute is emitted in the actual beam. Scatter from fluoroscopy can average 100 mrem per minute. Minimizing the length of time that the fluoroscope is activated and the distance from the primary beam greatly decreases the amount of exposure.

Monitoring Devices

Monitoring devices record the amount of radiation received during radiographic procedures. These devices are worn during every radiographic procedure and then are sent to an approved laboratory to be processed. The amount of radiation each badge receives is recorded under the individual's Social Security number. This allows a cumulative radiation dose to be recorded for each individual, which is totaled for a lifetime dose.

The four main types of monitoring devices used in veterinary medicine are film badges, thermoluminescent dosimeters (TLDs), optically stimulated luminescence (OSL) badges, and ion chambers (Figure 7-1). Film badges, TLDs, and OSL badges contain three or four elements of filtration, an open window, plastic, aluminum, and copper. Each element measures varying degrees of radiation exposure. The open window records the lowest exposure, and the copper records the highest. Each badge type differs in how the radiation dose is recorded and how it is read out.

Film badges are the most common method of monitoring ionizing radiation. Each badge contains a small piece of film enclosed in a lightproof envelope. This envelope is placed in a plastic carrier, such as a ring, wristband, or a clip-on for the collar. The badge is worn for a specified amount of time and is then returned to an approved laboratory for evaluation. The film is developed, and a value in mrem is correlated by the degree of blackness on the film. The amount of radiation received is proportional to the degree of blackness on the film.

Thermoluminescent dosimeters contain lithium fluoride or calcium fluoride crystals. These crystals store the energy produced by radiation exposure. When sent to a laboratory for evaluation, the crystals undergo heat processing, and a light is emitted. The amount of light is proportional to the amount of radiation that dosimeter received. Thermoluminescent crystals record greater amounts of energy than the film badge. This means the badge can be worn for a longer period before it must be sent to the laboratory for evaluation.

Optically stimulated luminescence badges use more advanced technology. A thin layer of aluminum oxide is sandwiched between three-element filters placed in a light-tight pack. On analysis, the aluminum oxide layer is stimulated with different frequencies of laser light. The stimulation causes the aluminum oxide to illuminate in proportion to the amount of radiation received. OSL badges are extremely sensitive to radiation, allowing even low-dose radiation exposures to be recorded.

The *ion chambers* are the most complex monitoring devices. They are the size of a fountain pen and can be clipped onto a pocket. An electrometer is used to charge the chamber before being worn. With each exposure to radiation, the ion chamber discharges. At the end of the procedure the amount of ion discharge is read. The amount of discharge of the ions is proportional to the amount of radiation received.

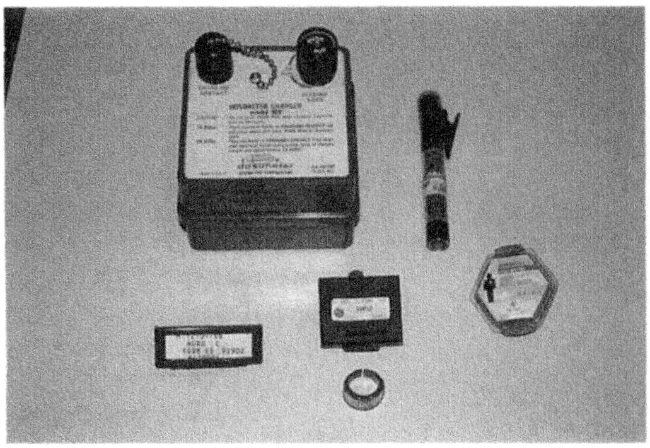

FIG. 7-1 Types of monitoring devices used to monitor staff exposure to radiation.

Minimizing Exposure

Time, distance, and shielding are methods for minimizing exposure to occupational radiation.

Lead Shielding

Lead shielding should be a requirement for all staff remaining in the room while exposure is being made. Lead gowns, gloves, and thyroid shields should all contain at least 0.5 mm of lead. Lead-based glasses can also be worn to protect the eyes.

Lead apparel is expensive, so it should be handled appropriately (Figure 7-2). Lead aprons should be draped over a rounded surface without folds or wrinkles to prevent cracks in the lead. Lead gloves can be

Lead apparel containing 0.5 mm of lead protects against scatter radiation.

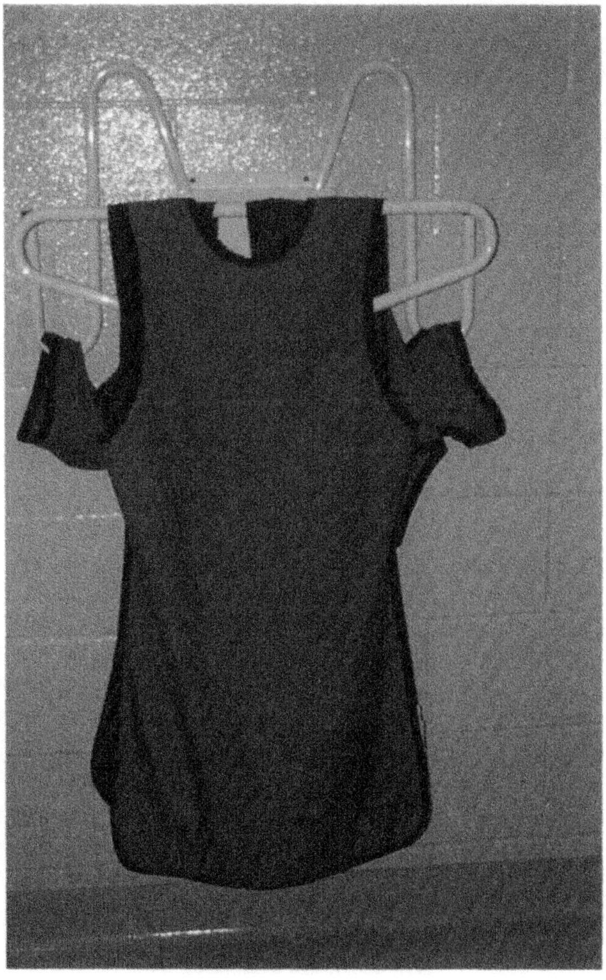

FIG. 7-2 Proper care of lead apparel is important. To prevent cracks in the lead, the gowns need to be stored on special racks or draped over a rounded surface.

stored with open-ended soup cans placed in them to prevent cracks and to provide air circulation to the liners (Figure 7-3). Gloves should be radiographed every 6 months. Lead gowns should be screened every 12 months to check for holes and cracks in the lead. A common technique for this procedure uses 5 mAs and 80 kVp. This can be adjusted as needed to attain the proper density in the radiographs.

Increased Distance

Staff exposure may also be decreased by increasing distance from the primary beam. The law of inverse squares states that x-ray beam intensity decreases to one fourth if the distance between the x-ray source and the operator is doubled.

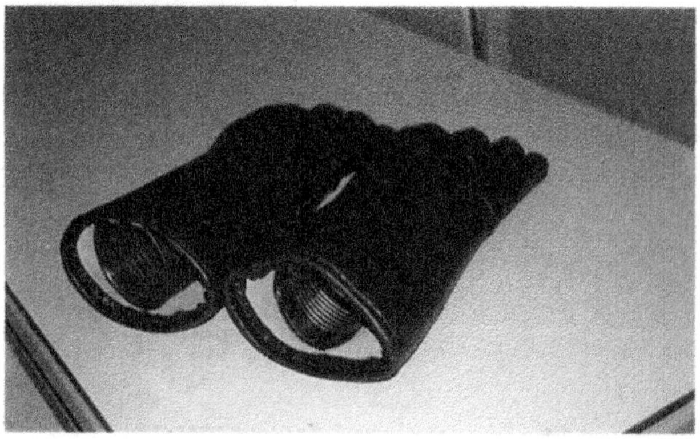

FIG. 7-3 Gloves need to be stored on special racks or with open-ended soup cans placed in them.

The staff restraining the animal should remain as far as possible from the x-ray source. During exposure, the restrainers should lean back and look away from the beam to protect their eyes (Figure 7-4). Staff should wear lead apparel properly to obtain full protection, unlike those pictured in Figure 7-5. Placing a glove over a hand for protection does not protect from scatter radiation. The scatter can come from any direction, including from under the tabletop.

Increasing the distance from the source of radiation decreases exposure to staff.

Increasing the distance also applies to large animal radiography. Usually during a large animal radiographic procedure, three people are necessary: one to hold the animal, one to hold the cassette, and one to set up the tube head. The person holding the cassette should have the cassette in a cassette holder that places the holder farther from the primary beam. The cassette should never be handheld, even with a gloved hand. The person positioning the x-ray tube should use the full length of the exposure cord. The x-ray machine should never be placed in the operator's lap and should not be handheld (Figure 7-6). Because a small amount of radiation is emitted from the bottom of the x-ray machine, increasing the distance from the x-ray tube decreases the amount of radiation significantly.

Reduced Time

Reduced time is also an important factor in reducing radiation exposure. Using the fastest film-screen combinations results

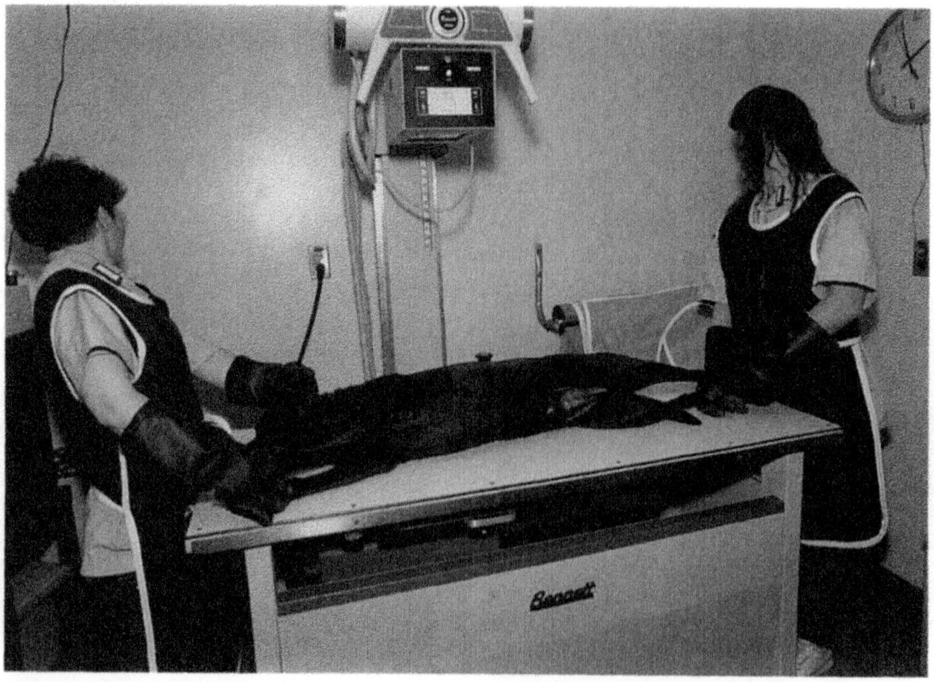

FIG. 7-4 Proper safety practices. The restrainers have increased their distance from the primary beam by leaning back. They are also protecting their eyes by looking away.

in reduced exposure time to patient and personnel. Proper darkroom practices and technique charts allow for consistent, high-quality films, reducing the number of retakes. The beam should be collimated down to the area of interest to reduce scatter radiation exposure to staff. Cones and diaphragms may also be attached to the tube window to increase detail and reduce scatter radiation. A 2-mm aluminum filter is used at the tube window to filter out soft rays too weak to penetrate the patient. If these rays are not filtered out, they scatter about the room, fogging the film and striking staff.

Each clinic should have a radiation control program. A proper radiation control program includes safe use of x-ray equipment, low-exposure techniques, shielding, and monitoring of radiation exposure to staff. The state government usually regulates x-ray equipment (e.g., State Board of Health). Regulations vary among states, so a particular state's policy regarding radiation-producing devices should be consulted before use. Box 7-1 indicates general radiation safety guidelines when operating radiation-producing devices.

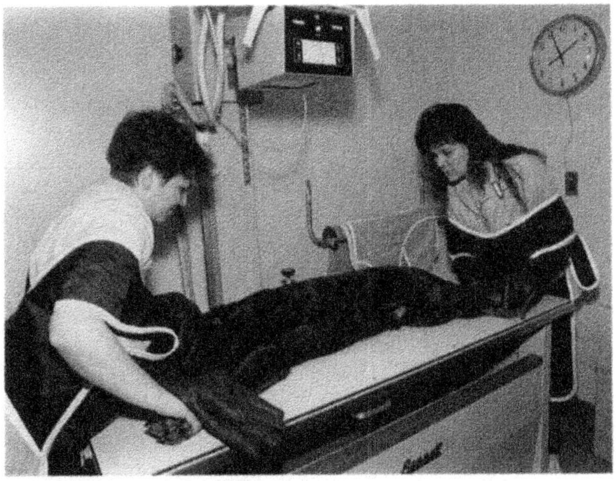

FIG. 7-5 Improper safety practices. The restrainers are leaning in and looking at the patient. Note that one hand is not properly gloved.

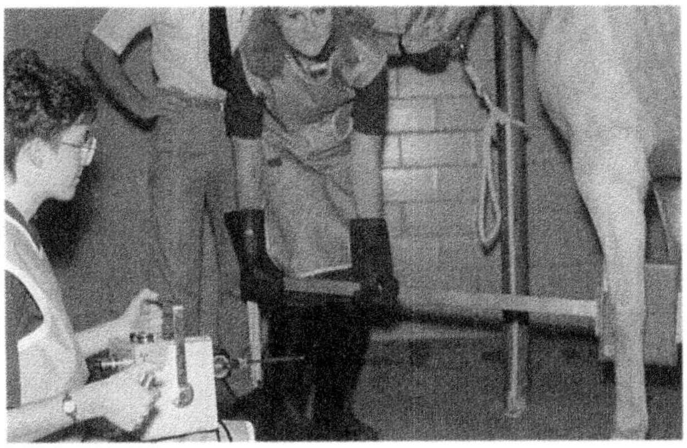

FIG. 7-6 Improper radiation safety practice during a large animal radiographic procedure. Note that the person is holding the x-ray machine in her lap and that the person holding the horse needs to be gowned.

BOX 7-1

GENERAL RADIATION SAFETY GUIDELINES

1. Always wear lead gloves and lead aprons when remaining in the room during radiography or fluoroscopy. Lead gowns and lead gloves must be worn by all individuals involved in the restraint of the animal.
2. Always wear a radiation-monitoring device on the collar outside the apron when working around x-ray equipment. NOTE: Badges should not be exposed to sunlight, dampness, or extreme temperatures. This could cause falsely high readings.
3. Never allow any part of the body to be exposed to the primary beam. Lead clothing does not protect against primary beam exposure.
4. Always look away from the x-ray beam during an exposure to protect the eyes. Lead-based glasses may be worn for protection.
5. Use alternative methods of restraint (e.g., drugs, tape, sandbags) when using high radiographic techniques.
6. Pregnant women and persons under the age of 18 years should *not* be involved in radiographic procedures.
7. Only the minimum number of people required for restraint should remain in the room when an exposure is being made.
8. Neither the x-ray machine nor the cassette should ever be handheld during a large animal x-ray procedure.

Recommended Reading

Frankel R: *Radiation protection for radiologic technologists,* New York, 1976, McGraw-Hill.

Hall EJ: *Radiobiology for the radiologist,* ed 4, Philadelphia, 1994, Lippincott.

Hendee WR, Edwards MF: Trends in radiation protection of medical workers, *Health Phys* 58:251, 1990.

Morgan JP, Silverman S: *Techniques of veterinary radiography,* ed 5, Davis, Calif, 1993, Veterinary Radiology Associates.

Noz ME, Maguire GQ: *Radiation protection in the radiologic and health sciences,* ed 2, Philadelphia, 1985, Lea & Febiger.

Pizzarello DJ, Witcofski RL: *Medical radiation biology,* ed 2, Philadelphia, 1982, Lea & Febiger.

Ryan GD: *Radiographic positioning of small animals,* Philadelphia, 1981, Lea & Febiger.

Ticer JW: *Radiographic technique in veterinary practice,* ed 2, Philadelphia, 1984, Saunders.

Widmer WR et al: Radiation biology and radiation safety, *Compend Contin Educ Pract Vet* 11:1237, 1989.

Wrigley RH, Borak TB: The effect of kVp on the dose equivalent from scattered radiation by radiography personnel, *Vet Radiol* 24:181, 1983.

8

Developing a Small Animal Radiographic Technique Chart

CHERYL HURD

CHAPTER OBJECTIVES

- Explain the importance of a technique chart for each x-ray machine.
- List the variables that must be consistent for a technique chart to remain unchanged.
- List the steps for constructing a technique chart.
- State why the first three trial exposures are made over the liver region.
- Explain how to derive a technique chart when minimum or maximum machine capabilities are a factor.
- Describe how to derive a technique chart when only one speed of intensifying screen is available.
- List the conversion factors when switching from high-speed to slow-speed screens.

One of the most valuable pieces of information in the field of radiology is a radiographic technique chart. A technique chart allows the production of radiographs of consistent quality with a reduced number of repeat exposures, which reduces radiation exposure to the patient and staff. The construction of a technique chart is simple when these step-by-step procedures are followed.

Preparation

Some important factors must be considered before starting. The animal used to develop the technique chart should not be overweight or underweight. A dog weighing approximately 40 pounds is ideal. The dog should be anesthetized when performing the chart development. The process moves faster if the animal does not have to be restrained.

Choose an animal that is not thin or obese.

The variables that can affect the radiographic density must be eliminated. Film-processing chemicals should be fresh, not several months old. The same brand of chemicals should be used after the technique chart has been established. Consistent processing times and chemical temperatures should be maintained. Increasing or decreasing the time or temperature affects the radiographic density.

A standard focal-film distance of 36 to 40 inches and consistent film-screen combination should be maintained. The safelights and darkroom should be checked for light leaks. This eliminates film fogging, which can decrease the quality of the radiograph. After the technique has been established, if any of these variables changes, adjustments in the technique chart are necessary.

Establishing the Baseline mAs Chart

Step 1 Construct an mAs matrix chart using the mA stations and exposure times available on the x-ray machine (Table 8-1).

Step 2 With the dog in lateral recumbency, measure the thickness of the abdomen in centimeters at the widest point, usually over the liver region. This measurement should be between 10 and 20 cm. It is also used to establish the variable kVp chart. Set the kVp for the three trial exposures according to the following measurements:

<10 cm = 60 kVp

10 to 20 cm = 70 kVp

>20 cm = 80 kVp

TABLE 8-1
mAs MATRIX CHART

TIME (IN SECONDS)	mA 50	100	150	200	300
0.0083	0.42	0.83	1.25	1.67	2.5
0.016	0.83	1.67	2.5	3.3	5
0.025	1.25	2.5	3.75	5	7.5
0.033	1.67	3.3	5	6.6	10
0.04	2.08	4.2	6.2	8.3	12.5
0.05	2.5	5	7.5	10	15
0.058	3	5.8	8.7	11.7	17.5
0.066	3.3	6.7	10	13.3	20
0.083	4.2	8.3	12.5	16.7	25
0.1	5	10	15	20	30
0.133	6.67	13.3	20	26.67	40
0.166	8.3	16.67	25	33.3	50

14" × 17" cassette

Exposure #1	Exposure #2	Exposure #3
1.67 mAs 70 kVp	3.3 mAs 70 kVp	5 mAs 70 kVp

FIG. 8-1 Technique settings for the three trial exposures.

Step 3 Divide a 14 × 17–inch cassette with lead blockers into three sections to make three trial exposures (Figure 8-1). Center each over the caudal thoracic and the liver region. Using one 14 × 17–inch cassette conserves film and reduces processing variables. Select a high-speed screen or the fastest-speed screen available for soft tissues. The cassette is placed on the tabletop for this first series of exposures, regardless of the thickness of the area. If these exact mAs choices are not available, use numbers that are as close as possible, employing the fastest times available.
Set the mAs for the three trial exposures at the following:

- 1 mAs for the first exposure
- 3 mAs for the second exposure
- 6 mAs for the third exposure

Step 4 Process the film.

Step 5 Choose the technique that allows the best visualization of the soft tissue structures. If none of the exposures is satisfactory, adjust the mAs accordingly and expose the entire abdomen. The technique chosen can be used as the tabletop abdominal technique. It can also be baseline mAs for the remainder of the technique chart.

> If any adjustments need to be made when first establishing the chart, adjust only the mAs.

Step 6 Using the selected mAs value as the tabletop abdominal technique with the following conversion factors, develop the remainder of the variable mAs chart (Table 8-2).

HIGH-SPEED SCREENS*

Tabletop abdomen	Selected value
Grid abdomen	Three times tabletop abdomen
Tabletop thorax	One half tabletop abdomen
Grid thorax	Three times tabletop thorax

SLOW-SPEED SCREENS

Tabletop bone	Four times tabletop abdomen
Grid bone	Three times tabletop detail

Step 7 Prepare a variable kVp chart using the following rules:

TABLE 8-2
VARIABLE mAs CHART

TECHNIQUE	mAs
HIGH-SPEED SCREENS	
Tabletop abdomen	3.3
Grid abdomen	9.9
Tabletop thorax	1.6
Grid thorax	4.8
SLOW-SPEED SCREENS	
Tabletop bone	13.2
Grid bone	39.6

*High-speed screens to slow speed → 4 times the high-speed mAs; high-speed screens to par speed → 2 times the high-speed mAs.

- *Rule 1*: Subtract 2 kVp from the initial kVp used for each centimeter decrease from the initial measurement.
- *Rule 2*: Add 2 kVp to the initial kVp used for each centimeter increase from the initial measurement. This is done up to 80 kVp.
- *Rule 3*: Add 3 kVp for each centimeter increase between 80 and 100 kVp.
- *Rule 4*: Add 4 kVp for each centimeter increase above 100 kVp.

See Table 8-3 for an illustration of this chart.

Step 8 Make one exposure for each of the calculated techniques (tabletop abdomen, grid abdomen, tabletop thorax, grid thorax, tabletop bone, and grid bone), using the variable mAs and kVp charts. If adjustments are necessary, adjust the mAs, leaving the kVp as it is, and test the techniques on large and small dogs, as well as cats.

Example of Technique Chart Development

Develop the mAs chart using the available mA stations and exposure times. Multiply each mA station and exposure time together to chart the mAs values available for that x-ray machine (see Table 8-1). When choosing an mAs, always use a setting with the highest mA station and the fastest time. This technique chart is calculated using an anesthetized 40-lb dog that measures 15 cm over the liver region.

Make three trial exposures centered over the liver region using 1.7, 3.3, and 5 mAs, all using 70 kVp. This area has been chosen because it allows visualization of each of the subject densities (Figure 8-2).

TABLE 8-3

VARIABLE kVp CHART

cm	kVp	cm	kVp	cm	kVp
RULE 1		RULE 2		RULE 4	
1	42	16	72	27	102
2	44	17	74	28	106
3	46	18	76	29	110
4	48	19	78	30	114
5	50	20	80		
6	52				
7	54	RULE 3			
8	56	21	83		
9	58	22	86		
10	60	23	89		
11	62	24	92		
12	64	25	95		
13	66	26	98		
14	68				
15	70				

The best tabletop abdominal technique is 3.3 mAs and 70 kVp. An mAs chart is calculated using 3.3 mAs as the tabletop abdomen mAs. If the exact mAs values are not available on the x-ray unit, use the closest choice that provides the highest mA station and the shortest exposure time. The kVp chart is calculated using 70 kVp at 15 cm (see Table 8-3).

kVp Charts for Machines with Maximum Capacity of 90 kVp

With low-output machines, Table 8-3 is not possible when the maximum kVp output is 90. A kVp chart can be developed that does not exceed 90 kVp. Because both mAs and kVp can affect the radiographic density, mAs can be increased to maintain the radiographic density while the kVp is lowered (Box 8-1).

Sparkle technique can be used when the radiograph has sufficient density but needs more detail. This is done by decreasing the kVp 16% and doubling the mAs. If this is not enough, the kVp can be decreased 16% again, and the mAs can be doubled.

This low-output kVp chart is calculated using the same anesthetized dog measuring 15 cm over the liver region as in the previous example. The variable mAs chart is figured the same way. The best tabletop abdominal technique was 3.3 mAs and 70 kVp (see Table 8-2).

When figuring the kVp chart for a low-output machine, it is necessary to adjust the technique once 90 kVp has been exceeded. This can be done by decreasing the kVp 16%. The following is an explanation of this adjustment, as well as Table 8-4:

- Exposure technique for a thorax measuring 20 cm → 4.8 mAs and 80 kVp
- Exposure technique for a thorax measuring 26 cm → 9.6 mAs and 82 kVp
- Exposure technique for a thorax measuring 30 cm → 19.2 mAs and 78 kVp

BOX 8-1

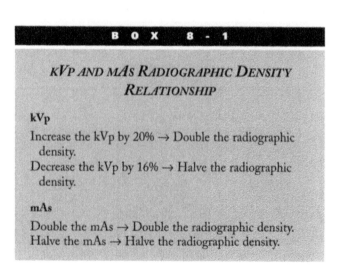

kVp and mAs Radiographic Density Relationship

kVp

Increase the kVp by 20% → Double the radiographic density.

Decrease the kVp by 16% → Halve the radiographic density.

mAs

Double the mAs → Double the radiographic density.

Halve the mAs → Halve the radiographic density.

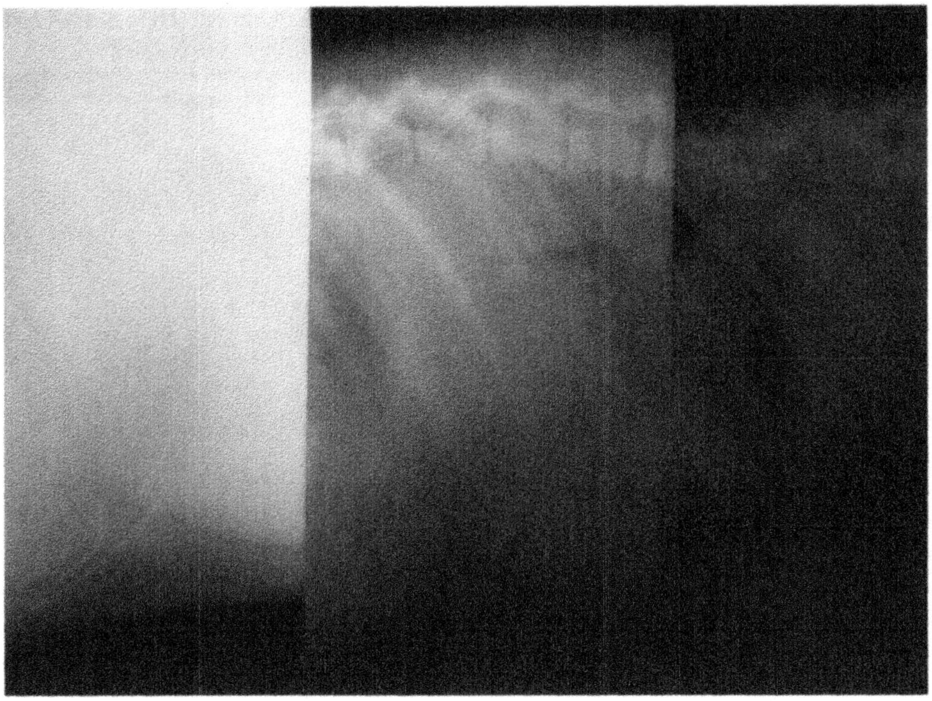

FIG. 8-2 Three trial exposures using a 14 × 17–inch cassette.

TABLE 8-4

VARIABLE kVp CHART WITH MAXIMUM 90 kVp OUTPUT

Examples are as follows:

cm	kVp	cm	kVp
1	42	16	72
2	44	17	74
3	46	18	76
4	48	19	78
5	50	20	80
6	52	21	83
7	54	22	86
8	56	23	89
9	58	24	77*
10	60	25	79*
11	62	26	82*
12	64	27	85*
13	66	28	88*
14	68	29	76†
15	70	30	78†

*At 24 cm, adding another 3 kVp to 89 exceeds the maximum kVp limits of the machine. The kVp is lowered to 77 by subtracting 16% of 92. Consequently, this decreases the radiographic density by one half. To compensate for the loss of density, the mAs must be doubled to return the radiograph to its original density.
†Again, adding 3 kVp exceeds the maximum 90-kVp limit. The kVp is once more decreased by 16%, resulting in one-half the radiographic density. To compensate, the mAs is doubled again.

Variable mA Chart for When Detail Cassettes Are Not Available

Some veterinary practices make images with only one speed of intensifying screens. Most of those practices use high-speed screens. The same 40-lb anesthetized dog is used. As in the previous example, the best tabletop abdominal technique was 3.3 mAs and 70 kVp. The mAs chart is figured in the same way as the other examples, except the tabletop bone technique is 1 mAs greater than the tabletop abdomen mAs (Table 8-5). That value is multiplied by 3 to establish the

TABLE 8-5

VARIABLE mAs CHART FOR USE WITHOUT DETAIL SCREENS

TECHNIQUE	mAs
HIGH-SPEED SCREENS	
Tabletop abdomen	3.3
Grid abdomen	9.9
Tabletop thorax	1.6
Grid thorax	4.8
Tabletop bone	4.3
Grid bone	12.9

grid bone mAs. The kVp chart is unaffected by having only one speed of intensifying screens and is set up the same as the first example.

Recommended Reading

Liebel-Flarsheim: *Characteristics and applications of x-ray grids*, Cincinnati, 1989, Liebel-Flarsheim.

Mendenhall A, Cantwell HD: *Equine radiographic procedures*, Philadelphia, 1988, Lea & Febiger.

Ticer JW: *Radiographic technique in veterinary practice*, ed 2, Philadelphia, 1984, Saunders.

9

Radiographic Artifacts

CONNIE HAN

CHAPTER OBJECTIVES

- Describe the artifacts that can be created before processing.
- Explain the artifacts that can be created during manual or automatic processing.

Artifacts are any unwanted radiographic densities in the form of blemishes arising from improper handling, exposure, processing, or housekeeping. Artifacts can mimic or mask a disease process or distract from the overall quality of the x-ray film.

Before radiographing an animal, check for external changes. Any dirt or mats in the coat should be removed. If the coat is wet, it should be dried off as much as possible. Any collars and leashes should be removed. Bandage material can be seen on the radiograph, so it should be removed if at all possible. This chapter identifies possible artifact problems.

Artifacts That Occur Before Radiographic Processing

1. Fogged film (overall gray appearance)
   - The film was exposed to excessive scatter radiation. The use of a grid is necessary when radiographing areas 10 cm or greater.
   - The film was exposed to radiation during storage.
   - The film was stored in an area that was too hot or humid.
   - The film was exposed to a safelight filter that was cracked or inappropriate for the type of film being used.
   - The film was exposed to a low-grade light leak in the darkroom.
   - The film has expired.
2. Black crescents or lines
   - Rough handling of the film occurred either before or after exposure (Figure 9-1).
   - Exposure resulting from static electricity is caused by low humidity (Figure 9-2).
   - The film surface was scratched either before or after exposure.
   - Fingerprint smudges result from too much pressure either before or after exposure.
3. Black areas
   - A black irregular border on one end of the film is caused by light exposure while still in the box or film bin.

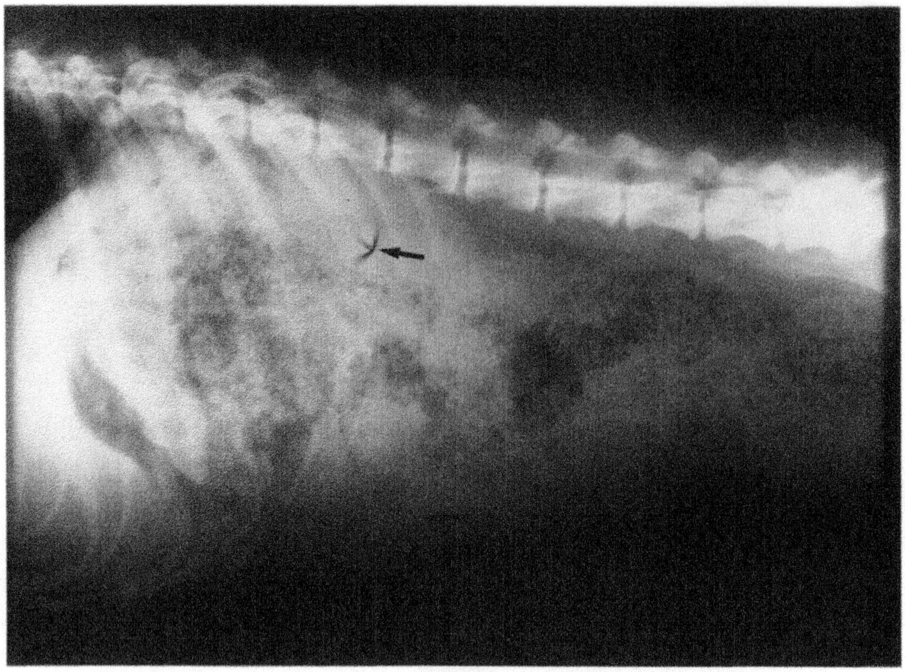

FIG. 9-1 Black crescent from rough handling of the film before or after exposure.

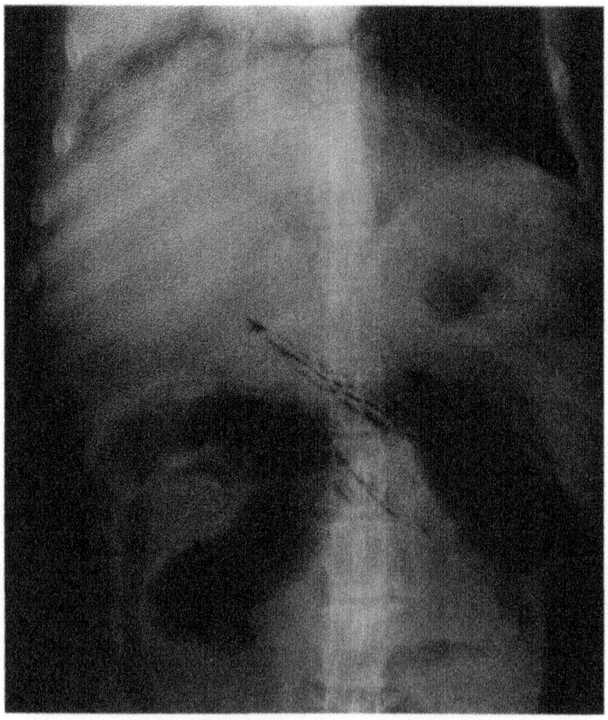

FIG. 9-2 Static electrical discharge.

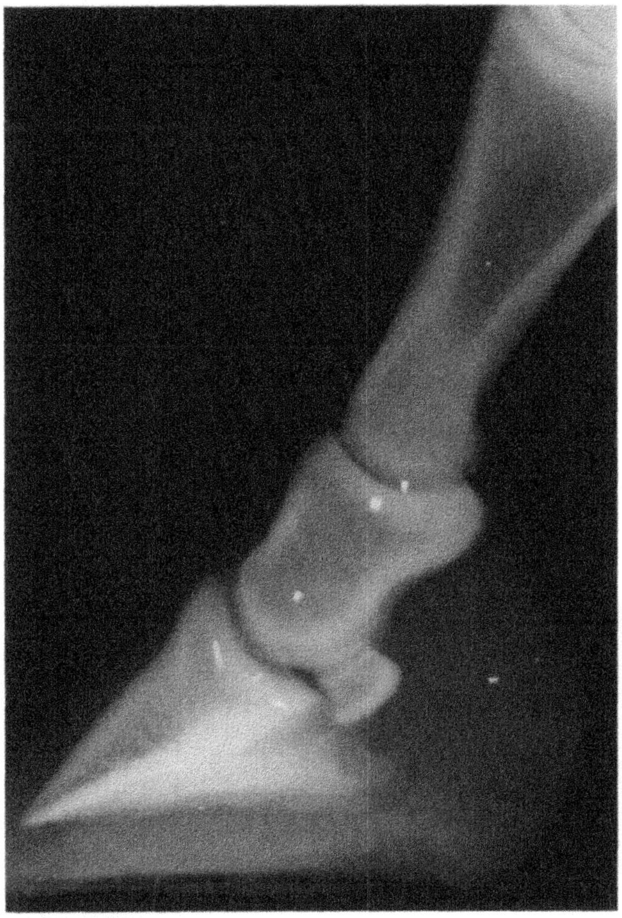

FIG. 9-3 Foreign material between the film and screen is blocking the light of the intensifying screen from exposing the film.

- A black irregular border occurring on multiple sides of the film is caused by felt damage in the cassette.

4. White areas
   - Foreign material exists between the film and screen (Figure 9-3).
   - Chemical spills on the screen cause permanent damage to the phosphor layer.
   - There is contrast medium on the patient, table, or cassette.
   - White fingerprints on the film result from oil or fixer on fingers before processing.
5. Visible grid lines
   - Grid lines on the entire film appear as a result of focal-film distance not being in the range of the grid's focus.
   - Grid lines that are more visible on one end of the film and an overall decrease in radiographic density are caused by the grid not being centered with the primary beam (Figure 9-4).
   - Grid lines on the entire film are caused by the grid not being perpendicular to the center of the primary beam.
   - Grid lines are visible in some areas more than others because of damage to the grid.
6. Decrease in detail
   - Patient motion (Figure 9-5).
   - Poor film-screen contact.
   - Increase in object-film distance.
   - Decrease in focal-film distance.

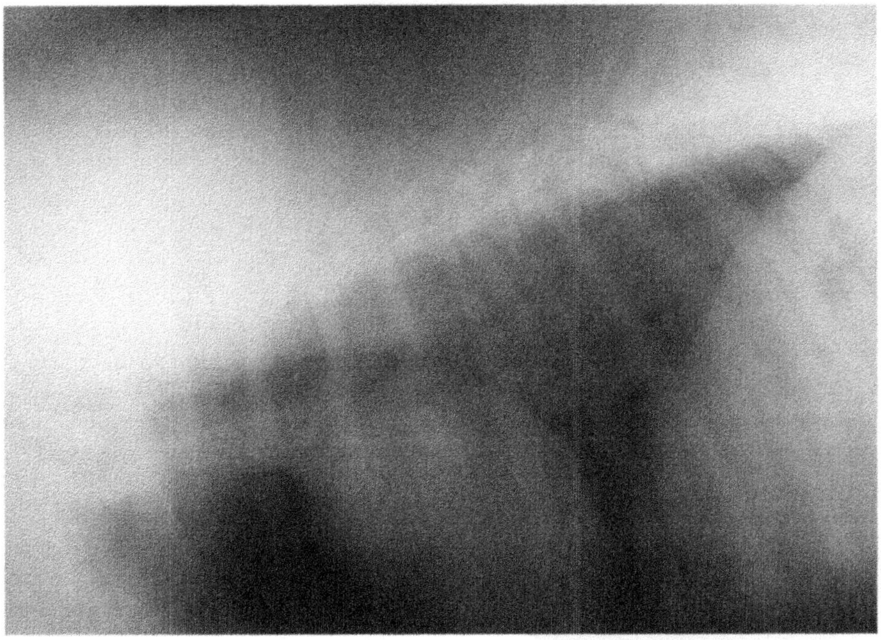

FIG. 9-4 Grid cutoff from the grid not being centered within the primary beam.

Artifacts That Occur During Manual or Automatic Processing

1. Increased radiographic density with poor contrast
   - The film was overdeveloped (longer than chemical's manufacturer recommends).
   - The film was developed in chemicals that were too hot. The correct temperature for manual tanks is 68° F (20° C) and for an automatic processor, 95° F (35° C).
   - The film was overexposed.
2. Decreased radiographic density with poor contrast
   - The film was underdeveloped (shorter then the chemical's manufacturer recommends).
   - The film was developed in chemicals that were too cold. The correct temperature for manual tanks is 68° F (20° C) and for an automatic processor, 95° F (35° C).
   - The film was processed in chemicals that were old or exhausted.
   - The film was underexposed.
3. Good radiographic density with poor contrast
   - Safelight fog from an improperly placed safelight (Figure 9-6).
   - Safelight fog from using the incorrect type of safelight filter for the film.
   - Safelight fog from a cracked safelight filter.
   - Low-grade light leak in the darkroom.

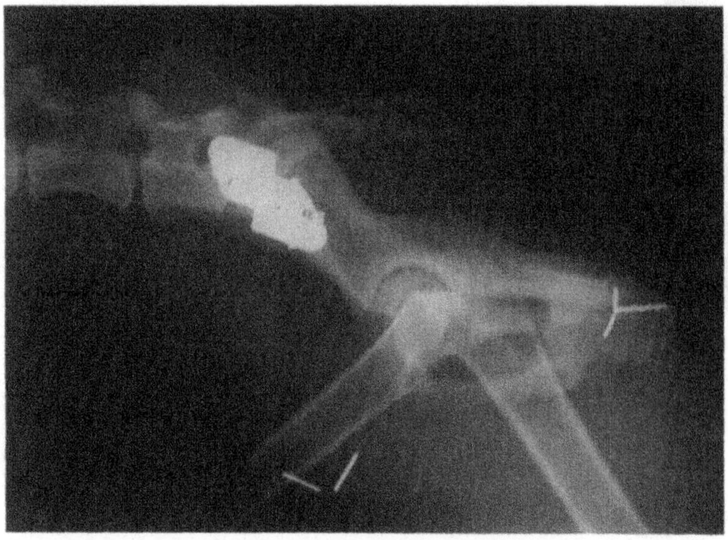

FIG. 9-5 Lack of patient cooperation or a panting patient combined with a long exposure time results in a blurred image.

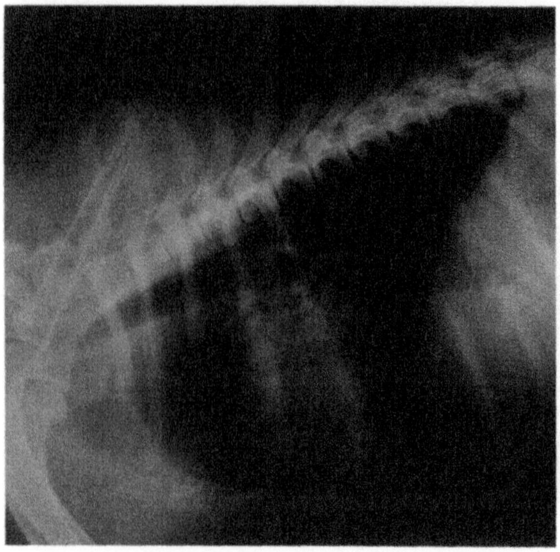

FIG. 9-6 Safelight fog created by a safelight that was placed too close to the workbench or by a cracked safelight filter. Note the light image of a person's hand over the heart. The area is light because the hand blocked the light from the safelight as the film was pushed into the automatic processor.

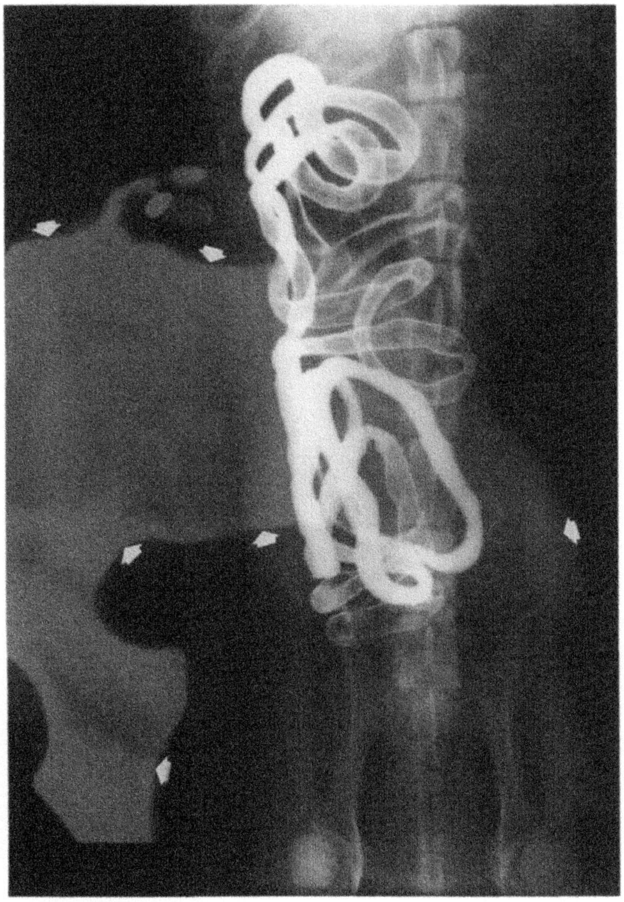

FIG. 9-7 This radiograph stuck to the side of the manual tank while in the developer. The arrows outline the artifact. A light image can still be seen because the film has emulsion on both sides of the film base. One side developed normally.

4. Uneven development
   - ◆ Unstirred chemicals that settle to the bottom of the tank.
   - ◆ Sight development.
   - ◆ Periodically viewing the film to determine the development time.
   - ◆ Uneven chemical levels.
5. Black areas, spots, or streaks
   - ◆ Identical black areas on two films that were processed together result from the films sticking to one another in the fixer and not being cleared correctly.
   - ◆ Black area on only one film occurs because it stuck to the side of the tank.
   - ◆ Well-defined spots or streaks result from developer splash before processing.
   - ◆ Linear black lines on the full length of the film and an equal distance apart result from pressure from rollers in the processor.

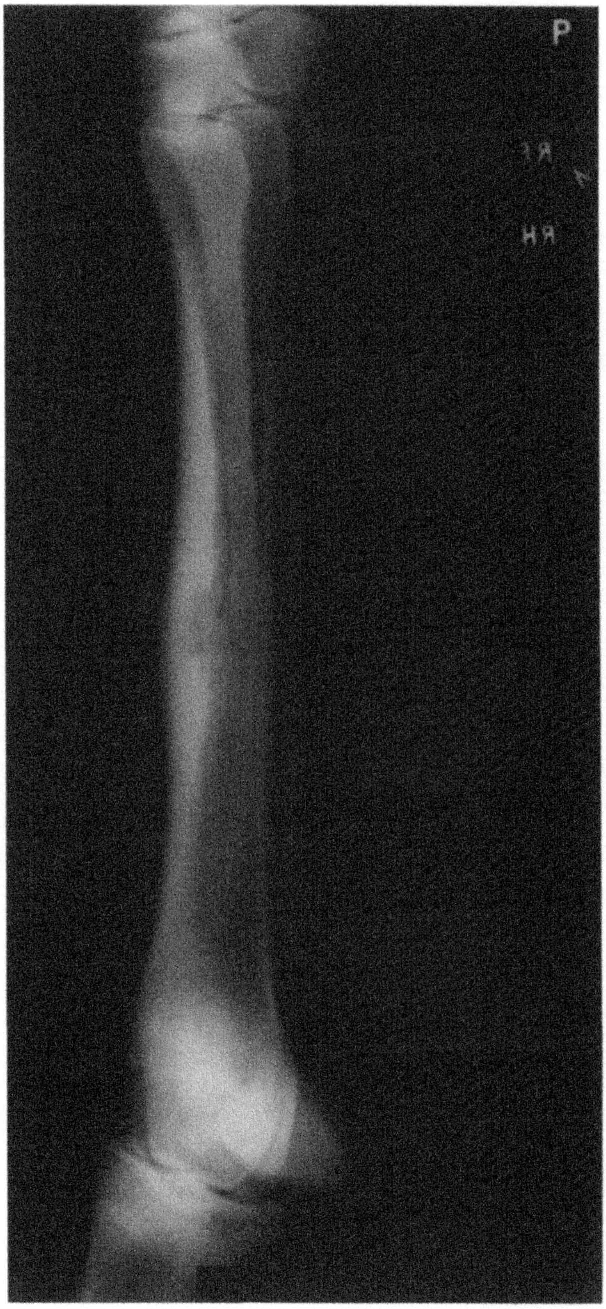

FIG. 9-8 Scratches on the film from a damaged roller in an automatic processor.

6. Defined areas of decreased radiographic density
   - ◆ Identical light areas on two films that were processed together result from the two films sticking together in the developer.
   - ◆ Light area on one film occurs because it stuck to the side of the tank during development (Figure 9-7).
   - ◆ Air bubbles clinging to the film during development.
   - ◆ Well-defined spots or streaks resulting from fixer splash before processing.

7. Clear areas or spots
   - Streaks occur where the emulsion has been scratched away.
   - Large areas of the film are clear because the film was left in the final wash too long, causing the emulsion to slide off the film base.
8. Defined white lines the length of the film
   - A damaged automatic processor roller caused scratches (Figure 9-8).
9. Entire film clear
   - There was no exposure.
   - The film was placed in the fixer before the developer.
10. Film turning brown in color
    - Final wash was conducted improperly.

Recommended Reading

Morgan JP, Silverman S: *Techniques of veterinary radiography*, ed 3, Davis, Calif, 1982, Veterinary Radiology Associates.

Ryan GD: *Radiographic positioning of small animals*, Philadelphia, 1981, Lea & Febiger.

Ticer JW: *Radiographic technique in veterinary practice*, ed 2, Philadelphia, 1984, Saunders.

PART TWO

Radiographic Positioning

10

Small Animal Radiography

CONNIE HAN

CHAPTER OBJECTIVES

- Define the terminology used to describe the positioning for radiographic procedures.
- Understand the oblique projections and how to label them.
- Read the written descriptions, look at the line drawing, and produce a diagnostic radiograph for any area of interest.

Proper patient positioning is as important as the radiograph itself. Misinterpretations can result from inaccurate positioning. This chapter serves as a reference for the radiographic procedures conducted in a veterinary hospital.

Directional Terminology

A basic knowledge of directional terminology is essential when describing radiographic projections. The American College of Veterinary Radiology (ACVR) has standardized the nomenclature for radiographic projections by using the currently accepted veterinary anatomic terms. The projections are described by the direction that the central ray enters and exits the part being imaged, as follows (Figure 10-1):

> Always take two views 90 degrees of one another.

1. **Ventral (V)**—The body area situated toward the underside of quadrupeds.
2. **Dorsal (D)**—The body area situated toward the back or topline of quadrupeds; opposite of ventral.
3. **Medial (M)**—The body area situated toward the median plane or midline.
4. **Lateral (L)**—The body area situated away from the median plane or midline.
5. **Cranial (Cr)**—Structures or areas situated toward the head (formerly *anterior).*
6. **Caudal (Cd)**—Structures or areas situated toward the tail (formerly *posterior).*
7. **Rostral (R)**—Areas on the head situated toward the nose.
8. **Palmar (Pa)**—Situated on the caudal aspect of the front limb, distal to the antebrachiocarpal joint.
9. **Plantar (Pl)**—Situated on the caudal aspect of the rear limb, distal to the tarsocrural joint.
10. **Proximal (Pr)**—Situated closer to the point of attachment or origin.

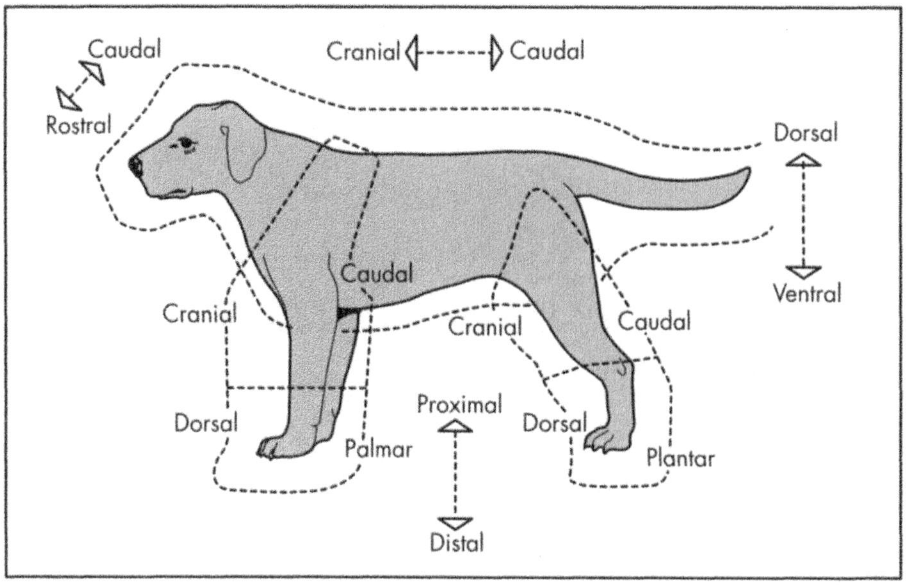

FIG. 10-1 Veterinary anatomic terminology.

11. **Distal (Di)**—Situated away from the point of attachment or origin.

Oblique Projections

Oblique projections are used to set off an area that would normally be superimposed over another area. When deciding what type of oblique projection is needed and how it is identified, follow these two guidelines:

1. Ensure that the area of interest is as close to the cassette as possible. This decreases magnification and increases detail.
2. Place a marker on the cassette during exposure to indicate the direction of entry and exit of the primary beam.

Positioning for Radiographs of The Skull

Correct positioning is most important when radiographing the skull. The symmetry of the skull is used when interpreting the films. Even a small deviation can cause misinterpretations.

General anesthesia is required for proper patient positioning. The number of radiographs made depends on the clinical signs exhibited by the patient. Always begin with *lateral* and *ventrodorsal* radiographs. Because the animal is under anesthesia and motion is not a factor, the grid is used to increase the detail and contrast on the radiograph. Positioning aids such as tape, sandbags, and clean, dry roll cotton or foam wedges are used to minimize personnel exposure.

Lateral Position

Place the patient in lateral recumbency, and position the head so the tympanic bullae and the rami of the mandibles are superimposed. This is accomplished by padding beneath the dependent mandible with rolled cotton or a clean foam wedge. Roll the head so that an imaginary line can be drawn superimposing one eye over the other, perpendicular to the table. Also pad under the nose so that an imaginary line can be drawn from the nose to between the eyes parallel to the table. Center the primary beam on the skull, making sure that the collimation light shows the tip of the nose, the top of the head, the base of the skull, and the mandible (Figures 10-2 and 10-3).

> When radiographing for a nasal problem, measure for the kVp slightly rostral to the highest point to avoid overexposing the air-filled nasal passages.

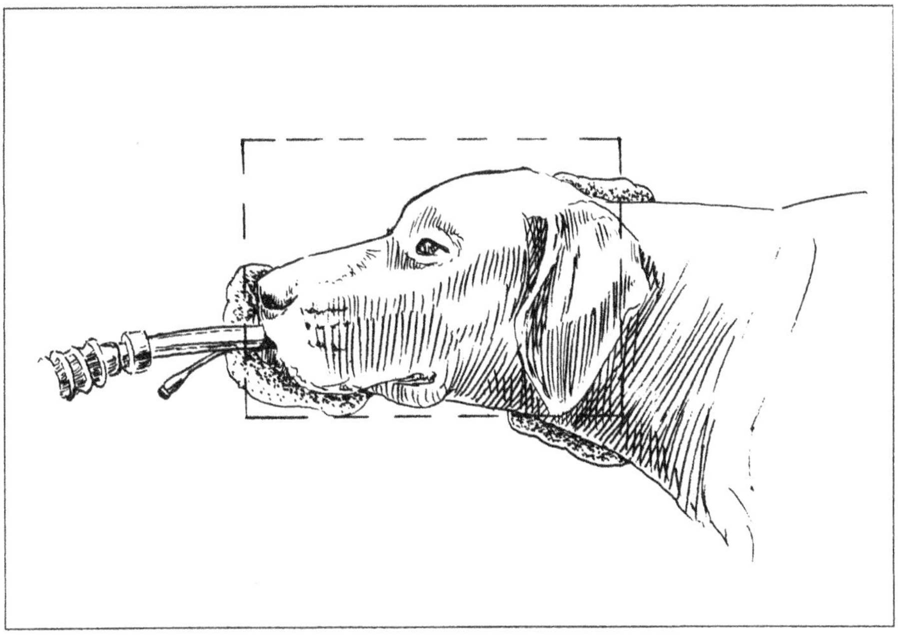

FIG. 10-2 Positioning for a lateral projection of the skull.

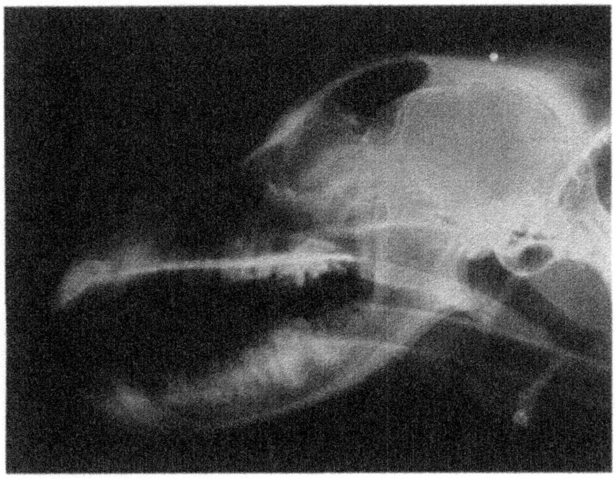

FIG. 10-3 Lateral projection of the skull.

Ventrodorsal Position

The patient is placed in ventrodorsal position with the front limbs extended caudally. The hard palate should be parallel to the table. This can be achieved by either taping across the incisor teeth from one side of the table to the other or placing roll cotton beneath the neck. Check the symmetry of the skull from the end of the table, making sure it is not oblique.

Center the primary beam on the skull, ensuring that the collimation light shows the tip of the nose, the base of the skull, and both right and left sides of the skull. Identify the left *(L)* or right *(R)* side. Before the exposure is made, remove the endotracheal tube to avoid superimposition over the skull (Figures 10-4 and 10-5).

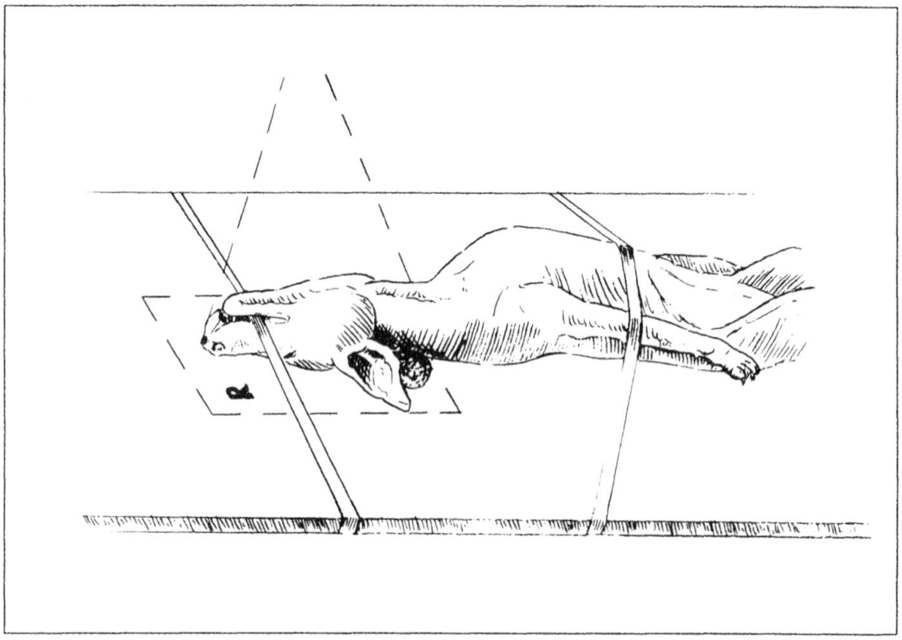

FIG. 10-4 Positioning for a ventrodorsal projection of the skull.

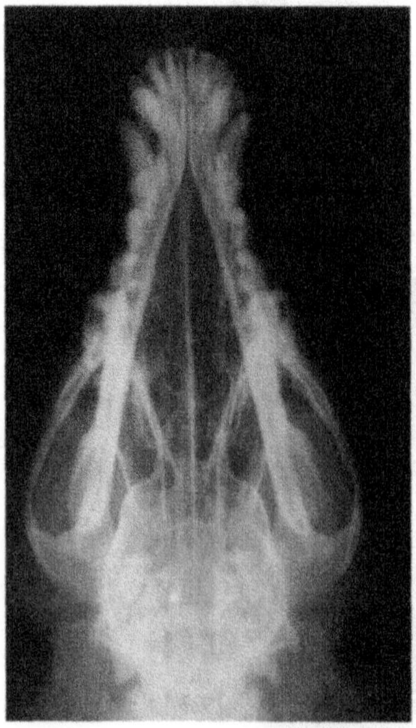

FIG. 10-5 Ventrodorsal projection of the skull.

Ventrodorsal Open Mouth (Maxillary) Position

Ventral 15 to 20 degrees/rostral-dorsocaudal oblique

This view shows the nasal and ethmoid regions without superimposition of the mandible. The patient is placed in ventrodorsal position with the front limbs extended caudally. Place tape across the incisor teeth to bring the hard palate parallel to the table, then place tape around the mandible, pulling it caudally and opening the mouth as wide as possible. Angle the x-ray tube rostral to caudal no more than 20 degrees. The degree of angle depends on how wide the mouth can be opened. Identify the left or right side. The tracheal tube does not need to be removed; include it in the tape pulling the mandible caudally (Figures 10-6 and 10-7).

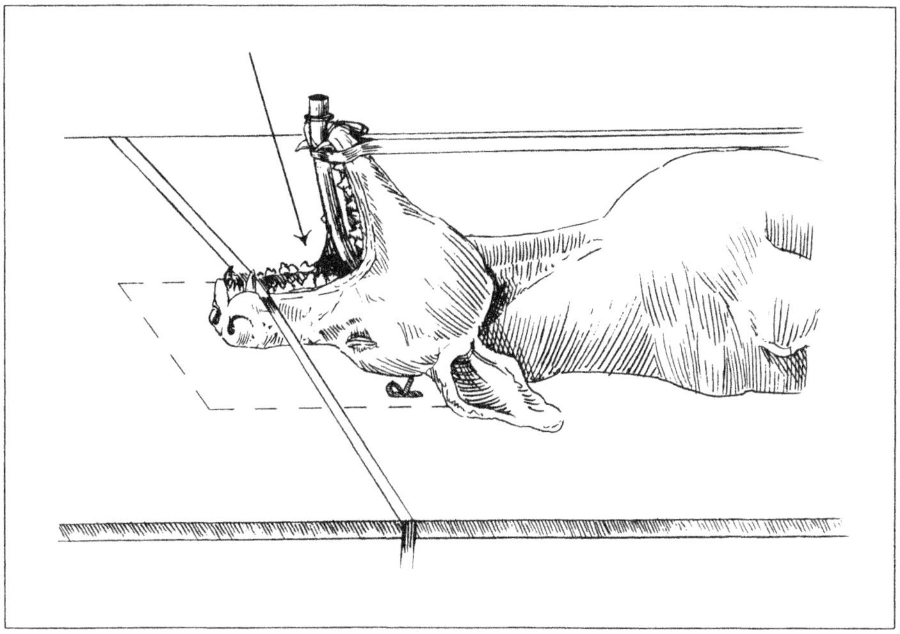

FIG. 10-6 Positioning for a ventrodorsal open mouth projection of the skull.

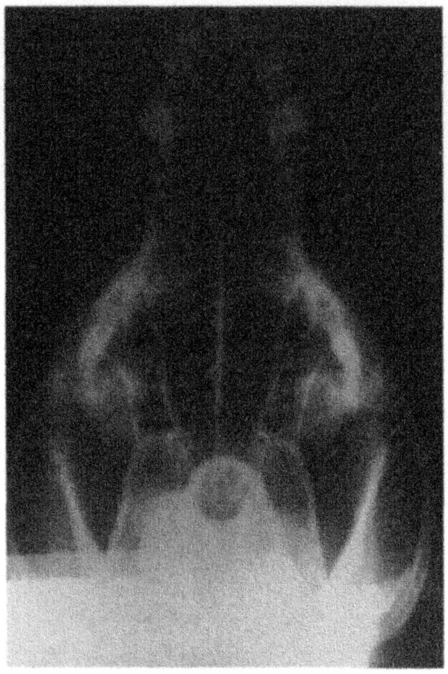

FIG. 10-7 Ventrodorsal open mouth projection of the skull.

Frontal 90 Degrees

Rostrocaudal

This view shows the frontal sinuses. The patient is placed in ventrodorsal position with the front limbs extended caudally. Place tape around the nose so that it can be pulled caudally. Position the nose so that the hard palate is perpendicular to the table. Center the primary beam on the frontal sinuses and collimate the beam. Measure the thickness for the kilovoltage peak (kVp) setting at the level of the sinuses, which is between the eyes. Identify the right or left side (Figures 10-8 and 10-9).

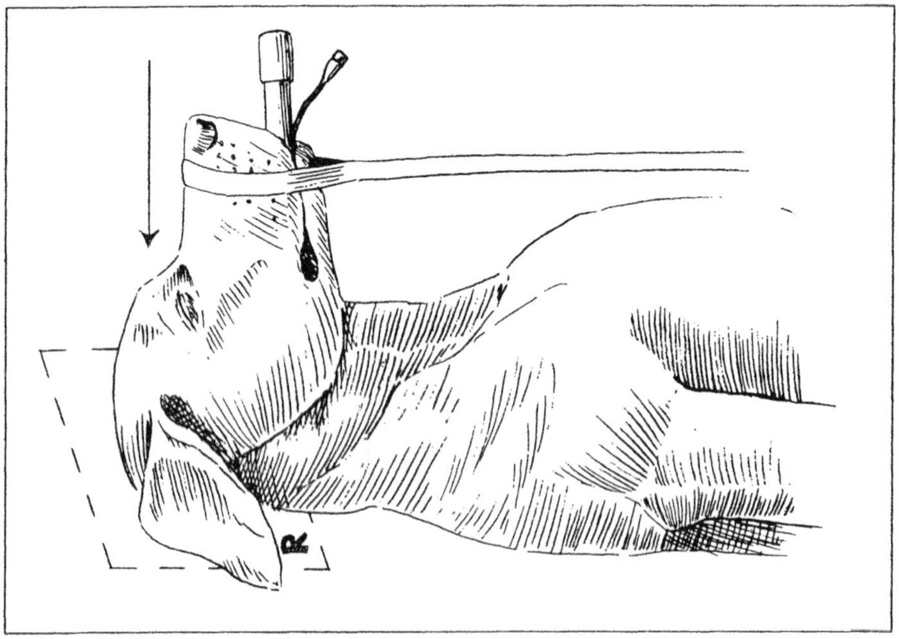

FIG. 10-8 Positioning for a frontal 90-degree projection of the skull.

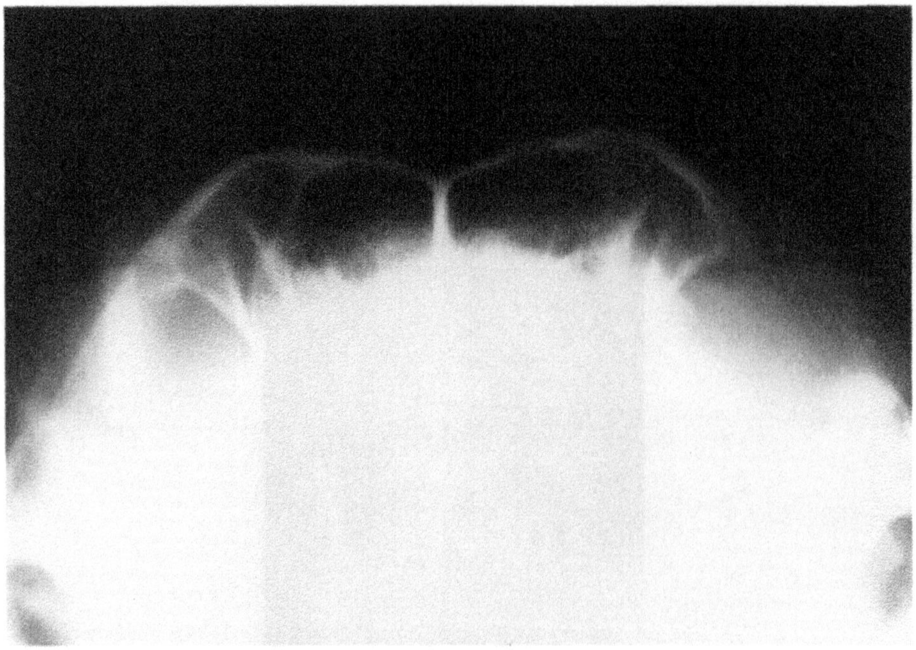

FIG. 10-9 Frontal 90-degree projection of the skull.

Frontal 15 to 20 Degrees

Rostral 15 to 20 degrees dorsal-caudoventral

This view shows the cranial vault, calvarium, and sagittal crest. The patient is placed in ventrodorsal position with the front limbs extended caudally. Place tape around the nose so that it can be pulled caudally. Position the skull so that the hard palate is pulled caudally 15 to 20 degrees from perpendicular. Measure thickness for the kVp setting at the level of the frontal sinuses. Identify the right or left side (Figures 10-10 and 10-11).

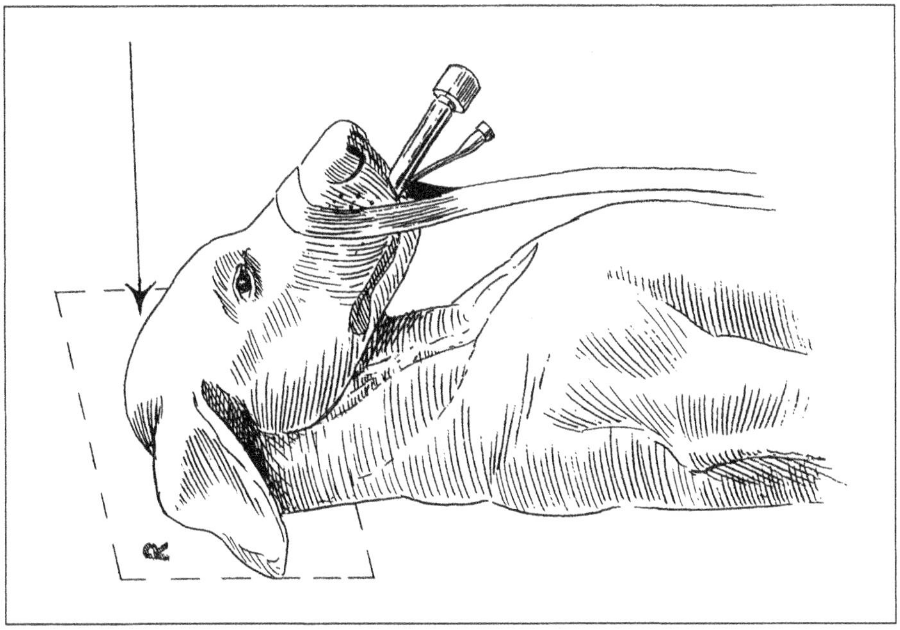

FIG. 10-10 Positioning for a frontal 15- to 20-degree projection of the skull.

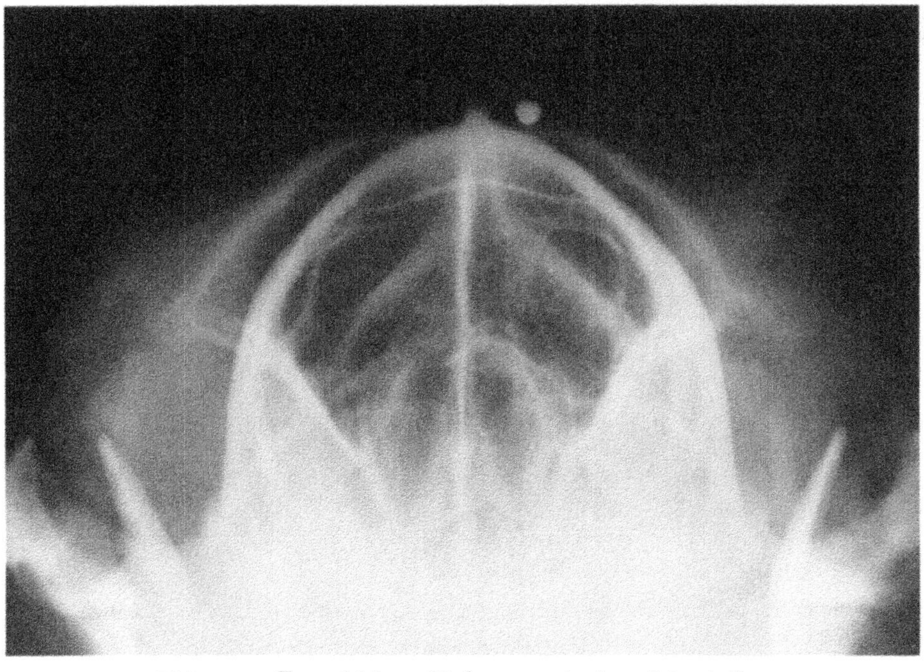

FIG. 10-11 Frontal 15- to 20-degree projection of the skull.

Open Mouth Tympanic Bulla

Rostral 30 degrees ventral-caudodorsal

This view shows the tympanic bulla with minimal superimposition of the petrous temporal bone. The patient is placed in ventodorsal position with the front limbs extended caudally. Place tape around the mandible, including the tongue and tracheal tube to keep the tube near the mandible and in the midline of the tongue. Using tape, pull the maxilla rostrally and the mandible caudally so that the primary beam is centered over the tympanic bulla perpendicular to the table. Measure for the kVp setting from the table to the commissure of the mouth. Collimate the beam and identify the right or left side (Figures 10-12 and 10-13).

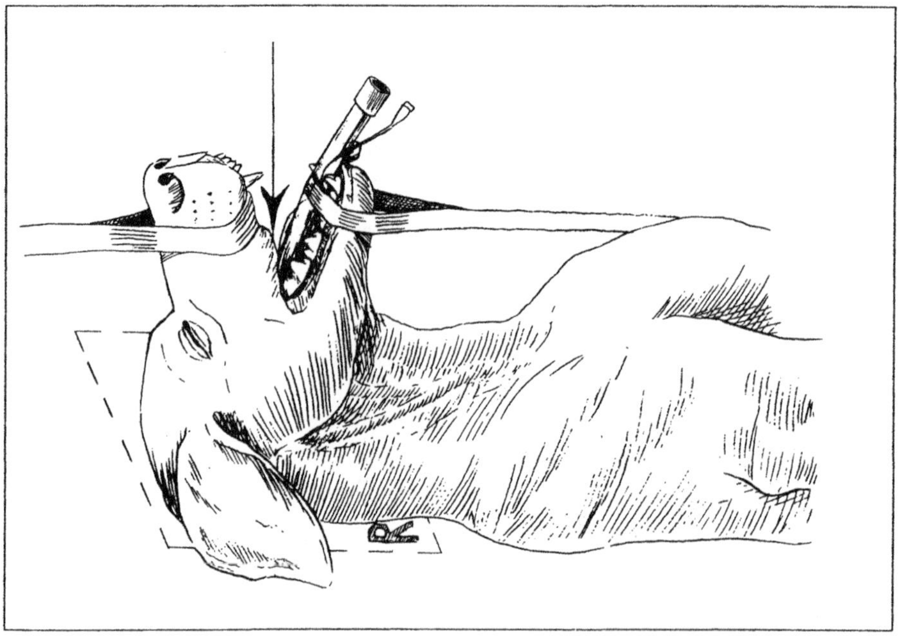

FIG. 10-12 Positioning for an open mouth tympanic bulla projection.

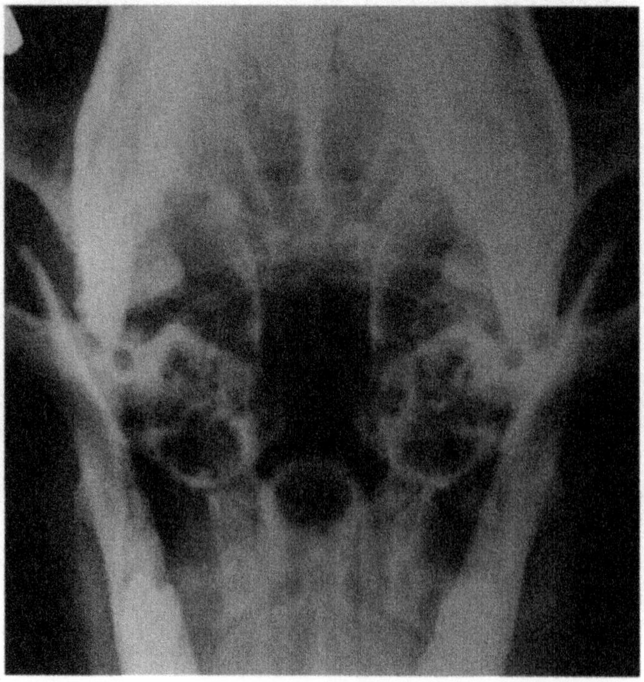

FIG. 10-13 Open mouth tympanic bulla projection.

Tympanic Bulla View for Cats

Rostral 10 degrees ventral-caudodorsal

This view shows the tympanic bulla in cats. The patient is placed in ventrodorsal position with the front limbs extended caudally. Position the skull so that the hard palate is pulled cranially 10 degrees from perpendicular. A small amount of padding can be wedged under the external occipital protuberance to maintain the 10-degree angle. Use the same kVp that was used for the ventrodorsal skull projection. Collimate the beam and identify the right or left side (Figures 10-14 and 10-15).

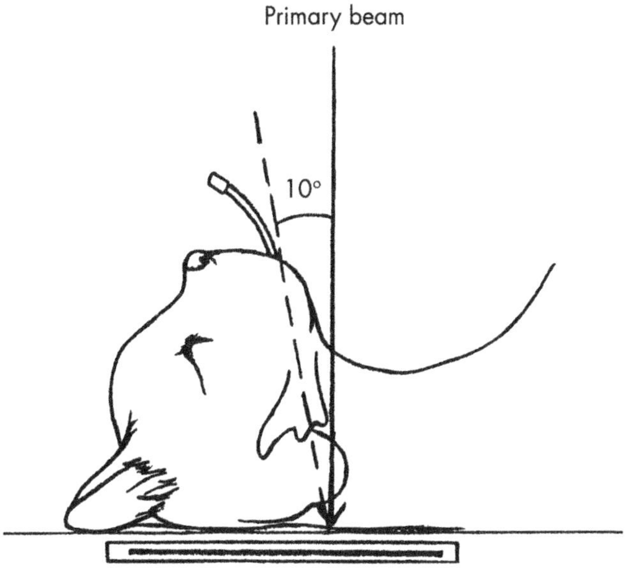

FIG. 10-14 Positioning for a tympanic bulla view on a cat.

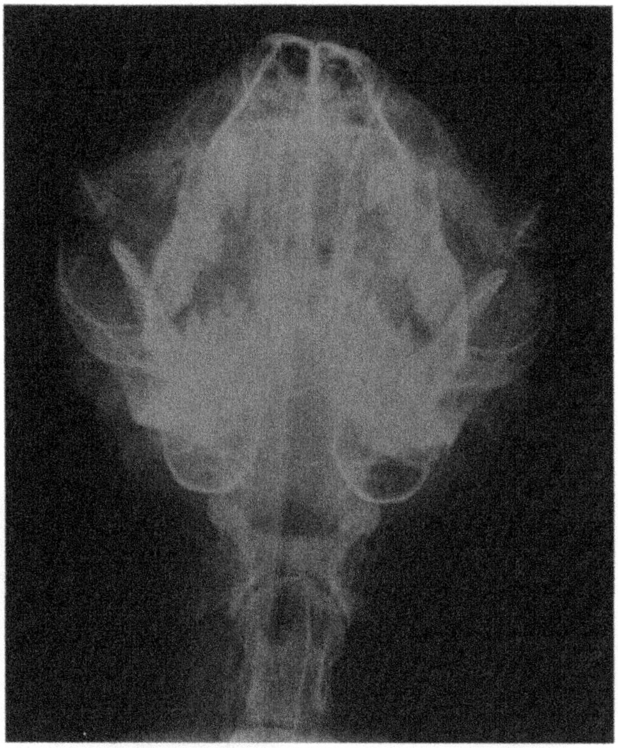

FIG. 10-15 Tympanic bulla projection on a cat.

Intraoral view

This view shows the rostral part of the mandible or maxilla without superimposition of the opposite dental arcade. The use of direct-exposure film is recommended to maximize the detail of the image. With either image, the skull needs to be in strict ventrodorsal or dorsoventral position.

MAXILLA

The patient is placed in sternal recumbency with the tracheal tube tied to the mandible. Place a corner of the direct-exposure film into the mouth as far as possible. Collimate and identify the right or left side (Figures 10-16 and 10-17).

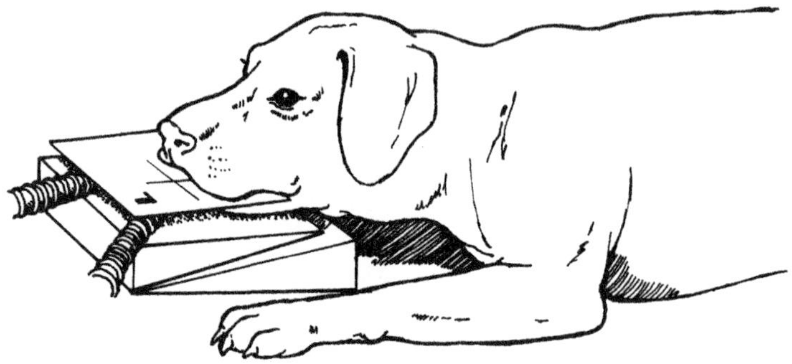

FIG. 10-16 Positioning for an intraoral image of the maxilla.

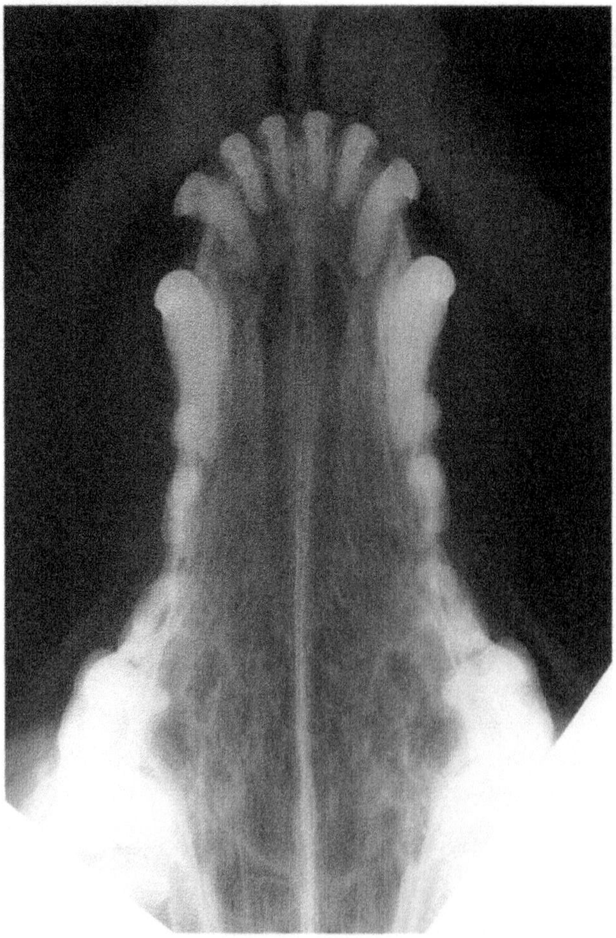

FIG. 10-17 Intraoral projection of the maxilla.

Mandible

The patient is placed in ventrodorsal position with the front limbs extended caudally. Place a corner of the direct-exposure film as far into the mouth as possible with the tongue down the center of the mandible. Collimate and identify the right or left side (Figures 10-18 and 10-19).

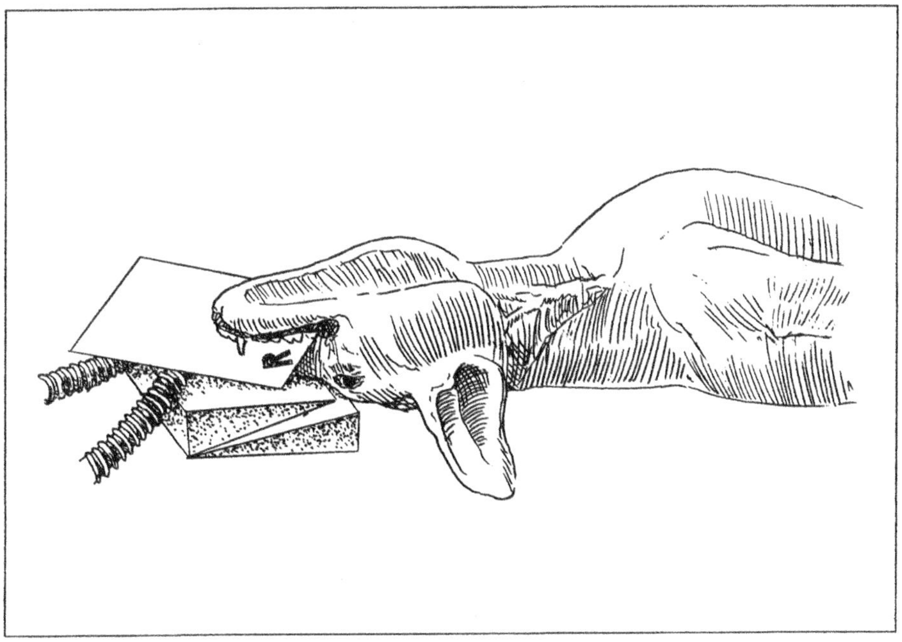

FIG. 10-18 Positioning for an intraoral image of the mandible.

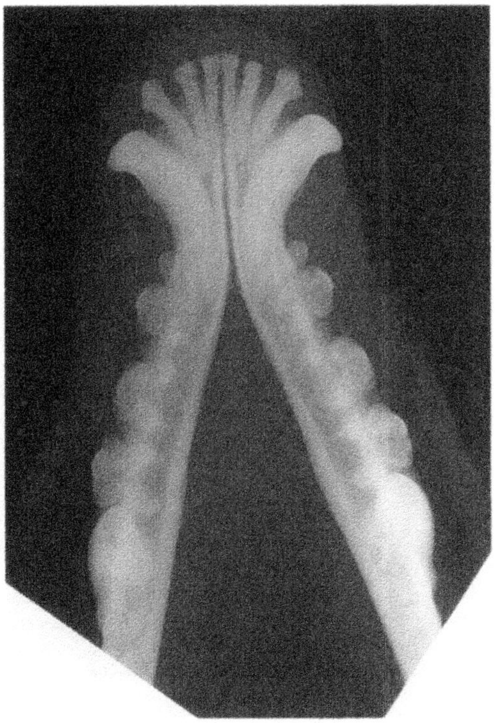

FIG. 10-19 Intraoral image of the mandible.

Lateral Oblique Positioning for the Maxillary Dental Arcade

Left 30 degrees ventral–right dorsal oblique; right 30 degrees ventral–left dorsal oblique

This projection allows visualization of the maxillary premolars and molars without superimposition of the other arcades. The patient is placed in right lateral recumbency to image the right maxillary arcade and in left lateral recumbency for the left maxillary arcade. Tie the endotracheal tube to the mandible. Prop the mouth open and oblique with the skull 30 degrees toward ventrodorsal position. Collimate and identify the oblique projection (Figures 10-20 and 10-21).

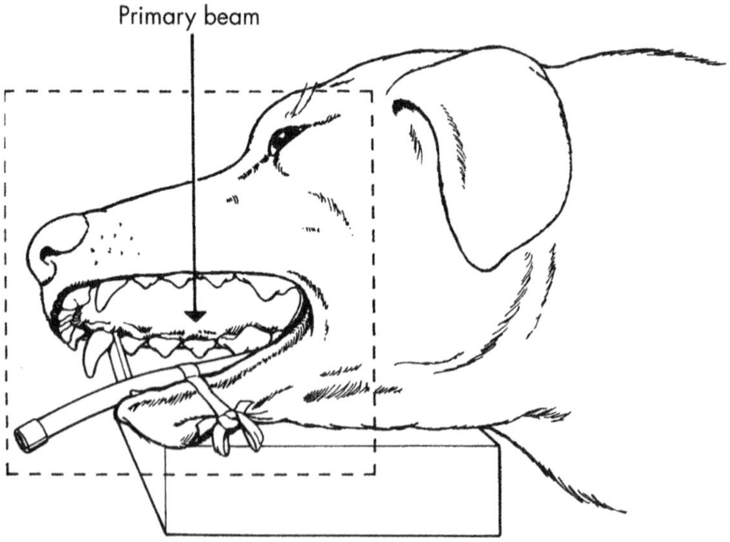

FIG. 10-20 Positioning for a lateral oblique view of the maxillary dental arcade.

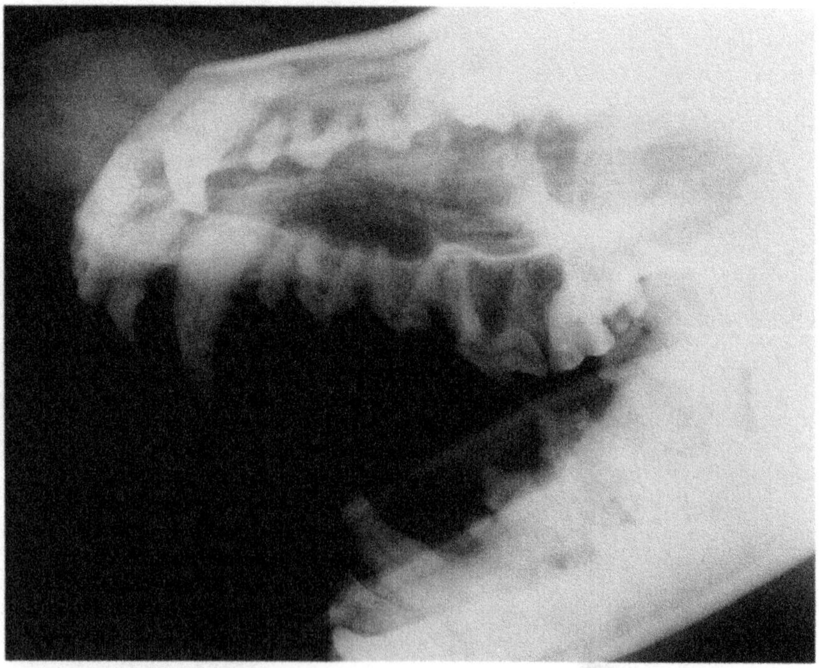

FIG. 10-21 Lateral oblique view of the maxillary dental arcade.

Lateral Oblique Positioning for the Mandibular Dental Arcade

Left 30 degrees dorsal–right ventral oblique; right 30 degrees dorsal–left ventral oblique

This projection allows visualization of the mandibular premolars and molars without superimposition of the other arcades. The patient is placed in right lateral recumbency to image the right mandibular arcade and in left lateral recumbency for the left mandibular arcade. Tie the endotracheal tube to the maxilla. Prop the mouth open and oblique with the skull 30 degrees toward dorsoventral position. Collimate and identify the oblique projection (Figures 10-22 and 10-23).

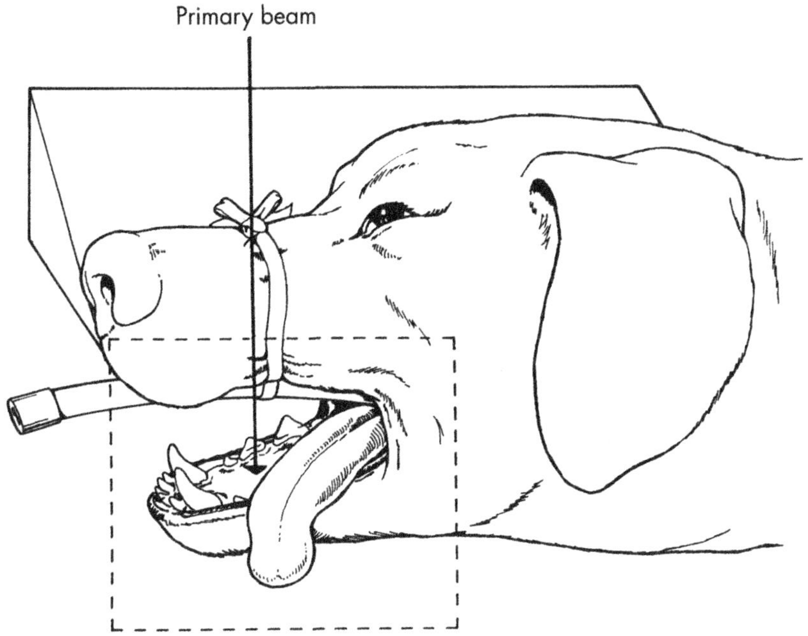

FIG. 10-22 Positioning for a lateral oblique view of the mandibular dental arcade.

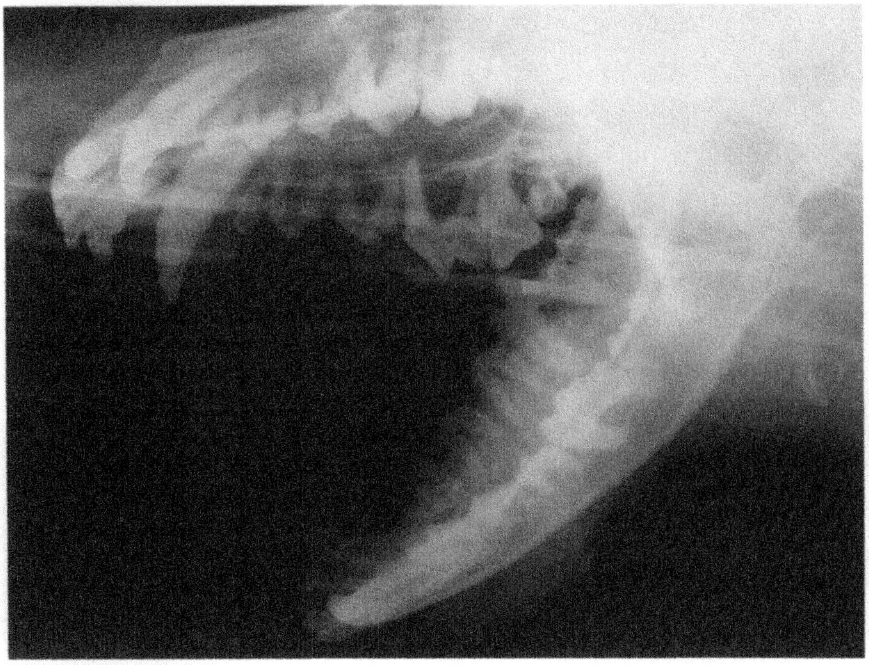

FIG. 10-23 Lateral oblique view of the mandibular dental arcade.

Lateral Oblique Positioning for the Tympanic Bullae and Temporomandibular Joints

Left 20 degrees ventral–right dorsal oblique; right 20 degrees ventral–left dorsal oblique

This projection separates the bullae and temporomandibular joints (TMJs). The patient is placed in right lateral recumbency to image the right bulla and TMJ and in left lateral recumbency for the left bulla and TMJ. Position the skull oblique 15 to 20 degrees toward ventrodorsal position, and raise the nose slightly (Figures 10-24 and 10-25).

> The oblique view for the TMJ can be achieved by positioning the animal with mouth propped open.

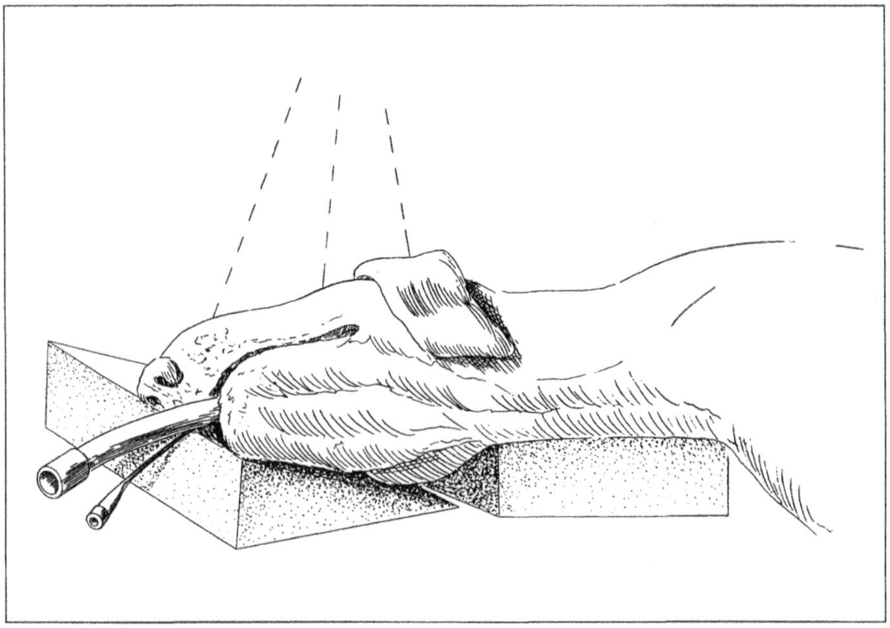

FIG. 10-24 Positioning for a lateral oblique view of the skull to image the tympanic bullae and temporomandibular joints.

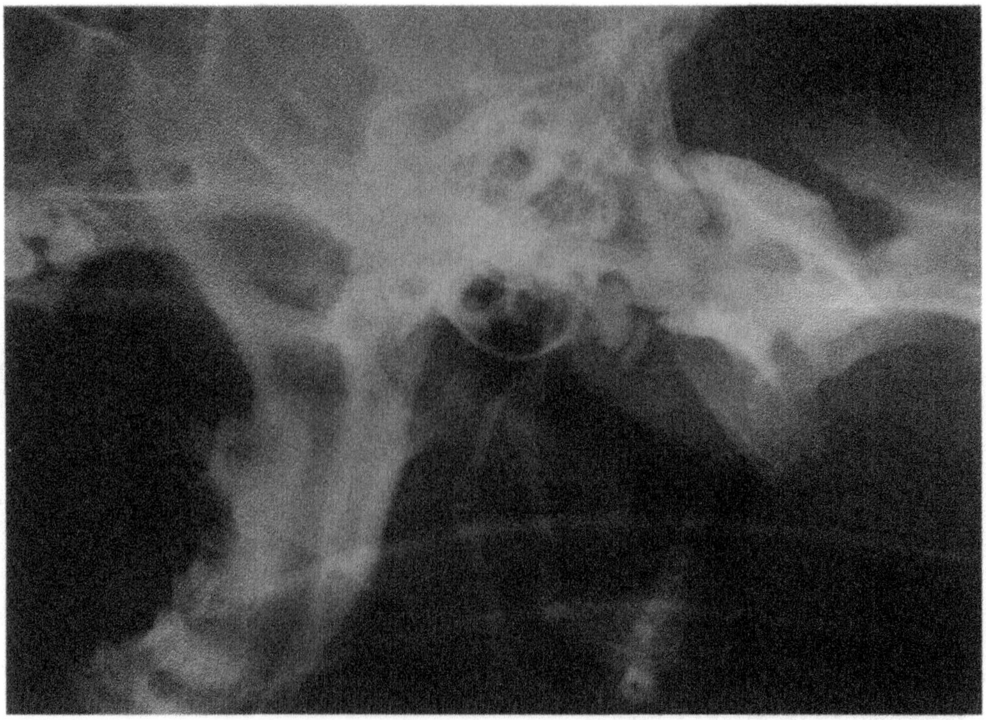

FIG. 10-25 Lateral oblique view of the skull projecting the tympanic bulla and temporomandibular joint.

Vertebral Column

General anesthesia is mandatory for obtaining quality radiographs of the vertebral column. If radiographs are made without anesthesia, false narrowing of the intervertebral disc spaces can result from muscle spasm. Since the patient is anesthetized and motion is not a factor, a grid is always used to increase the detail and contrast of the radiograph. With all radiographic procedures involving the vertebral column, place the longitudinal center of the primary beam on the vertebrae and collimate the width of the beam to increase the detail. Clean and dry padding should always be used. The use of tape or sandbags also aids in positioning the limbs.

Cervical Vertebrae

Lateral Position

Place the patient in lateral recumbency with the front limbs extended caudally. Do not overextend the limbs because rotation of the spine can occur. Pad beneath the mandible to superimpose the wings of the atlas. Padding may also be needed under the neck so that the spine does not sag in the middle, causing a false narrowing. However, too much padding can cause the spine to bulge, also producing a false narrowing. The cranial landmark is the base of the skull and the caudal landmark is the spine of the scapula. Place the wings of the atlas and the center of the spine of the scapula in the longitudinal center of the primary beam. Measure over the spine of the scapula for the kVp setting (Figures 10-26 and 10-27).

> The topographic landmark for the caudal cervical vertebrae is the center of the spine of the scapula.

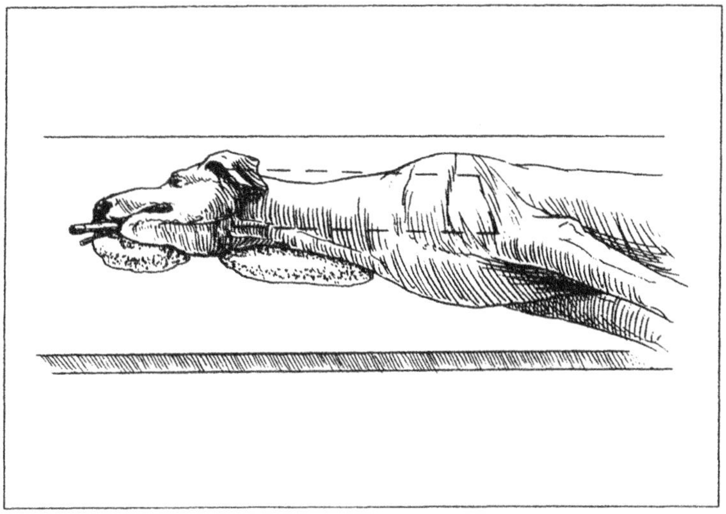

FIG. 10-26 Positioning for a lateral projection of the cervical vertebrae.

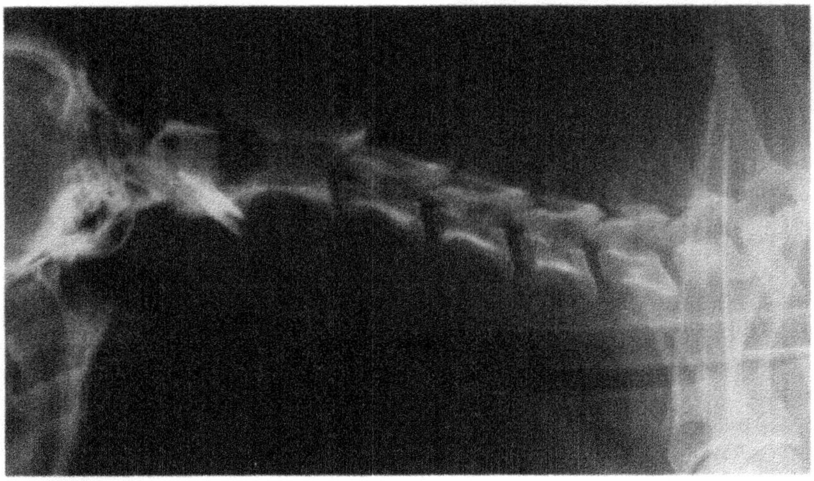

FIG. 10-27 Lateral projection of the cervical vertebrae.

Ventrodorsal Position

Place the patient in ventrodorsal position with the front limbs extended caudally. Ensure that the head and spine are placed in a natural position without padding and are not oblique. The cranial landmark is the base of the skull, and the caudal landmark is the spine of the scapula. Measure at the manubrium for the kVp setting. Remove the tracheal tube before making the exposure (Figures 10-28 and 10-29).

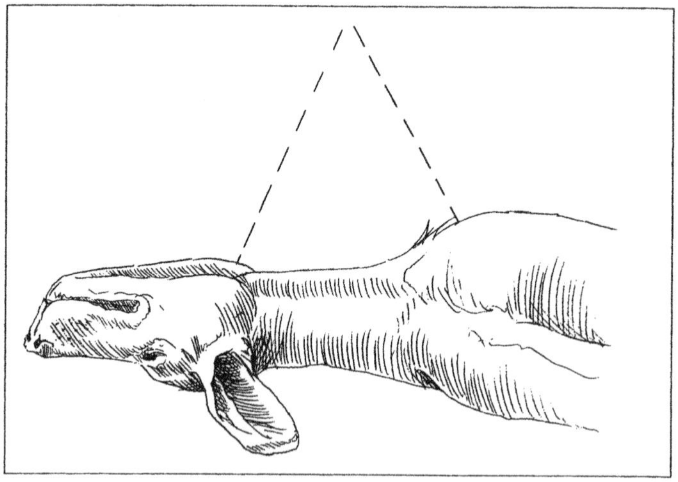

FIG. 10-28 Positioning for a ventrodorsal projection of the cervical vertebrae.

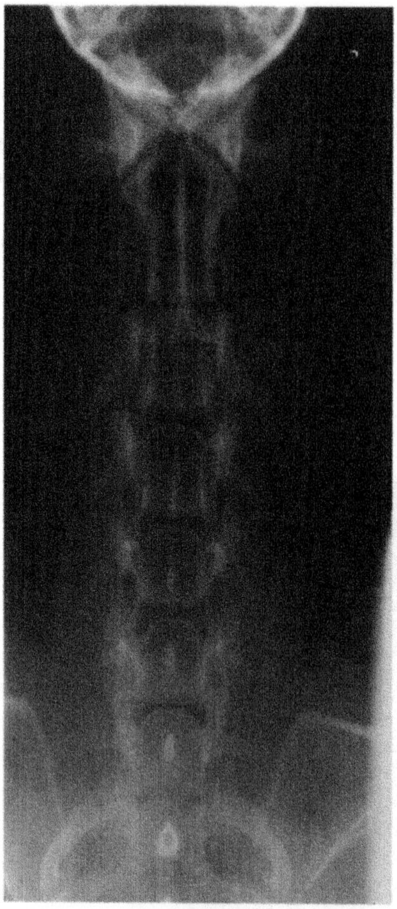

FIG. 10-29 Ventrodorsal projection of the cervical vertebrae.

Dorsoventral Position

For the dorsoventral position, place the patient in sternal recumbency. Pad under the head, keeping the vertebrae parallel to the table and not oblique. The cranial landmark is the base of the skull, and the caudal landmark is the spine of the scapula. Measure at the manubrium for the kVp setting. Remove the tracheal tube before making the exposure (Figure 10-30).

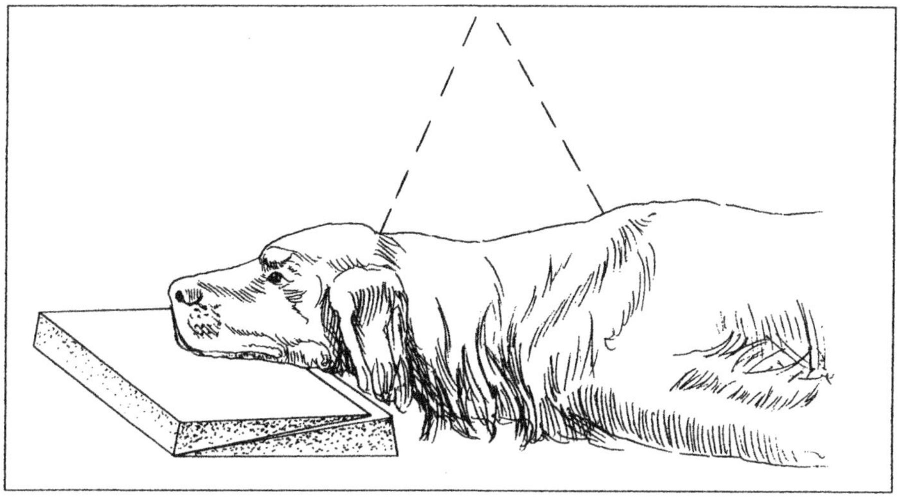

FIG. 10-30 Positioning for a dorsoventral projection of the cervical vertebrae.

Oblique Projection

The purpose for this view is to help localize a myelographic lesion observed on the lateral and ventrodorsal projections. Position the patient in lateral recumbency with the front limbs extended slightly caudal. Place padding under the cranial thorax to obtain a 45-degree oblique projection. Pad the head so that it is also at a 45-degree angle. Both oblique projections should be made for comparison (Figure 10-31).

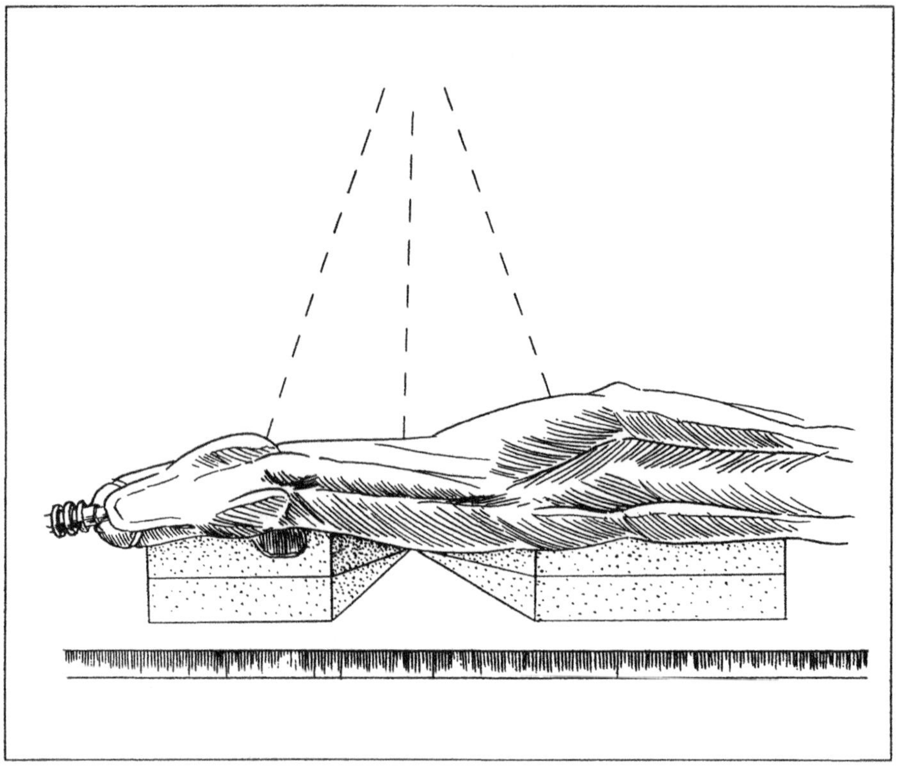

FIG. 10-31 Positioning for a 45-degree oblique view of the cervical vertebrae.

Flexed Lateral Position

This view is sometimes made during myelography to visualize spinal cord impingement by extradural changes associated with vertebral instability. Position the patient in lateral recumbency with the front limbs extended slightly caudal. Place a thin rope or tape around the lower canine teeth, and flex the head and neck ventrally and caudally. It is important to flex the fifth and sixth cervical vertebrae (C5-6) as much as C2-3 (Figure 10-32).

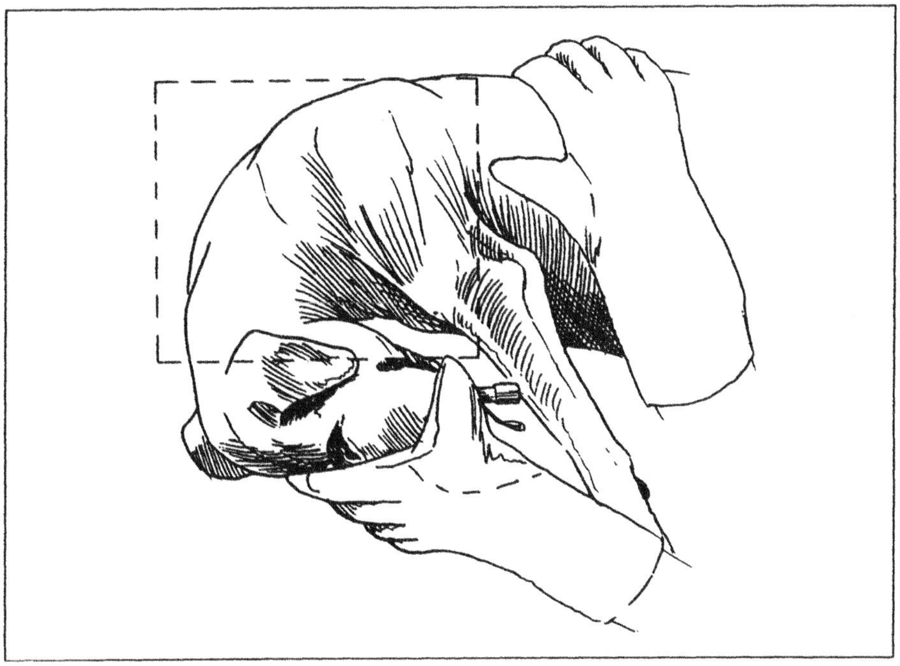

FIG. 10-32 Positioning for a flexed lateral view of the cervical vertebrae.

Extended Lateral Position

This view is sometimes made during myelography to visualize spinal cord impingement by extradural changes associated with vertebral instability. Position the patient in lateral recumbency with the front limbs extended slightly caudal. With sandbags, hyperextend the head and neck dorsally and caudally. The cranial landmark is the base of the skull, and the caudal landmark is the spine of the scapula (Figure 10-33).

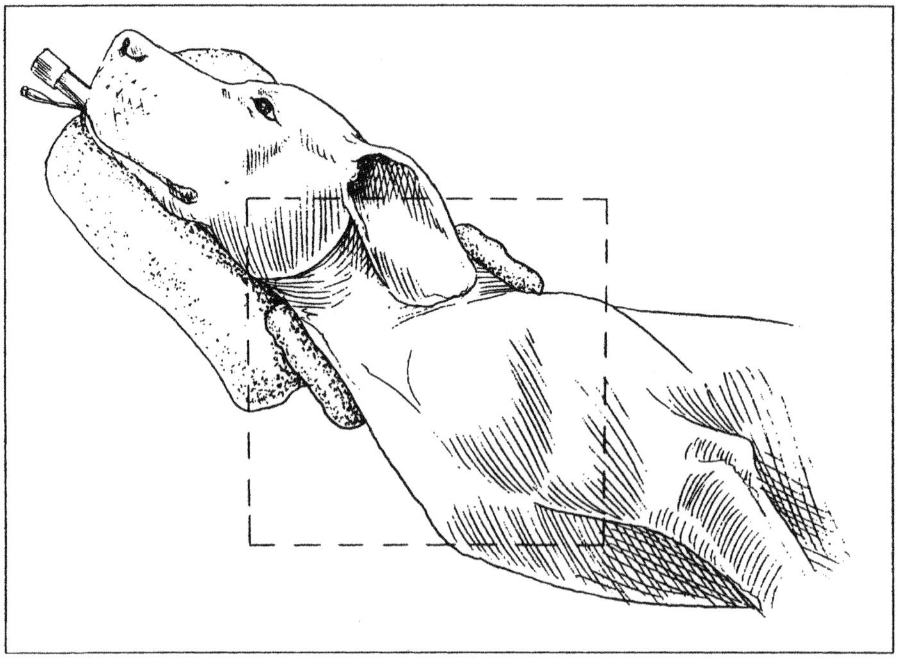

FIG. 10-33 Positioning for an extended lateral view of the cervical vertebrae.

Thoracic Vertebrae

Lateral Position

Place the patient in lateral recumbency with the front limbs extended cranially. Pad under the sternum or the spine to position the sternum and the spinous processes in a plane parallel to the table. This superimposes the ribs over one another, providing better visualization of the intervertebral disc spaces. The cranial landmark is the spine of the scapula. The caudal landmark is halfway between the xiphoid and the last rib and dorsal to the vertebrae. Measure at the highest point of the thorax for the kVp setting (Figures 10-34 and 10-35).

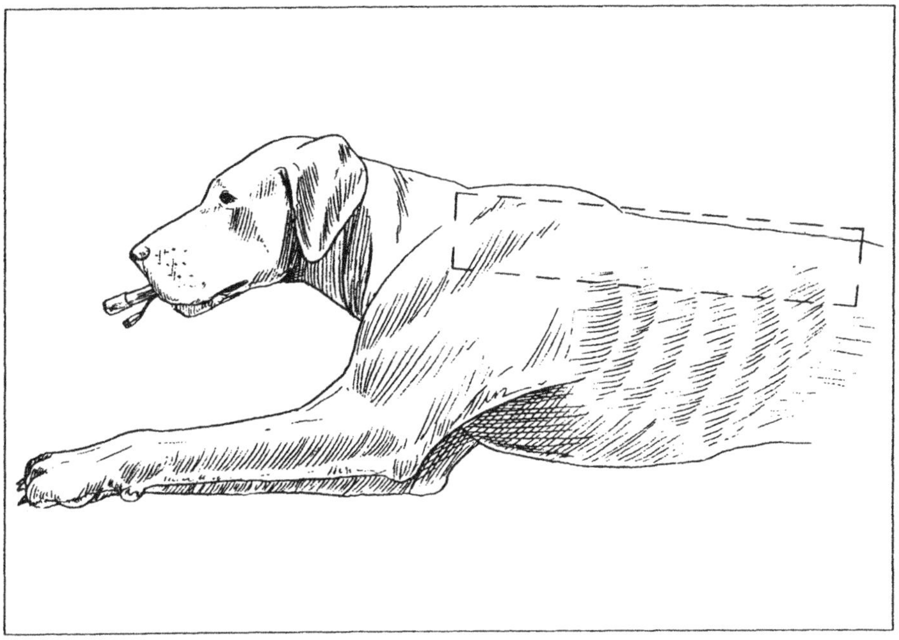

FIG. 10-34 Positioning for a lateral projection of the thoracic vertebrae.

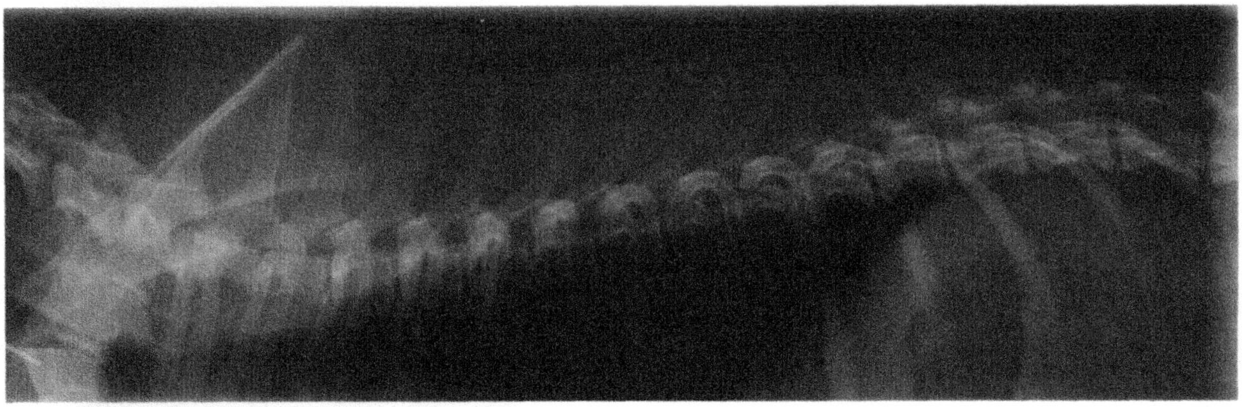

FIG. 10-35 Lateral projection of the thoracic vertebrae.

Ventrodorsal Position

Place the patient in ventrodorsal position with the front limbs extended cranially. Position the patient so the sternum and vertebrae are superimposed in a plane perpendicular to the table. The cranial landmark is the spine of the scapula. The caudal landmark is halfway between the xiphoid and the last rib and dorsal to the vertebrae. Measure at the highest point of the thorax for the kVp setting (Figures 10-36 and 10-37).

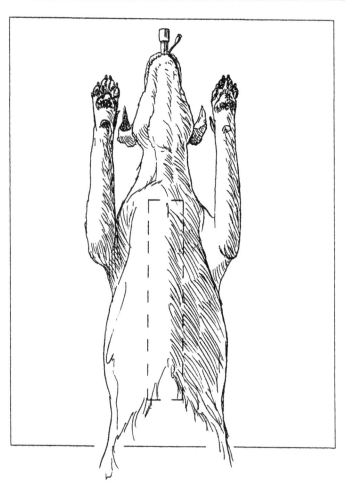

FIG. 10-36 Positioning for a ventrodorsal projection of the thoracic vertebrae.

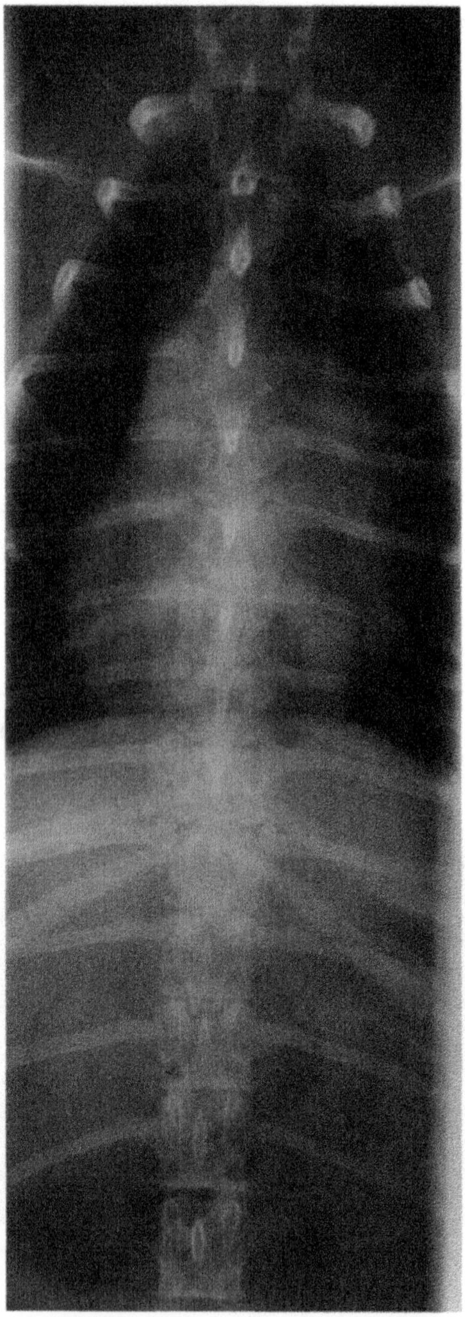

FIG. 10-37 Ventrodorsal projection of the thoracic vertebrae.

Thoracolumbar Vertebrae

Lateral Position

Place the patient in lateral recumbency. Center the primary beam on the thoracolumbar (T-L) junction by finding the point halfway between the xiphoid and the last rib and dorsal to the vertebrae. Pad under the sternum or the spine to position the sternum and the spinous processes in a plane parallel to the table. This superimposes the ribs over one another, providing better visualization of the intervertebral disc spaces. Measure at the highest point for the kVp setting (Figures 10-38 and 10-39).

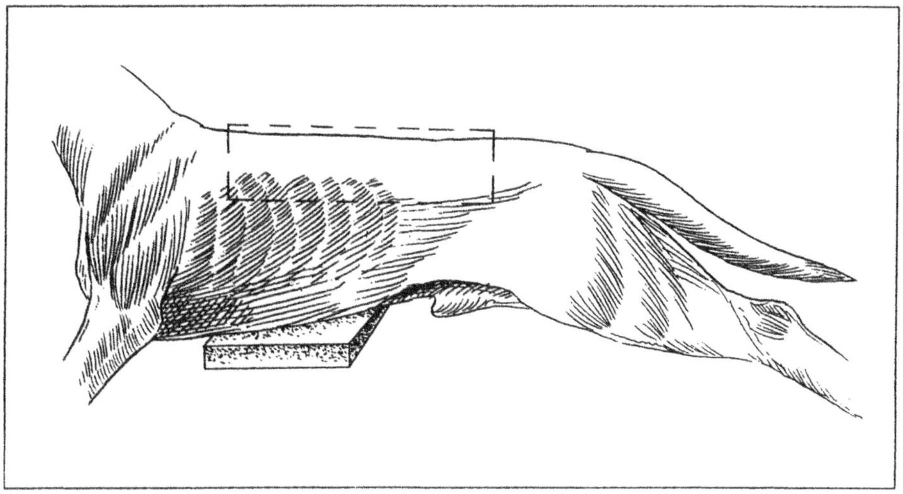

FIG. 10-38 Positioning for a lateral projection of the thoracolumbar vertebrae.

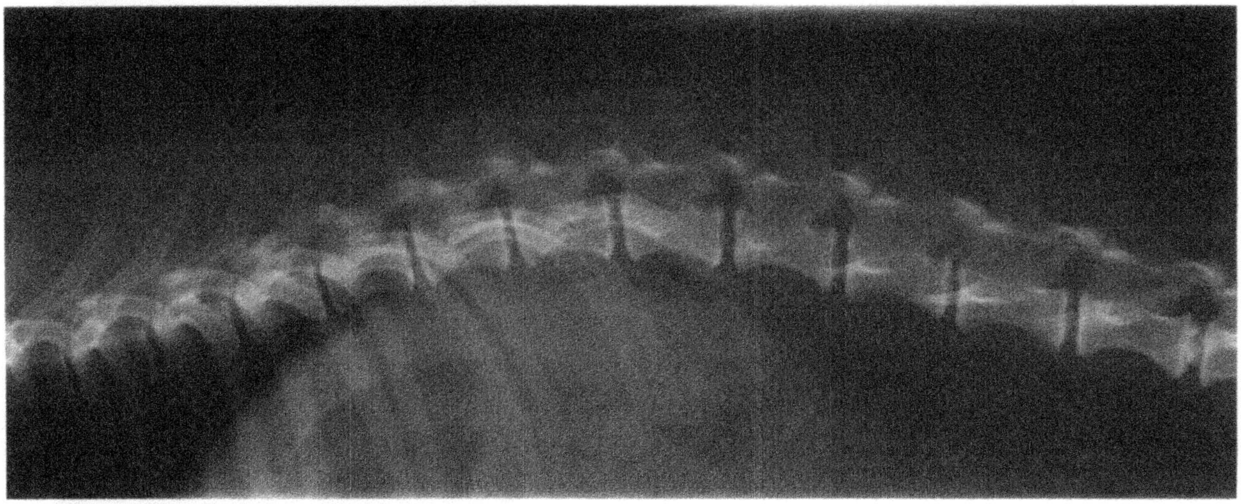

FIG. 10-39 Lateral projection of the thoracolumbar vertebrae.

Ventrodorsal Position

Place the patient in the ventrodorsal position with the front limbs extended cranially. Position the patient so the sternum and vertebrae are superimposed in a plane perpendicular to the table. Center the primary beam on the T-L junction by finding the point midway between the xiphoid and the last rib and dorsal to the spine. Measure at the highest point for the kVp setting (Figures 10-40 and 10-41).

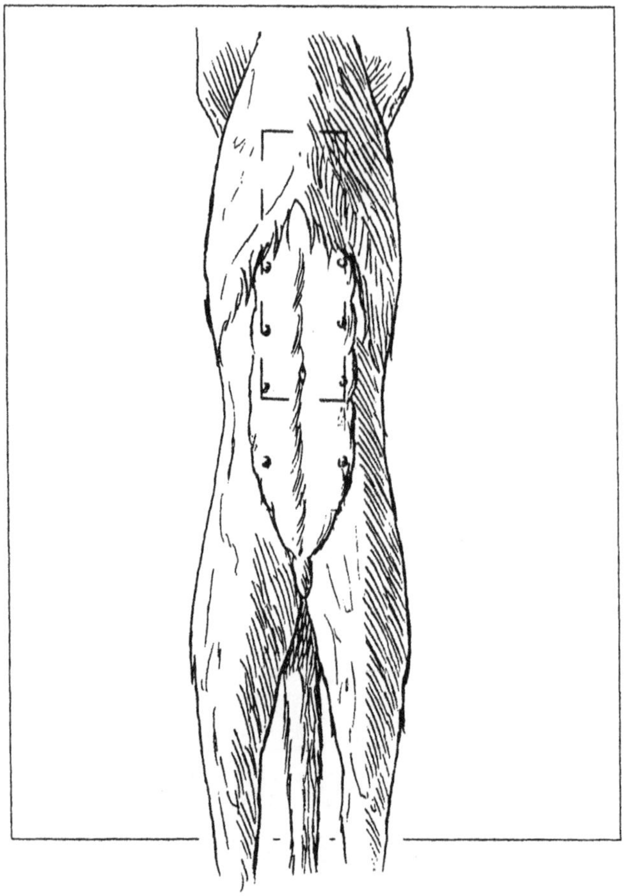

FIG. 10-40 Positioning for a ventrodorsal projection of the thoracolumbar vertebrae.

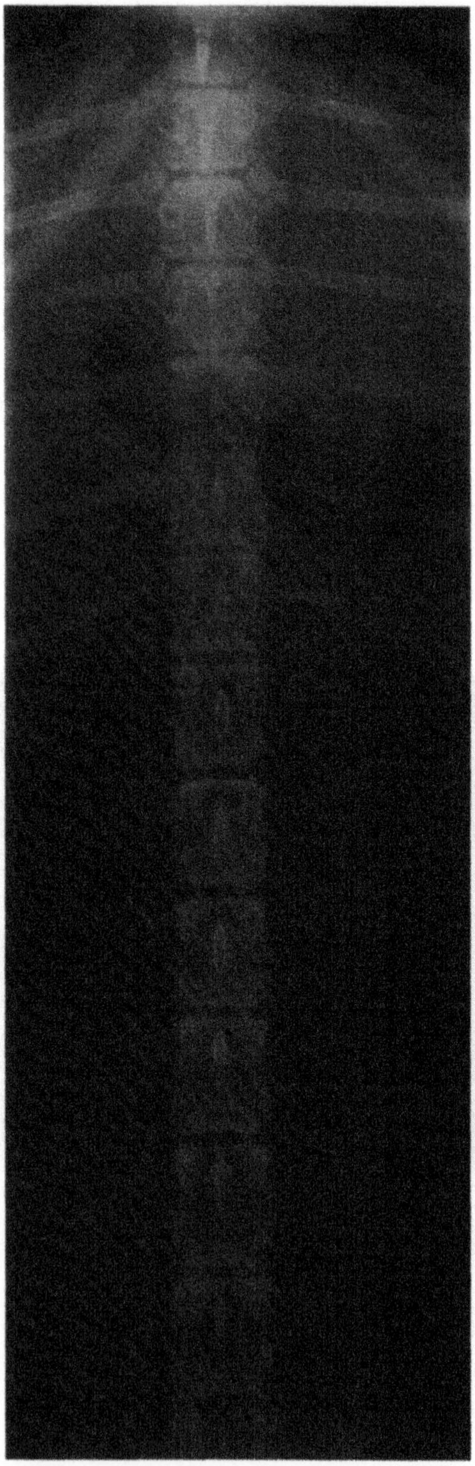

FIG. 10-41 Ventrodorsal projection of the thoracolumbar vertebrae.

Lumbar Vertebrae

Lateral Position

Place the patient in lateral recumbency with the rear limbs extended caudally. Position the patient so that the sternum and the spinous processes are in a plane parallel to the table and the wings of the ilium are superimposed. Padding may be required in the midlumbar area to prevent sagging of the vertebral column. The cranial landmark is halfway between the xiphoid and the last rib and dorsal to the vertebrae. The caudal landmark is the wings of the ilium. Measure over the T-L junction for the kVp setting (Figures 10-42 and 10-43).

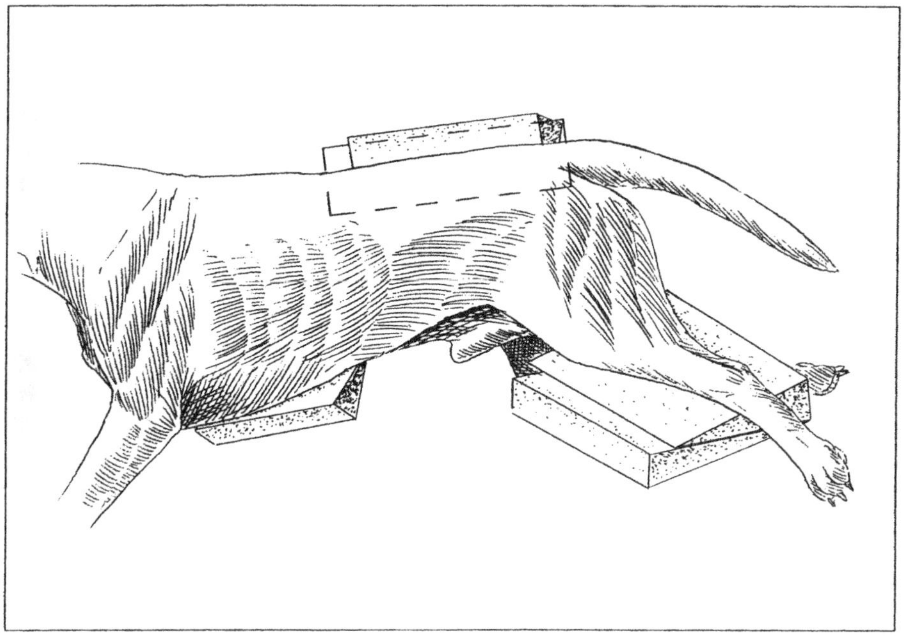

FIG. 10-42 Positioning for a lateral projection of the lumbar vertebrae.

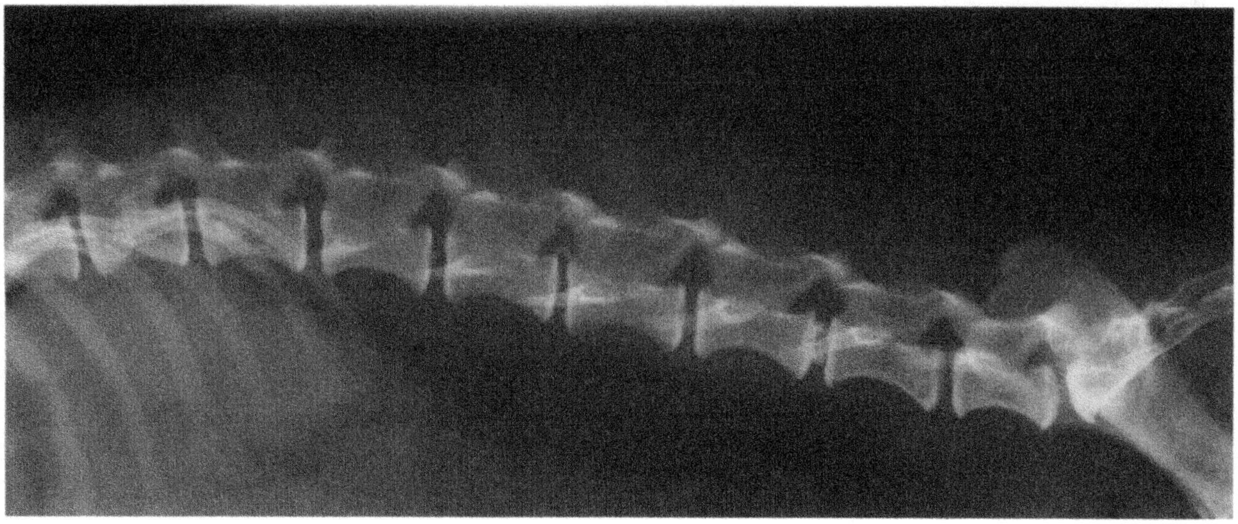

FIG. 10-43 Lateral projection of the lumbar vertebrae.

Ventrodorsal Position

Place the patient in the ventrodorsal position with the front limbs extended cranially. Position the patient so that the sternum and vertebrae are superimposed in a plane perpendicular to the table, with the wings of the ilium also in a plane parallel to the table. The cranial landmark is midway between the xiphoid and the last rib and dorsal to the vertebrae. The caudal landmark is the wings of the ilium. Measure over the T-L junction for the kVp setting (Figures 10-44 and 10-45).

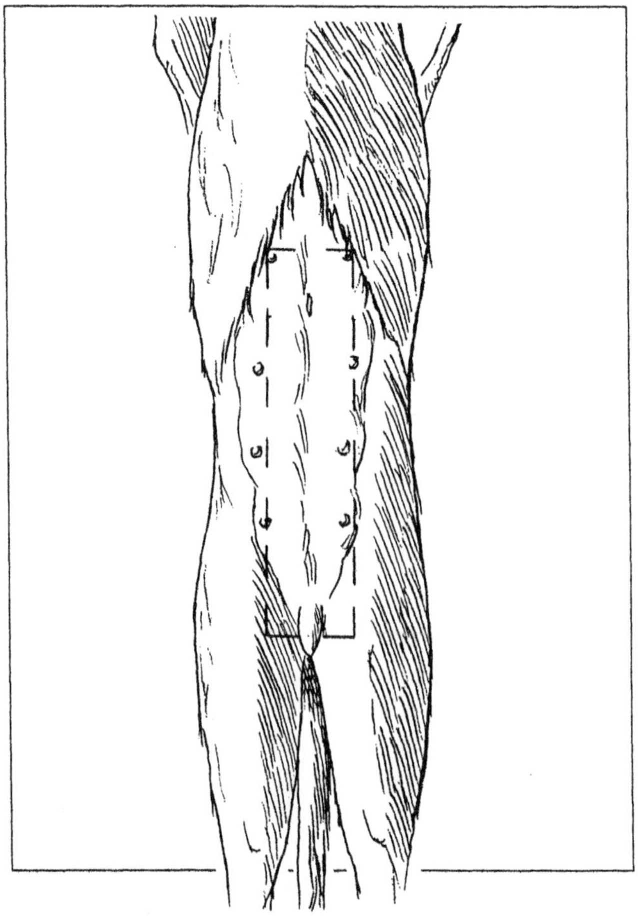

FIG. 10-44 Positioning for a ventrodorsal projection of the lumbar vertebrae.

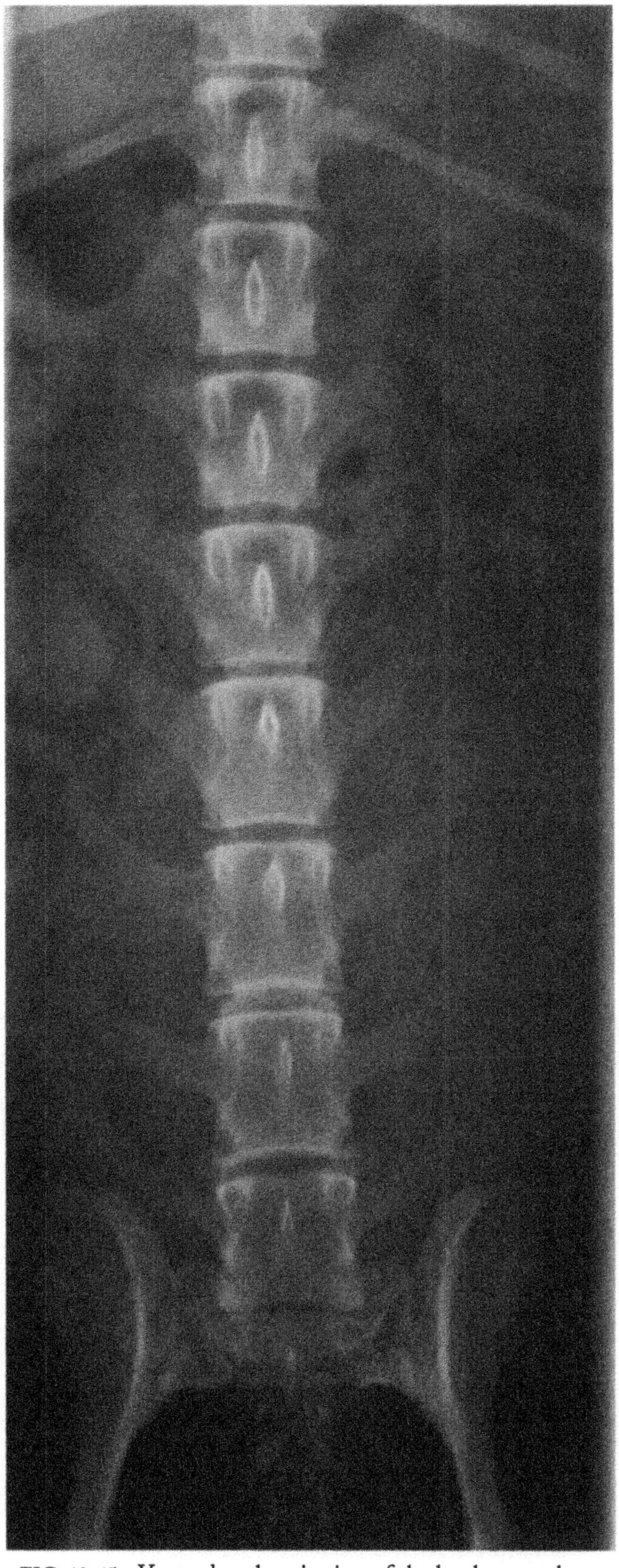

FIG. 10-45 Ventrodorsal projection of the lumbar vertebrae.

Lumbosacral Vertebrae

Some patient preparation is necessary before making lumbosacral radiographs. Give cleansing enemas 1 to 2 hours before imaging to evacuate the colon of feces. On the ventrodorsal view the colon is superimposed over the vertebral column. Excessive amounts of feces can make visualization difficult.

> Enemas may be necessary when radiographing the lumbosacral vertebrae.

Lateral Position

Place the patient in lateral recumbency with the rear limbs extended caudally. Position the animal so that the wings of the ilium are superimposed by padding under the nondependent limb. Place the center of the primary beam on the wings of the ilium. Measure at the highest point for the kVp setting. Sometimes the kVp needs to be increased because of the thick density of the subject (Figures 10-46 and 10-47).

> Increase 6 to 8 kVp when imaging the lumbosacral vertebrae in the lateral position.

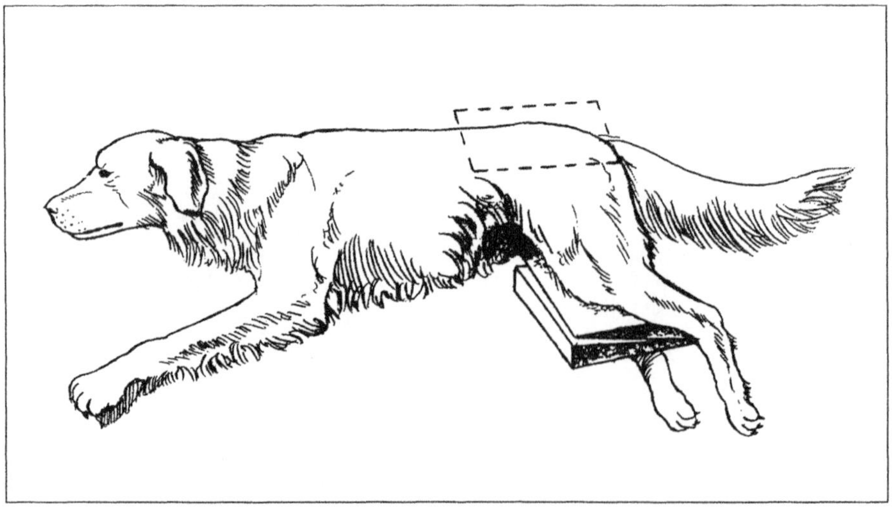

FIG. 10-46 Positioning for a lateral projection of the lumbosacral vertebrae.

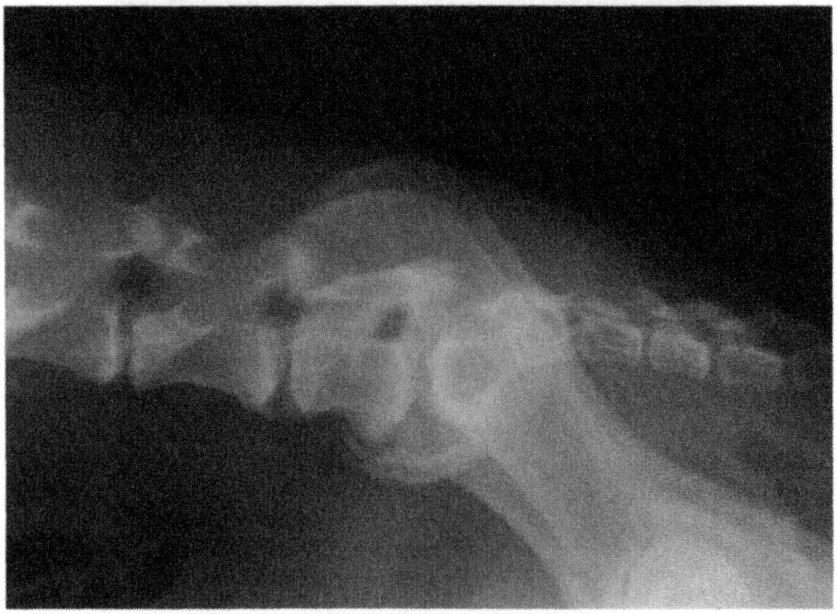

FIG. 10-47 Lateral projection of the lumbosacral vertebrae.

Ventrodorsal Position

Place the patient in ventrodorsal position with the front limbs extended cranially. Position the animal so that the wings of the ilium are in a plane parallel to the table. Center the primary beam on the wings of the ilium, and angle the beam 20 degrees caudal to rostral. This is necessary to open up the lumbosacral joint space. Measure at the highest point for the kVp setting (Figures 10-48 and 10-49).

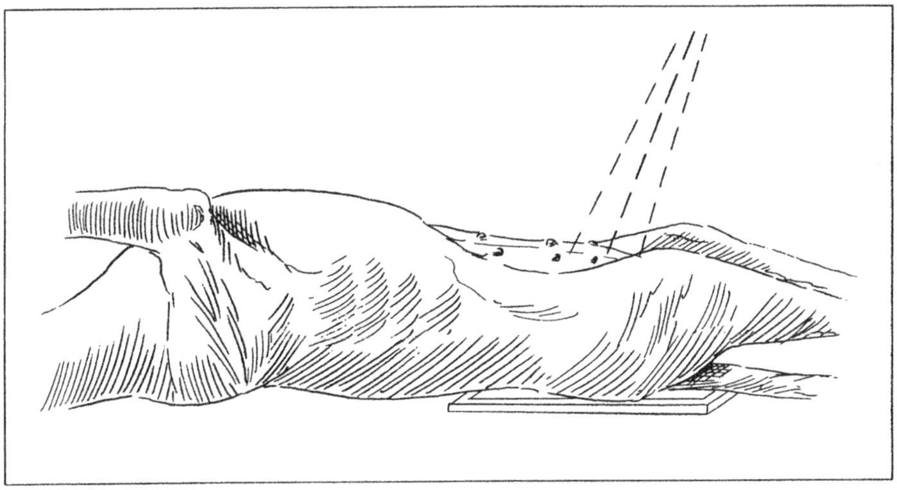

FIG. 10-48 Positioning for a ventrodorsal projection of the lumbosacral vertebrae.

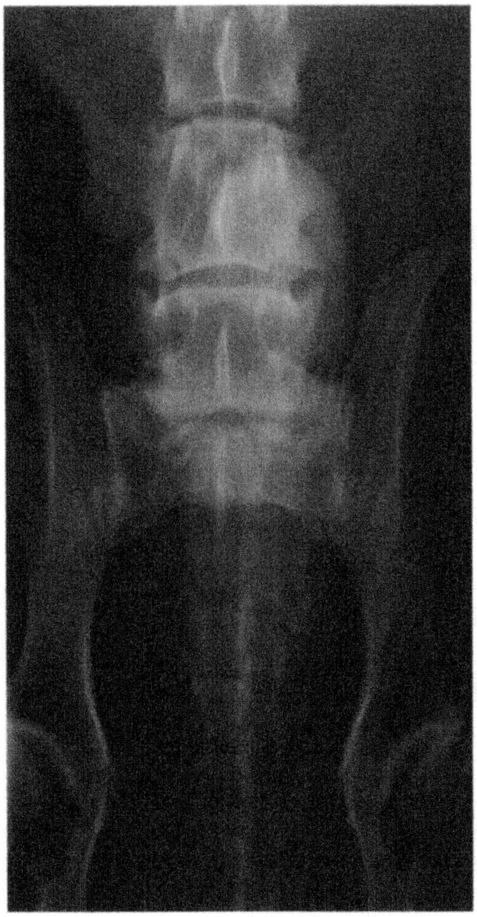

FIG. 10-49 Ventrodorsal projection of the lumbosacral vertebrae.

Metacarpus and Digits

Mediolateral Position

Place the patient in lateral recumbency with the area of interest closest to the table. Extend the unaffected limb caudally and out of the way. Center the primary beam on the metacarpus and collimate to include the carpal joint and digits. Place a right or a left marker on the dorsal side of the limb. Sometimes the usefulness of a lateral projection is limited because of the superimposition of the digits. To open a space between each metacarpal, slightly angle the limb obliquely. To image just the digits, tape each digit so that it is not superimposed over the others (Figures 10-50 and 10-51).

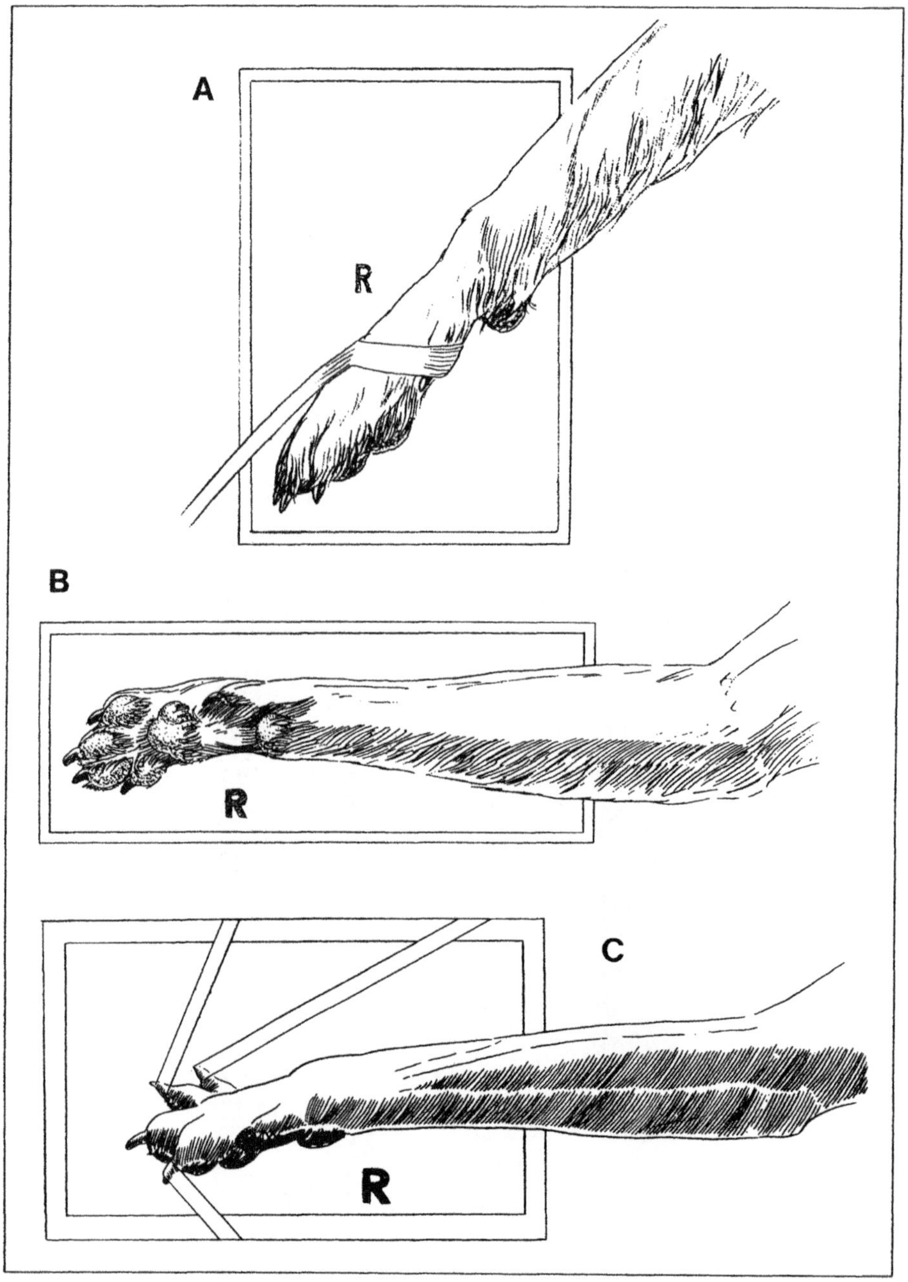

FIG. 10-50 **A,** Positioning for a mediolateral projection of the metacarpus and digits. **B,** Positioning for a lateral oblique view of the metacarpus. This sets off each metacarpal without the others being superimposed. **C,** Positioning for a lateral projection of the digits.

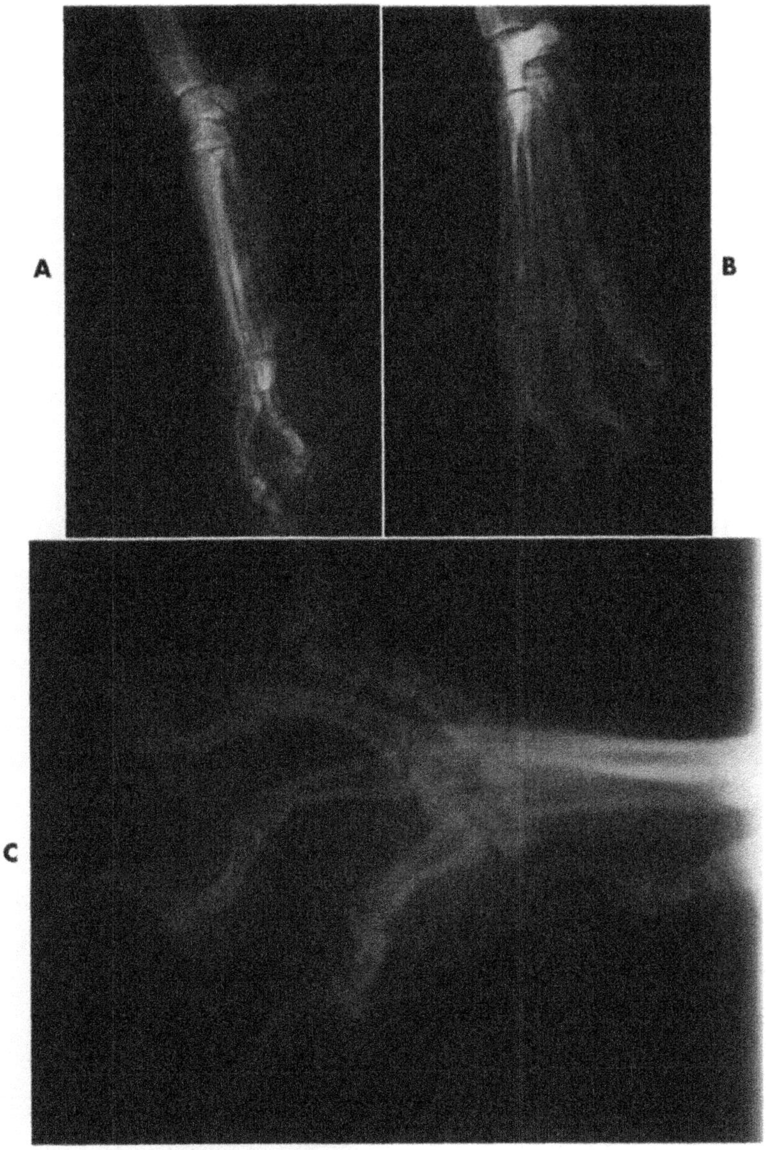

FIG. 10-51 **A,** Lateral projection of the metacarpus and digits. **B,** Lateral oblique view of the metacarpus. **C,** Lateral projection of the digits using tape to separate the digits.

Dorsopalmar Position

For the dorsopalmar position, place the patient in sternal recumbency with the affected limb extended cranially. Move the patient's body to the right and left to position the limb accurately. Center the primary beam on the metacarpus and collimate to include the carpal joint and digits. Place a right or left marker on the lateral side of the limb (Figures 10-52 and 10-53).

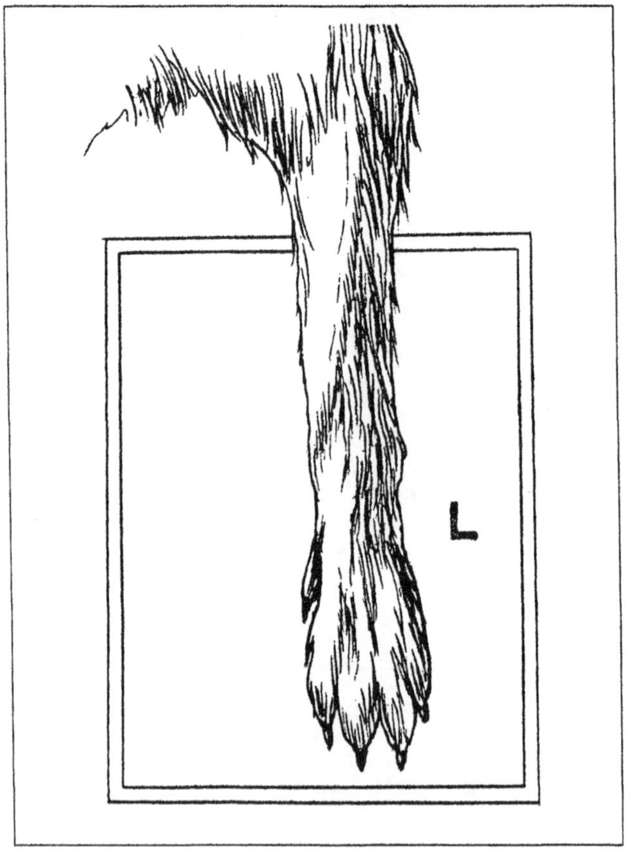

FIG. 10-52 Positioning for a dorsopalmar projection of the metacarpus and digits.

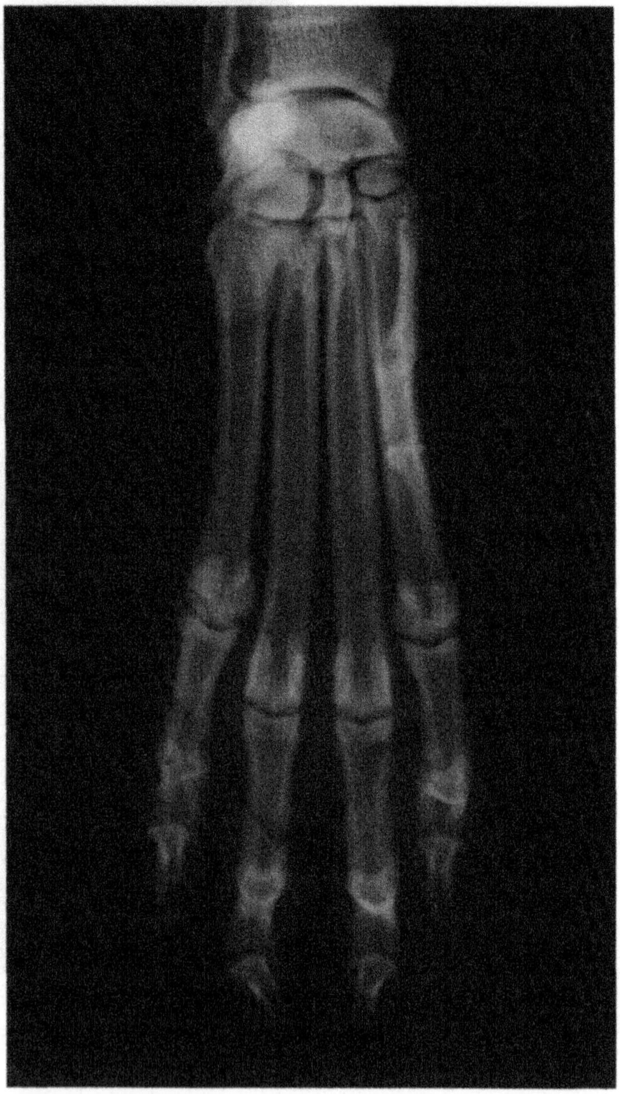

FIG. 10-53 Dorsopalmar projection of the metacarpus and digits.

Carpus

Mediolateral Position

Place the patient in lateral recumbency with the limb of interest closest to the table. Extend the unaffected limb caudally and out of the way.

When imaging any joint, be sure the joint is in the center of the primary beam, then collimate.

Place tape on the metacarpus and extend forward. Center the primary beam on the carpus and collimate. Place a right or left marker on the dorsal side of the limb (Figures 10-54 and 10-55).

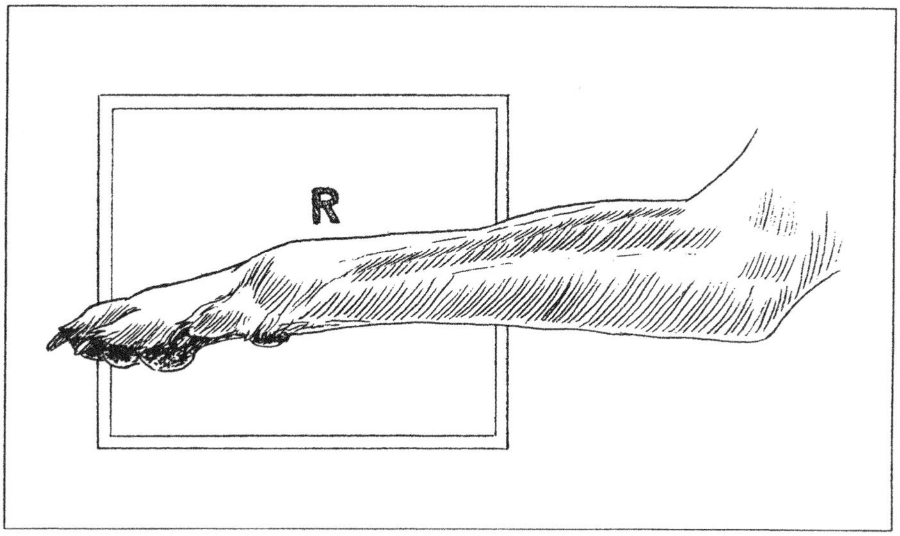

FIG. 10-54 Positioning for a mediolateral projection of the carpus.

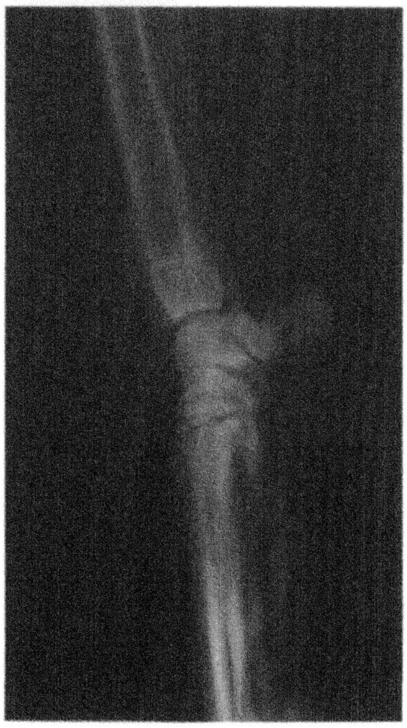

FIG. 10-55 Mediolateral projection of the carpus.

Dorsopalmar Position

Place the patient in sternal recumbency with the affected limb extended cranially. Move the patient's body to the right and left to position the carpus for dorsopalmar projection. Center the primary beam on the carpus and collimate. Place a right or left marker on the lateral side of the limb (Figures 10-56 and 10-57).

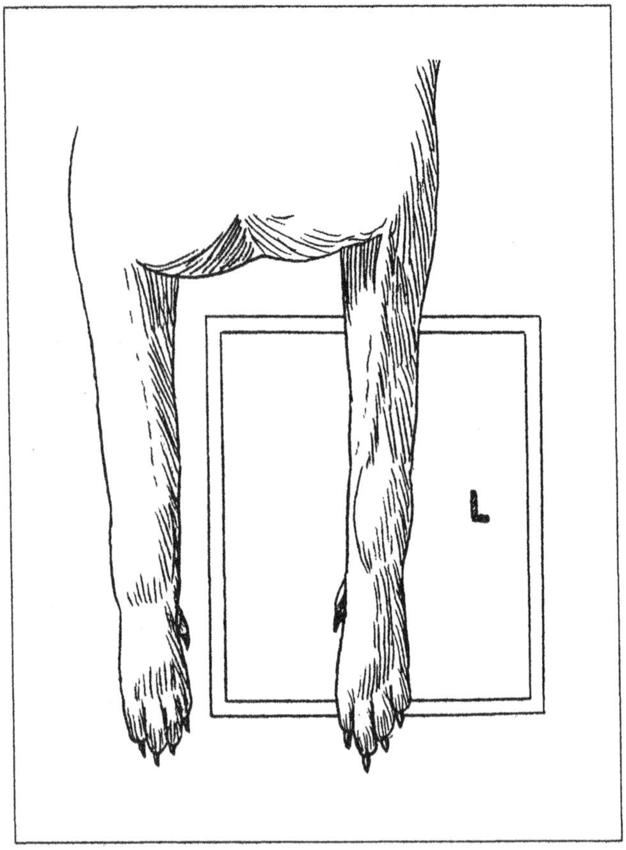

FIG. 10-56 Positioning for a dorsopalmar projection of the carpus.

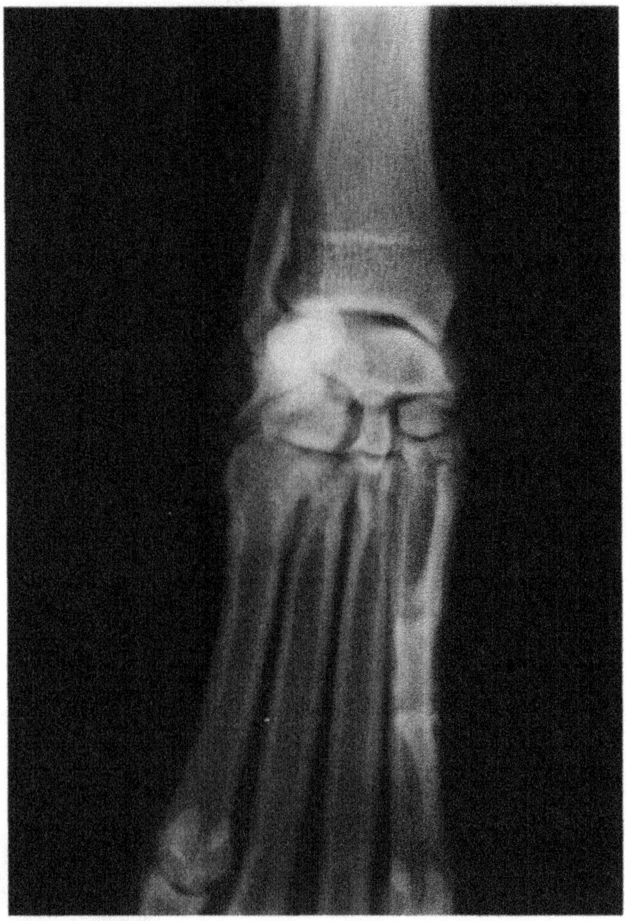

FIG. 10-57 Dorsopalmar projection of the carpus.

Radius and Ulna

Mediolateral Position

Place the patient in lateral recumbency with the limb to be imaged closest to the table. Extend the unaffected limb caudally and out of the way. Extend the metacarpus cranially with tape. Center the primary beam on the center of the radius and collimate to include carpal and elbow joints. Place a right or left marker on the cranial side of the limb (Figures 10-58 and 10-59).

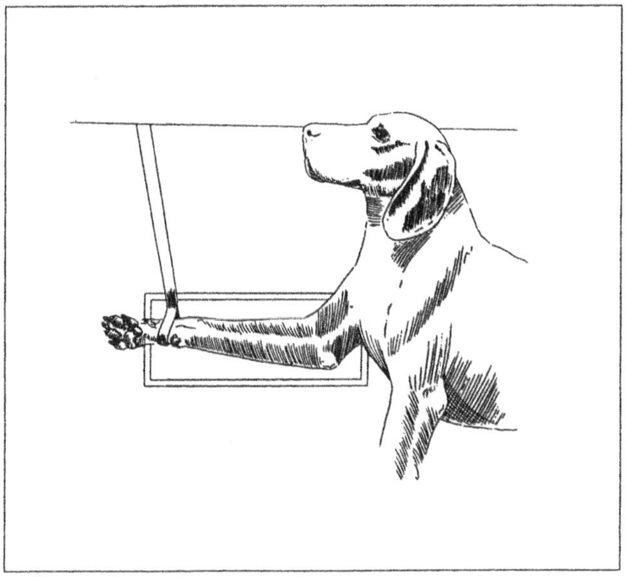

FIG. 10-58 Positioning for a mediolateral projection of the radius and ulna.

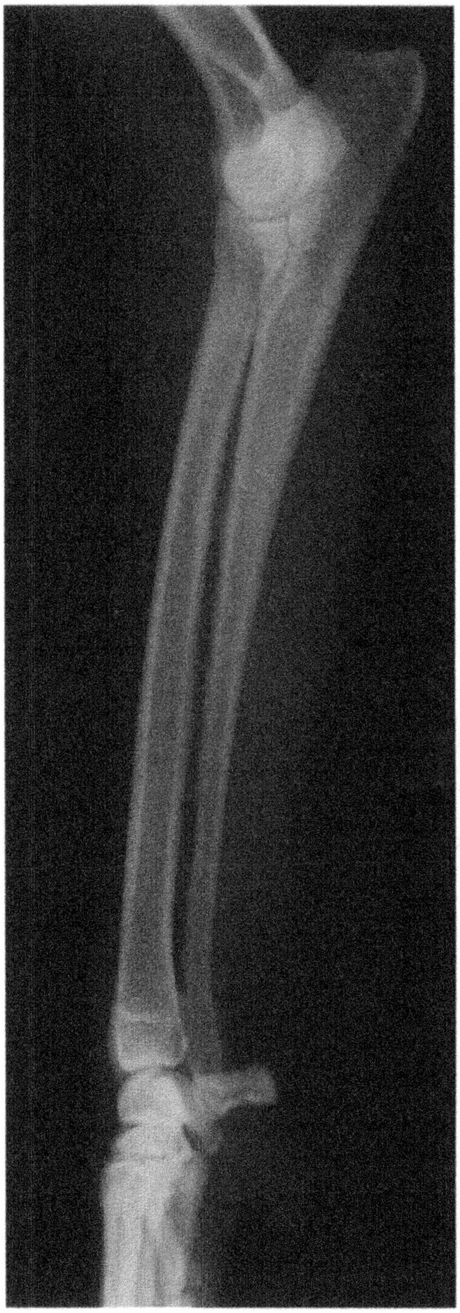

FIG. 10-59 Mediolateral projection of the radius and ulna.

Craniocaudal Position

Place the patient in sternal recumbency with the affected limb extended cranially. Move the patient's body to the right and left so that the olecranon of the ulna palpates in the center of the joint. Center the primary beam on the center of the radius and collimate to include carpal and elbow joints. Place a right or left marker on the lateral side of the limb (Figures 10-60 and 10-61).

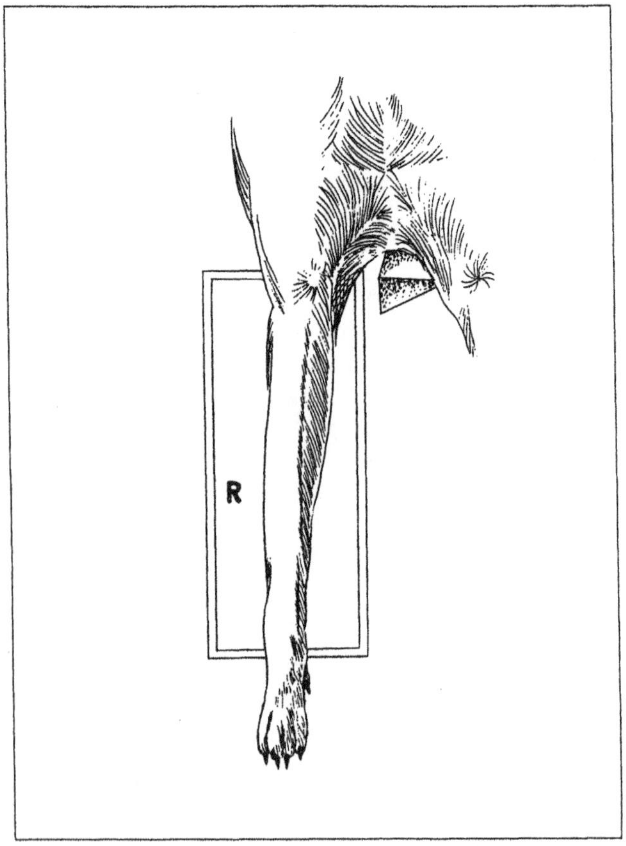

FIG. 10-60 Positioning for a craniocaudal projection of the radius and ulna.

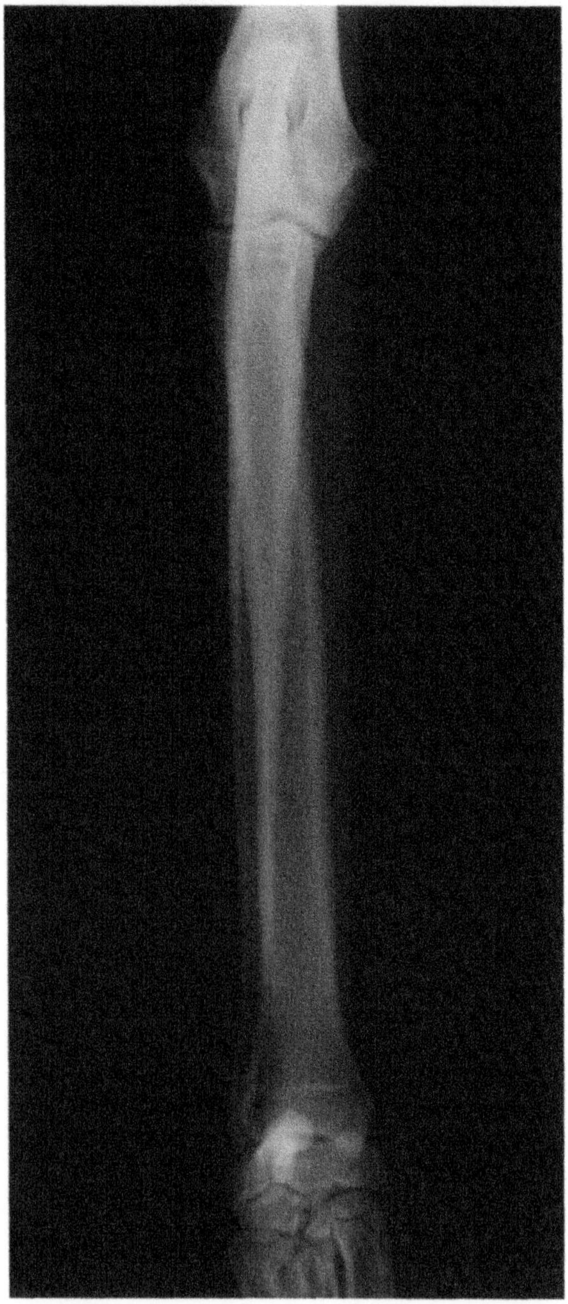

FIG. 10-61 Craniocaudal projection of the radius and ulna.

Elbow Joint

Mediolateral Position

Place the patient in lateral recumbency with the limb of interest closest to the table. Extend the unaffected limb caudally. Place tape around the metacarpus and extend the limb cranially. Center the primary beam on the elbow and collimate to include only the region of the joint. A flexed mediolateral position may be necessary to better evaluate the joint. Position the flexed limb the same as for the standard mediolateral projection, except flex the limb as much as possible. Place a right or left marker on the cranial side of the limb (Figures 10-62 and 10-63).

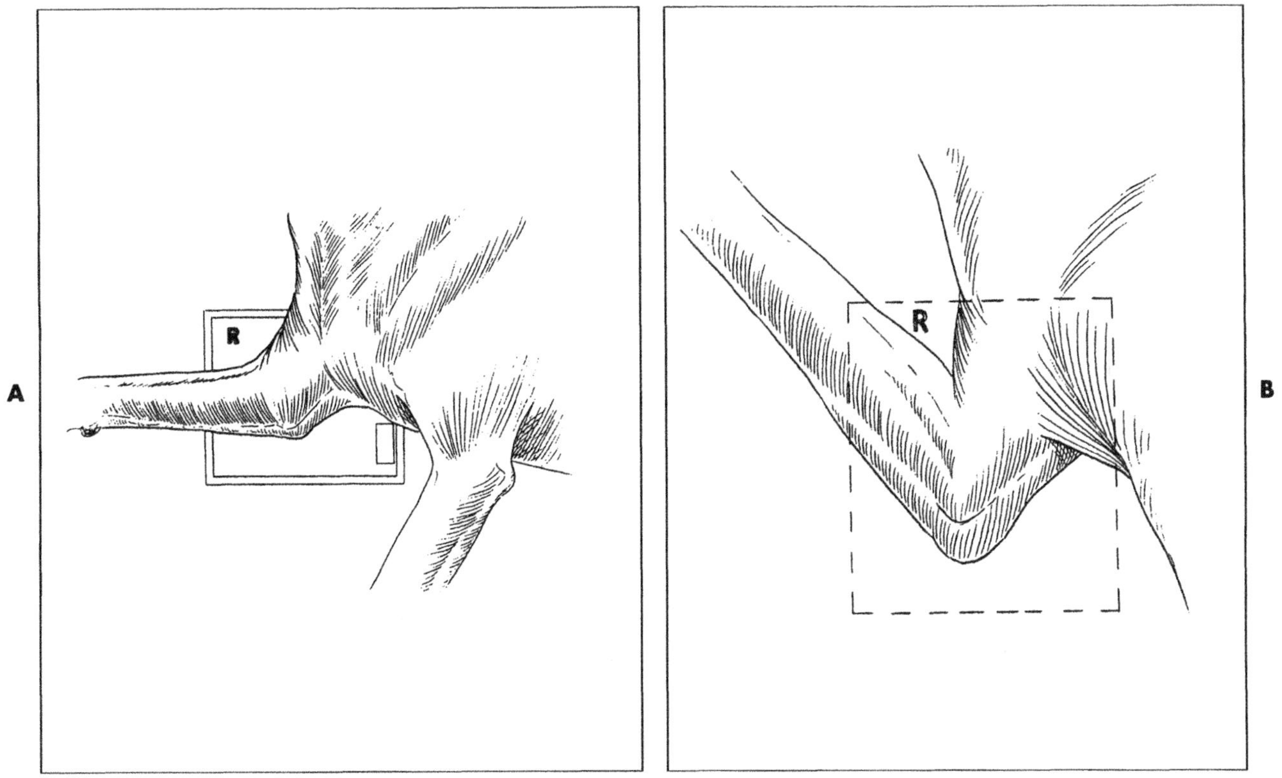

FIG. 10-62 **A,** Positioning for a mediolateral projection of the elbow. **B,** Positioning for a mediolateral projection of the elbow in the flexed position.

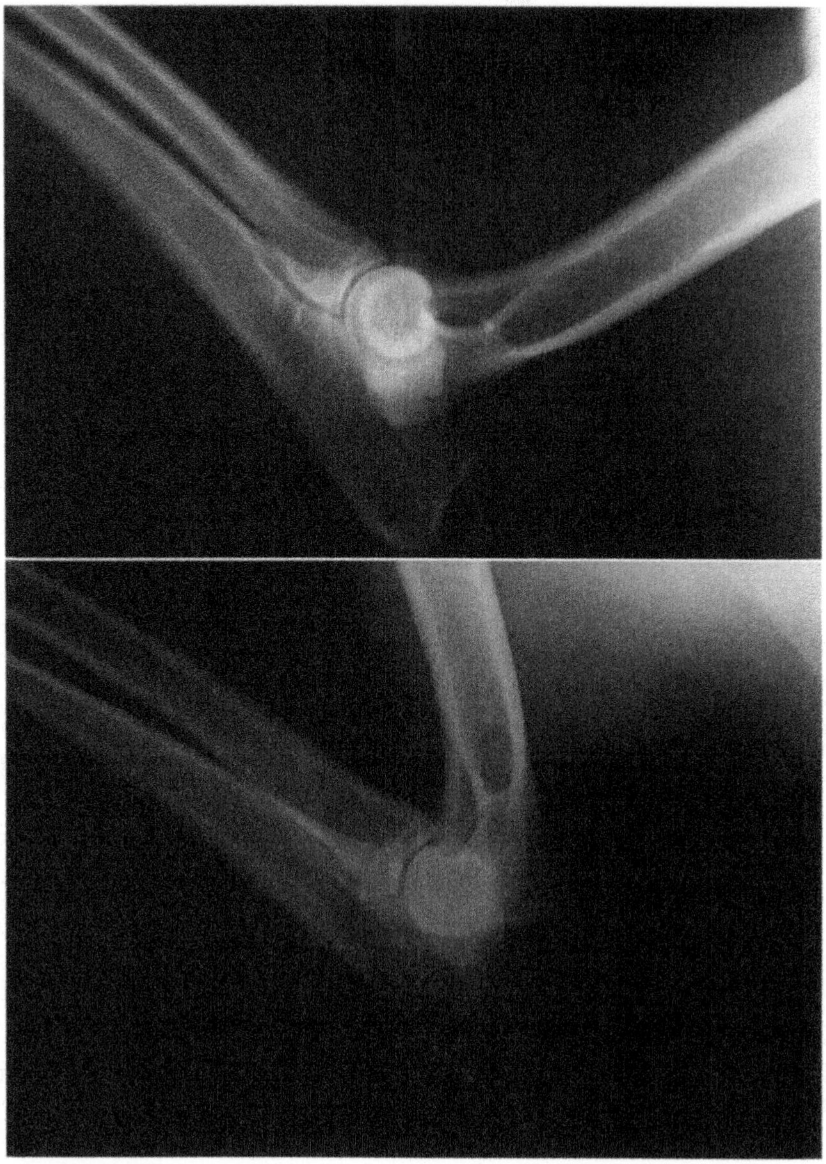

FIG. 10-63 **A,** Mediolateral projection of the elbow. **B,** Mediolateral projection of the elbow in the flexed position.

Lateromedial Position

> An LM projection of the elbow is used to demonstrate a fragmented coronoid process.

Place the patient in lateral recumbency with the limb of interest up (further from the table). Extend the other front limb caudally. Place the cassette on the table with the elbow joint in the center of the cassette. Pull the affected limb distally and down to the table. This creates a slightly oblique projection of the limb, from proximal to distal. An increase in kVp is necessary compared with the mediolateral technique. The lateromedial view is used to demonstrate a fragmented coronoid process (Figures 10-64 and 10-65).

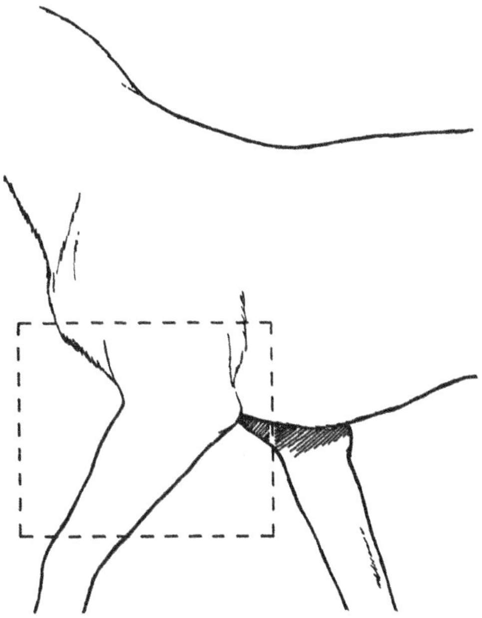

FIG. 10-64 Positioning for a lateromedial projection of the elbow.

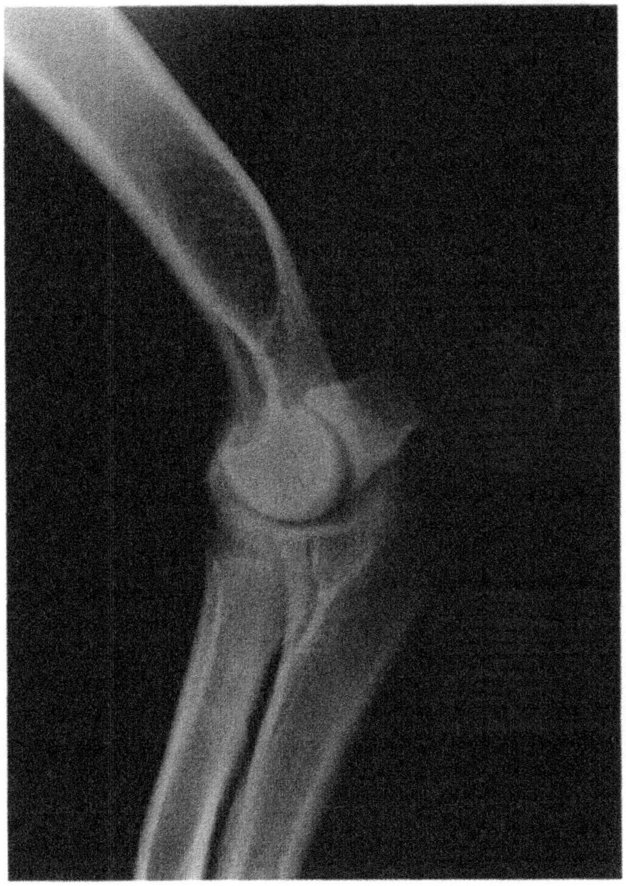

FIG. 10-65 Lateromedial projection of the elbow.

Craniocaudal Position

Place the patient in sternal recumbency with the limb of interest extended cranially. Bring the head up and slightly caudal to shift the soft tissues of the chest and neck away from the elbow area. Move the patient's body to the right and left so that the olecranon of the ulna palpates in the center of the joint. Center the primary beam on the elbow and collimate to include only the region of the joint. Place a right or left marker on the lateral side of the limb (Figures 10-66 and 10-67).

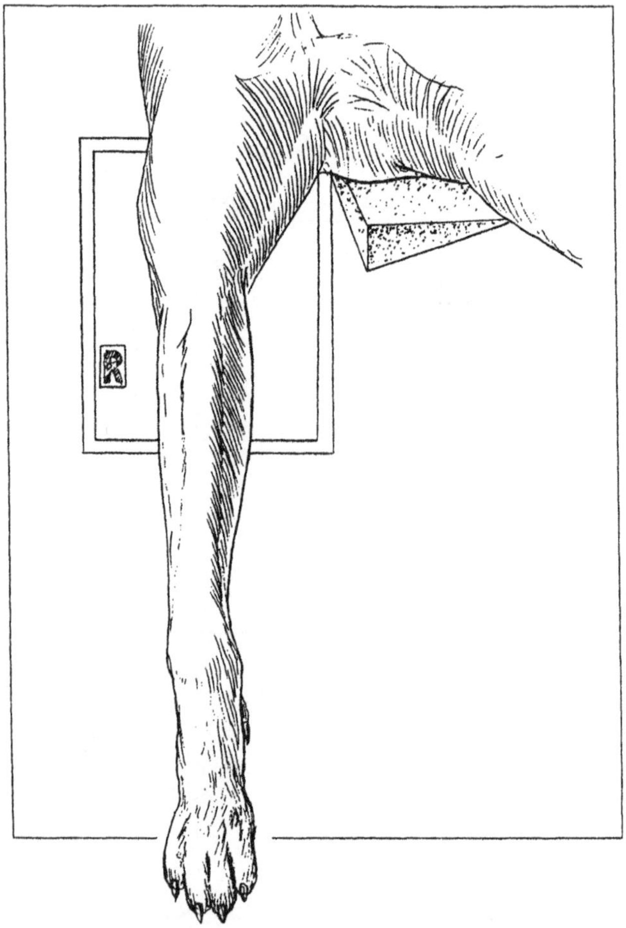

FIG. 10-66 Positioning for a craniocaudal projection of the elbow.

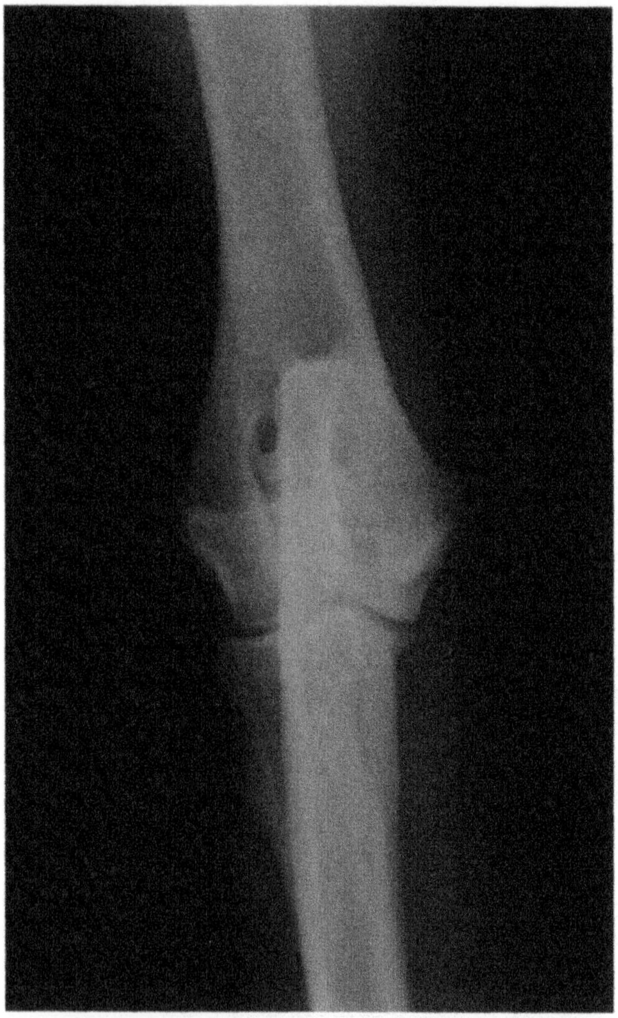

FIG. 10-67 Craniocaudal projection of the elbow.

Humerus

Mediolateral Position

Place the patient in lateral recumbency with the limb of interest closest to the table. Extend the unaffected limb caudally. Extend the metacarpus cranially, securing with tape. Center the primary beam on the humeral shaft and collimate, making sure the shoulder and elbow joints are included. Place a right or left marker on the cranial side of the limb (Figures 10-68 and 10-69).

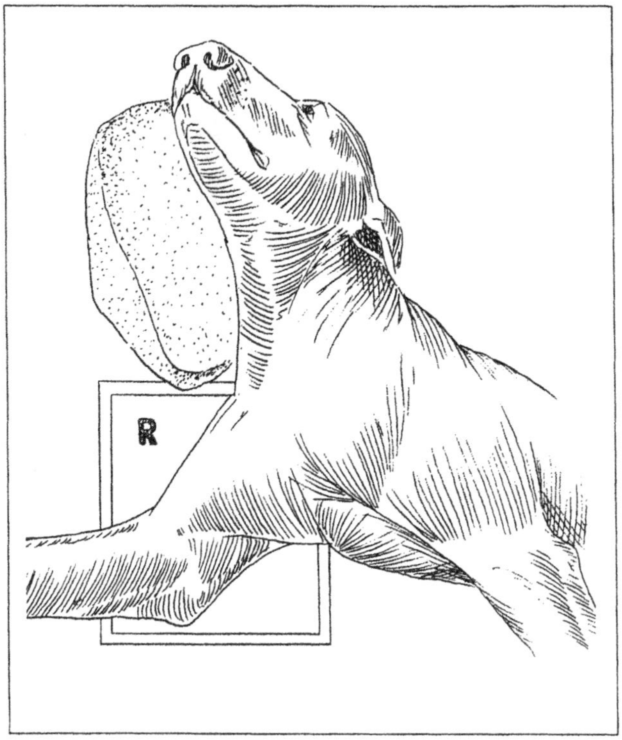

FIG. 10-68 Positioning for a mediolateral projection of the humerus.

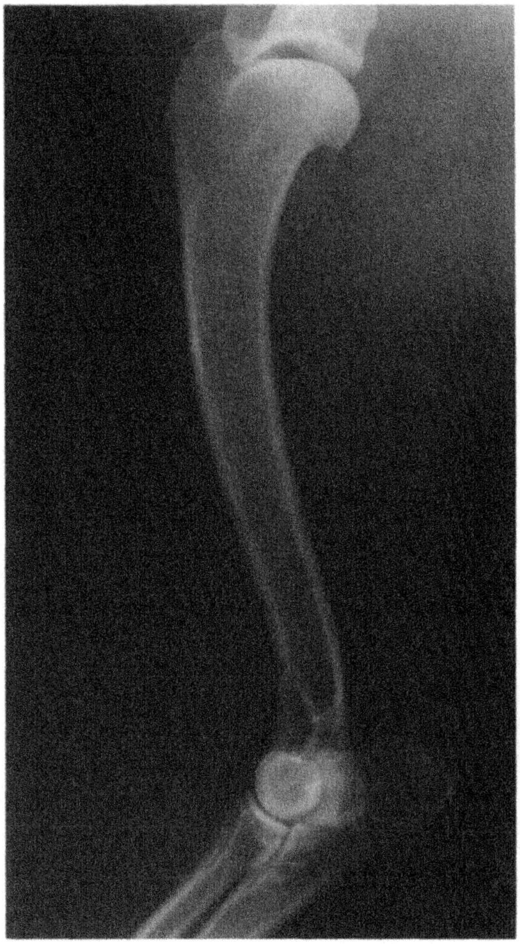

FIG. 10-69 Mediolateral projection of the humerus.

Caudocranial Position

Because of the structure of the humerus, it is impossible in the caudocranial position to extend it cranially and parallel to the cassette. This causes foreshortening of the limb, altering the true length and shape of the bone. There are two methods for positioning the humerus for caudocranial projection. The *cross-table projection* involves positioning the patient in lateral recumbency with the limb to be imaged nondependent (Figure 10-70). Place the cassette cranial to the limb and perpendicular to the table. Keep the cassette close to the limb and parallel to the humerus. Abduct the limb by rotating the elbow. Move the x-ray tube head down toward the table, and angle the primary beam perpendicular to the humerus. Center the primary beam on the center of the humeral shaft, making sure the elbow and shoulder joints are included. The *ventrodorsal extended projection* involves placing the patient in ventrodorsal position (Figure 10-71). Pull the limb of interest cranially to position the humerus parallel to the table. With this method, the increase in object-film distance (OFD) causes magnification and a decrease in detail. Place a right or left marker on the lateral side of the limb (Figure 10-72).

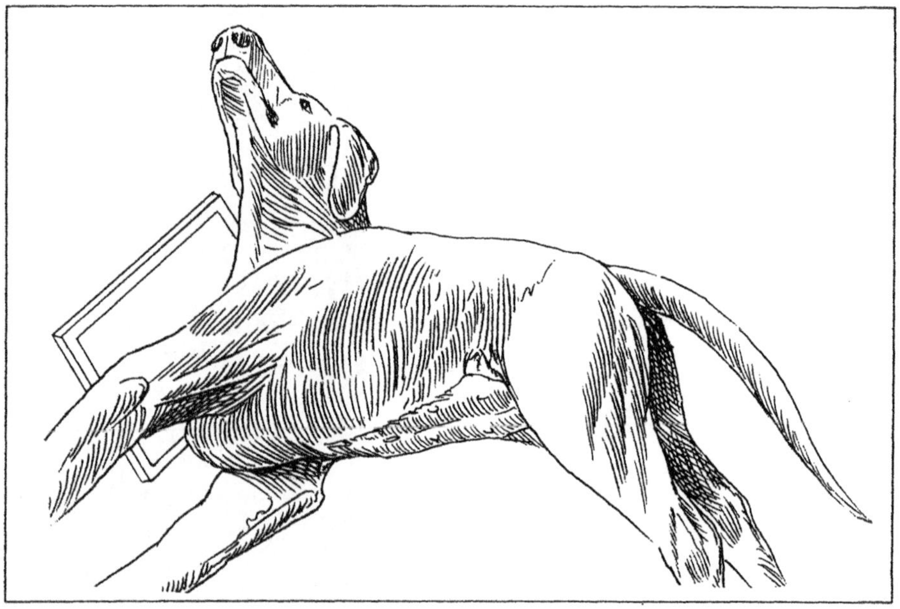

FIG. 10-70 Positioning for a caudocranial projection of the humerus using cross-table projection.

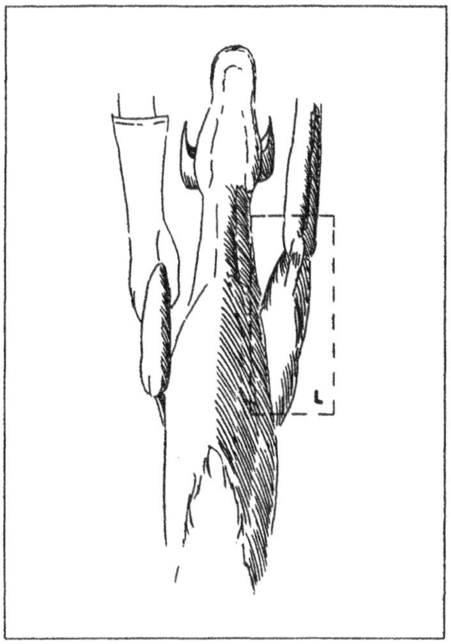

FIG. 10-71 Positioning for a caudocranial projection of the humerus using ventrodorsal extended projection.

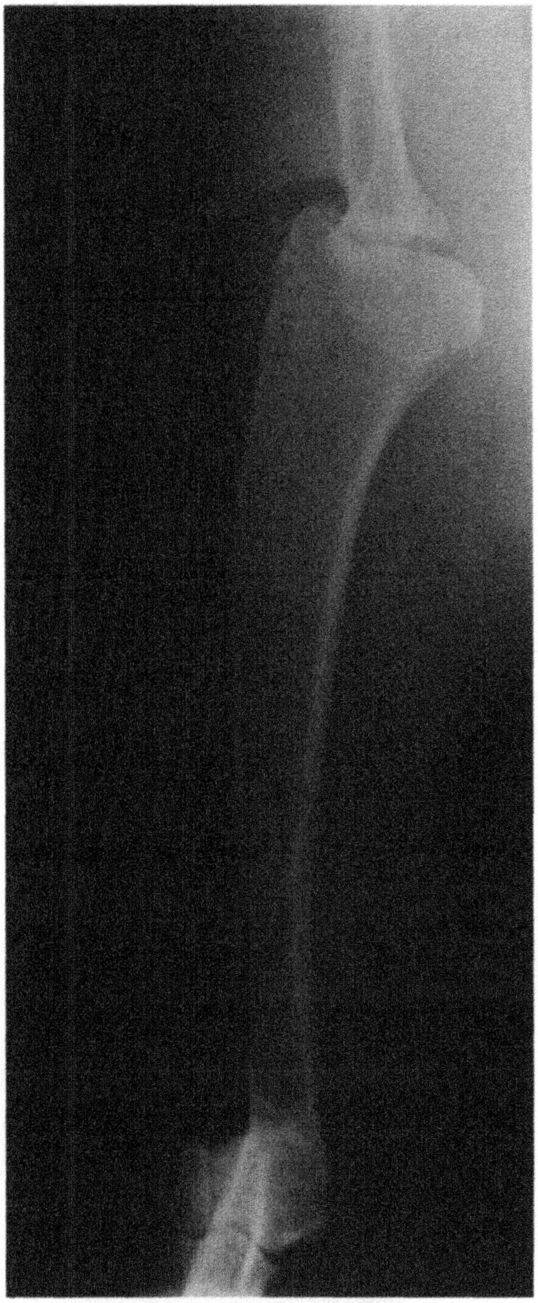

FIG. 10-72 Caudocranial projection of the humerus.

Shoulder Joint

Mediolateral Position

Place the patient in lateral recumbency with the joint of interest nearest to the table. The unaffected limb is pulled caudally to prevent superimposition of the manubrium over the joint. Extend the head dorsally and caudally to prevent superimposing the trachea over the joint. The affected limb is extended cranially. Center the primary beam on the shoulder joint and collimate to include only this joint. Place a right or left marker on the cranial side (Figures 10-73 and 10-74).

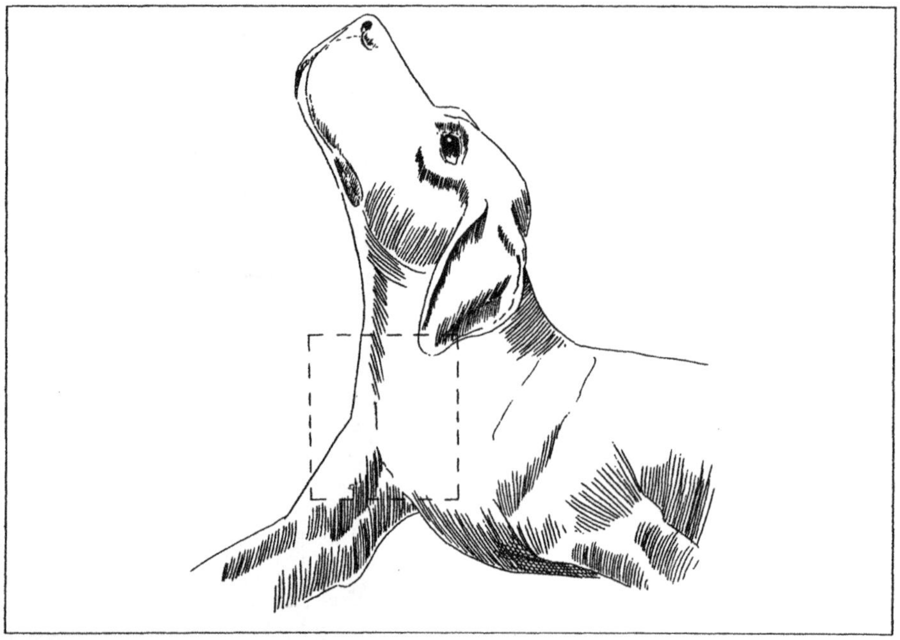

FIG. 10-73 Positioning for a mediolateral projection of the shoulder joint.

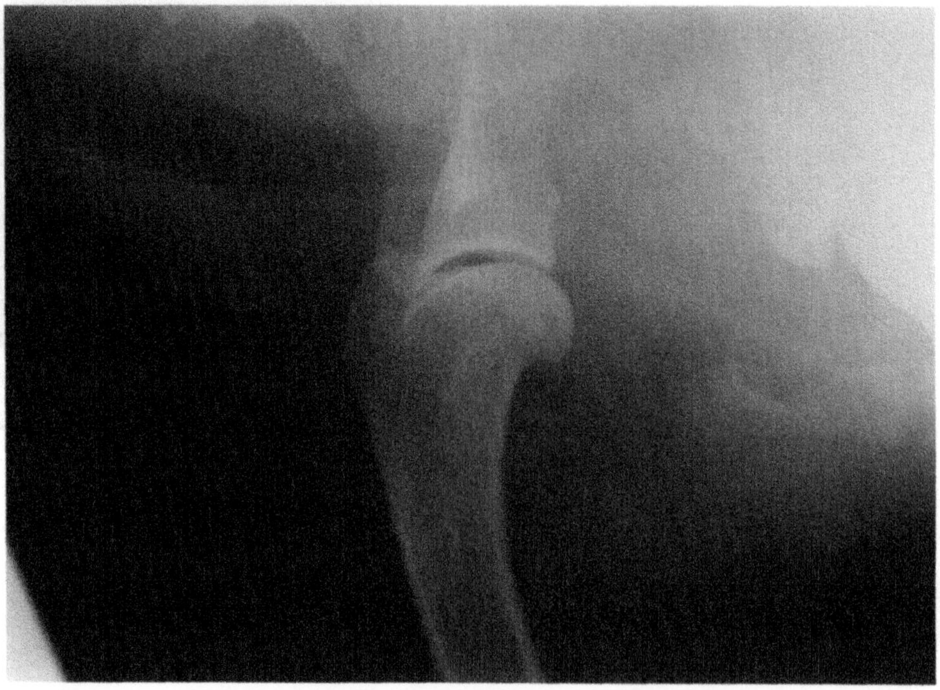

FIG. 10-74 Mediolateral projection of the shoulder joint.

Caudocranial Position

Place the patient in ventrodorsal position and extend the limb of interest cranially. Slightly roll the sternum away from the limb being imaged to prevent superimposition over the body wall. Center the primary beam on the shoulder joint and collimate to include only this joint. Place a right or left marker on the lateral side (Figures 10-75 and 10-76).

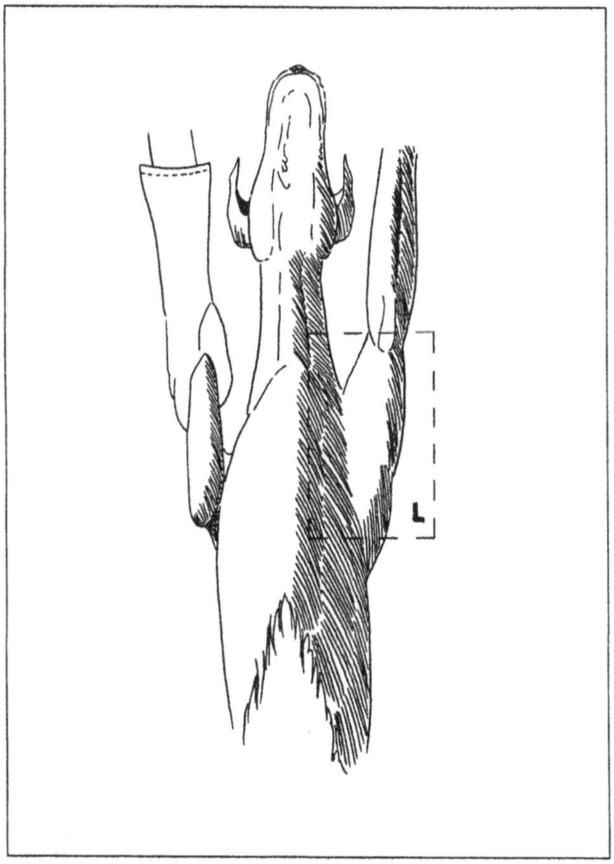

FIG. 10-75 Positioning for a caudocranial projection of the shoulder joint.

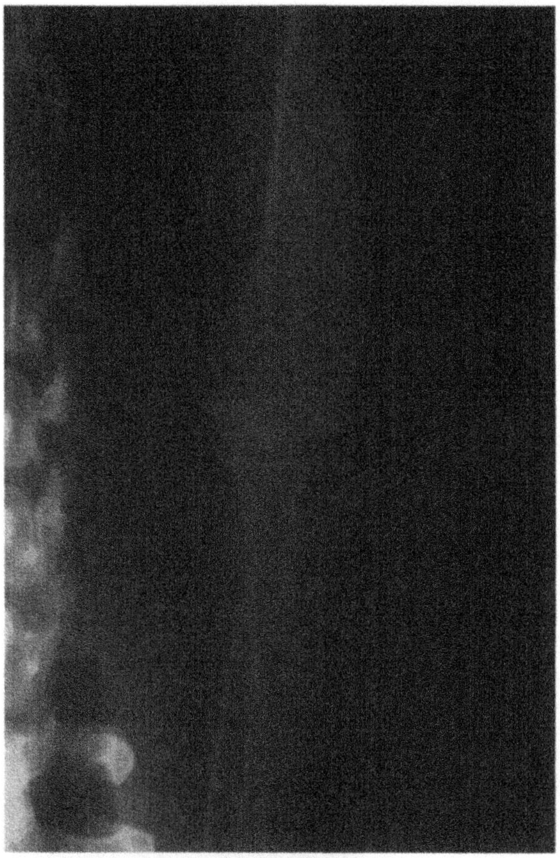

FIG. 10-76 Caudocranial projection of the shoulder joint.

Scapula

Mediolateral Position

Place the patient in lateral recumbency with the limb to be imaged nearest to the table. Pull the unaffected limb caudally, and extend the head dorsally and caudally. Extend the affected limb cranially. Center on the scapula, making sure the shoulder joint and the dorsal border of the scapula are included on the image. Place a right or left marker on the cranial side (Figures 10-77 and 10-78).

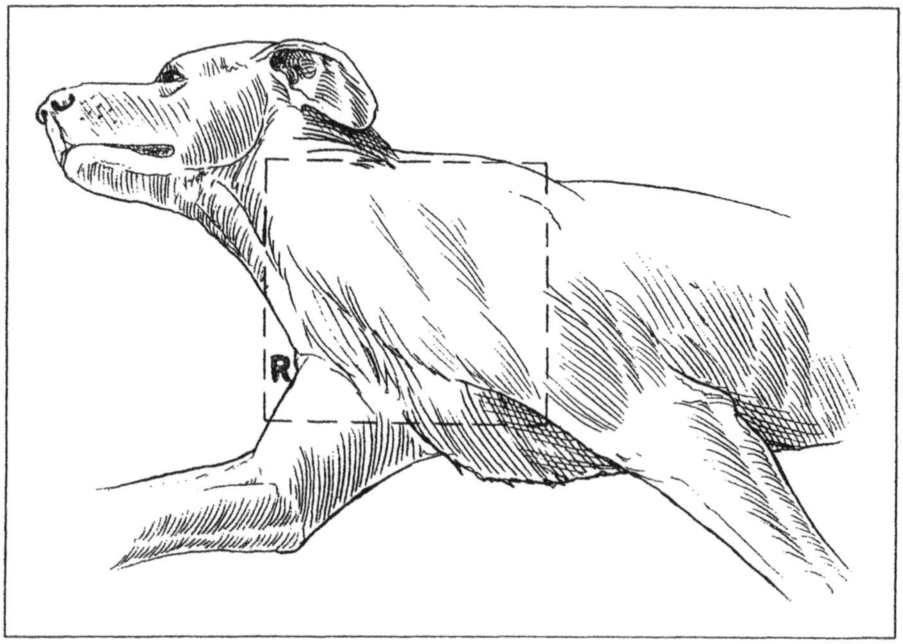

FIG. 10-77 Positioning for a mediolateral projection of the scapula.

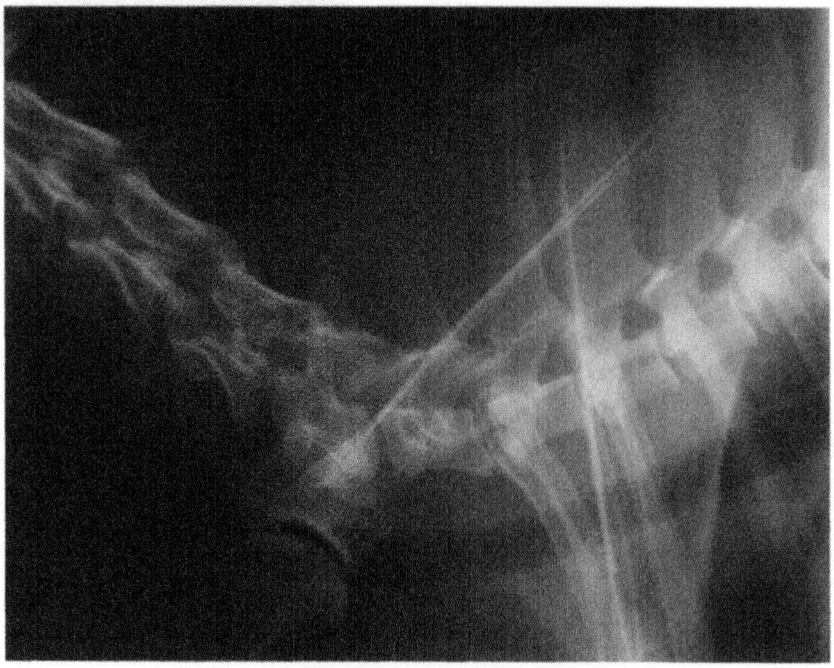

FIG. 10-78 Mediolateral projection of the scapula.

Caudocranial Position

Place the patient in ventrodorsal position with the limb of interest extended cranially. Slightly roll the sternum away from the limb being imaged to prevent superimposition over the body wall. Center on the scapula, making sure the shoulder joint and the dorsal border of the scapula are included on the image. Measure from the table to the sternum for the kVp. Place a right or left marker on the lateral side (Figures 10-79 and 10-80).

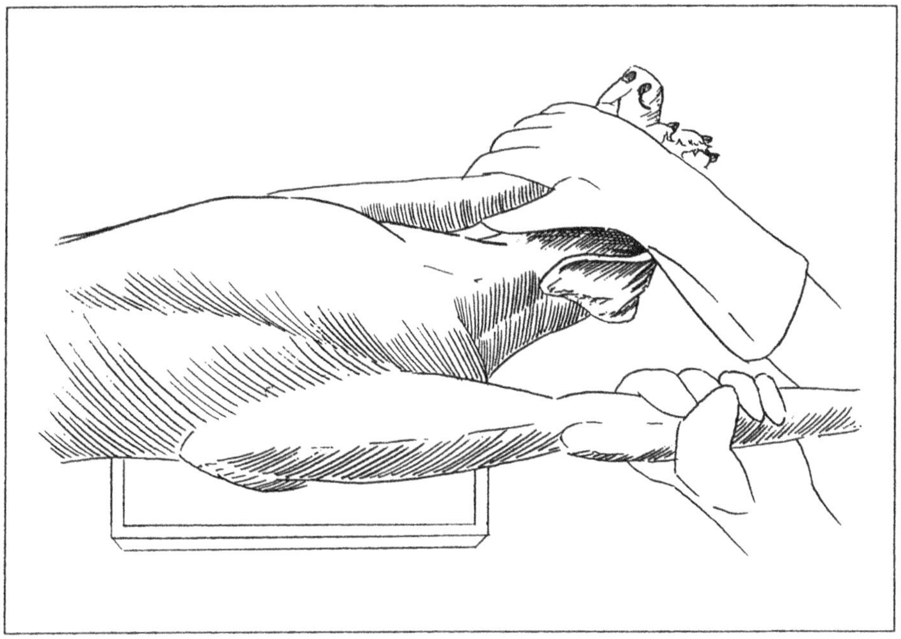

FIG. 10-79 Positioning for a caudocranial projection of the scapula.

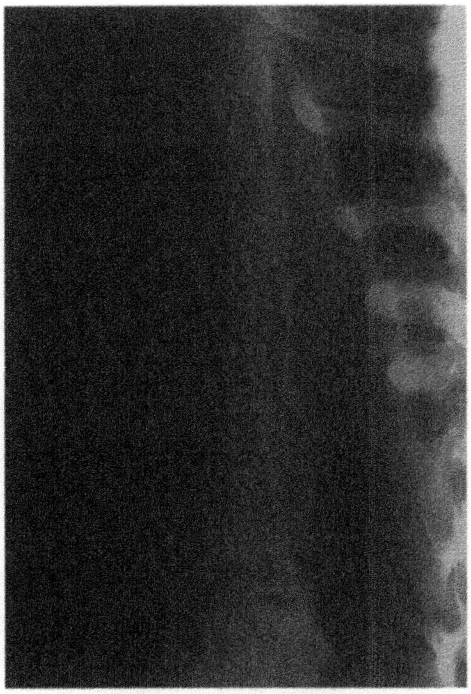

FIG. 10-80 Caudocranial projection of the scapula.

Thorax

Lateral Position

> Radiograph the thorax at peak inspiration.

Place the patient in right lateral recumbency with the front limbs extended cranially to avoid superimposing the triceps muscles on the cranial part of the lung field. The neck should be in a neutral position to prevent misinterpretation of the tracheal position.

The cranial landmark is the manubrium, and the caudal landmark is halfway between the xiphoid and the last rib. Use padding to keep the sternum and the dorsal spinous processes in a plane parallel to the table. Measure at the highest point for the kVp setting. Make the exposure during peak inspiration. If the thorax is being examined for metastasis, imaging the right and left lateral thorax is helpful (Figures 10-81 and 10-82).

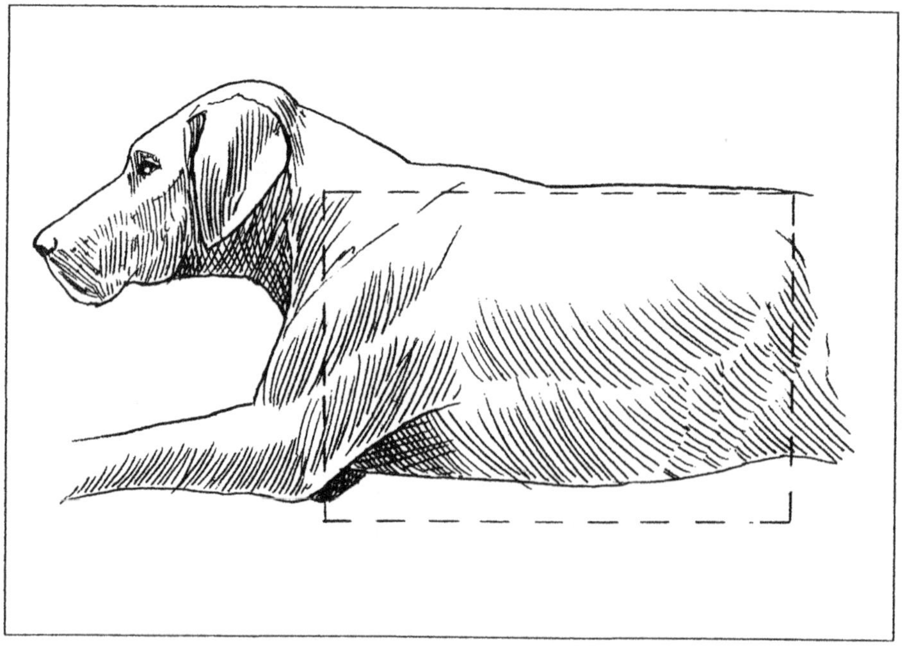

FIG. 10-81 Positioning for a lateral projection of the thorax.

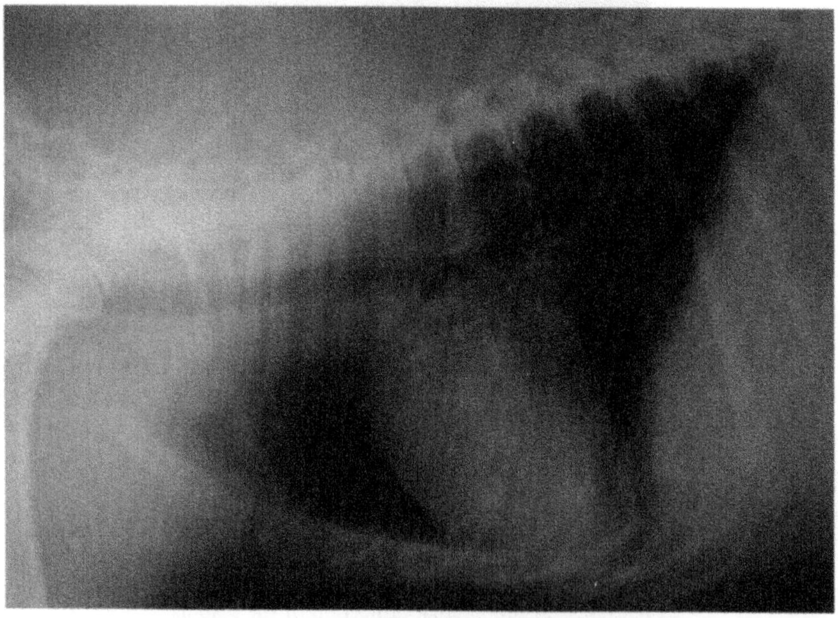

FIG. 10-82 Lateral projection of the thorax.

Ventrodorsal Position

Place the patient in ventrodorsal position with the front limbs extended cranially. The cranial landmark is the manubrium, and the caudal landmark is halfway between the xiphoid and the last rib. Position the thorax so that the sternum and vertebrae are superimposed in a plane perpendicular to the table. Measure at the highest point for the kVp setting. Make the exposure during peak inspiration (Figures 10-83 and 10-84).

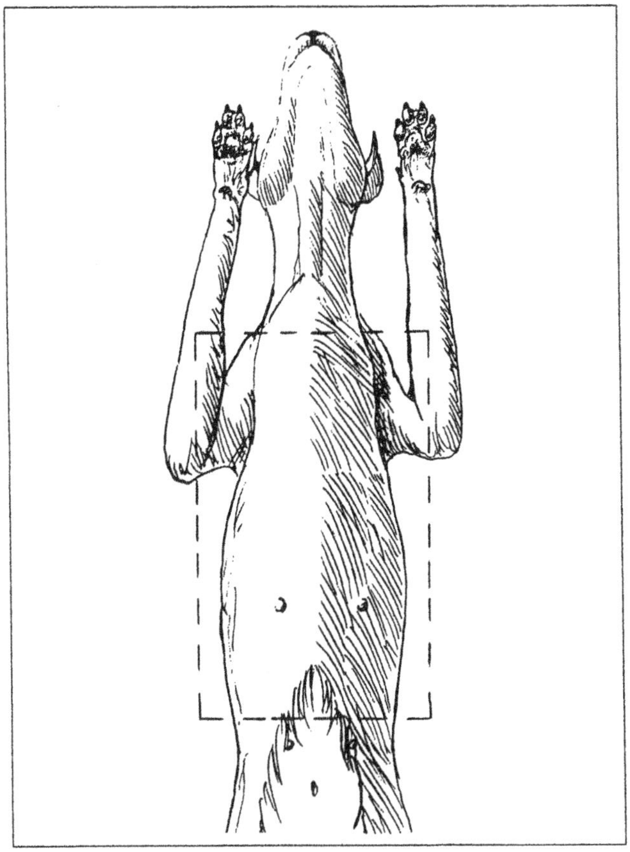

FIG. 10-83 Positioning for a ventrodorsal projection of the thorax.

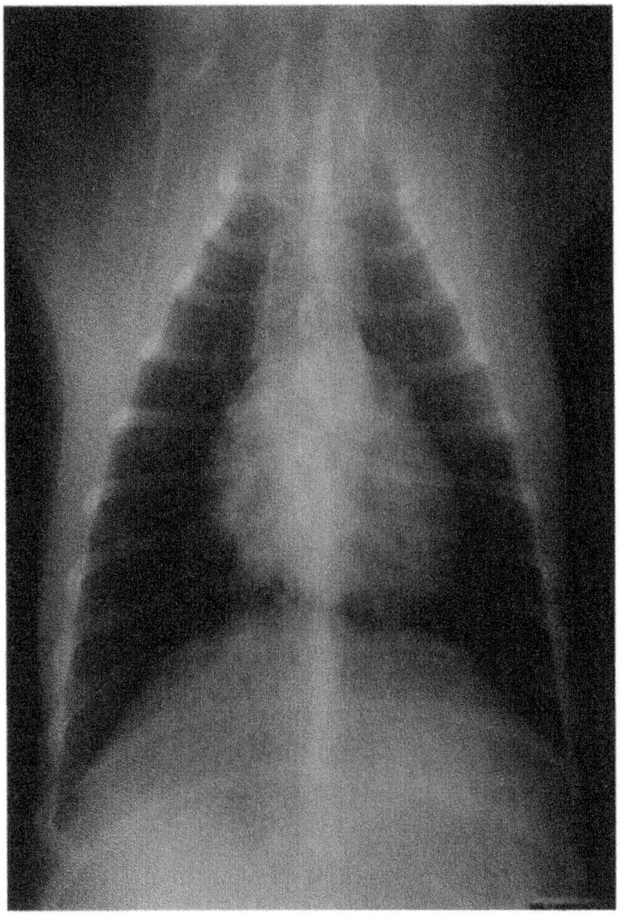

FIG. 10-84 Ventrodorsal projection of the thorax.

Dorsoventral Position

This view is helpful for evaluating pneumothorax. Place the patient in dorsoventral position with the front limbs extended cranially. The cranial landmark is the manubrium, and the caudal landmark is halfway between the xiphoid and the last rib. Position the thorax so that the sternum and vertebrae are superimposed in a plane perpendicular to the table. Measure at the highest point for the kVp setting. Make the exposure during peak inspiration (Figure 10-85).

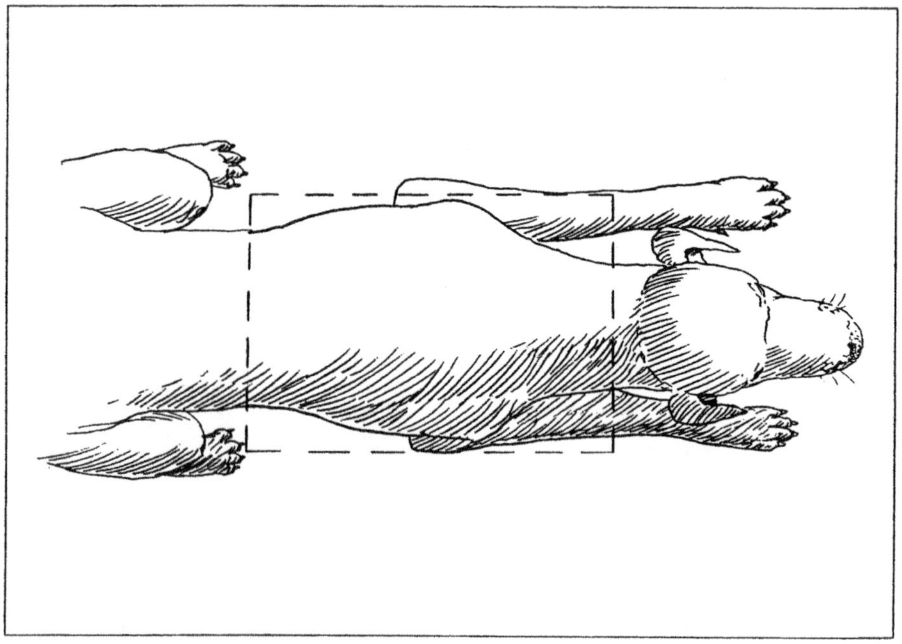

FIG. 10-85 Positioning for a dorsoventral projection of the thorax.

Abdomen

Lateral Position

Place the patient in right lateral recumbency with the hind limbs extended caudally. The cranial landmark is three rib spaces cranial to the xiphoid, and the caudal landmark is the greater trochanter of the femur. Use padding to keep the sternum and the dorsal spinous processes in a plane parallel to the table. Measure at the highest point for the kVp setting. Make the exposure during peak expiration (Figures 10-86 and 10-87).

Radiograph the abdomen at peak expiration.

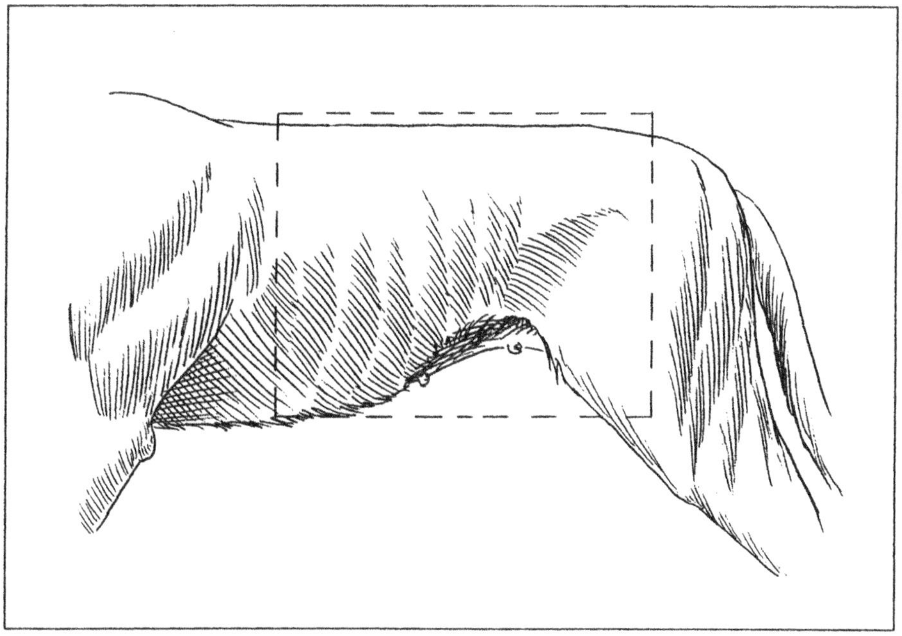

FIG. 10-86 Positioning for a lateral projection of the abdomen.

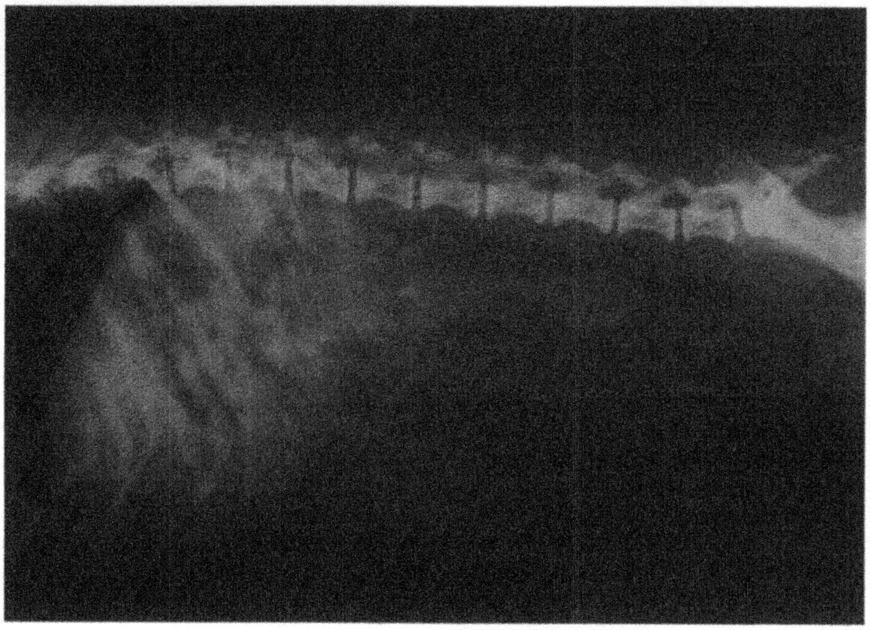

FIG. 10-87 Lateral projection of the abdomen.

Ventrodorsal Position

Place the patient in ventrodorsal position with the hind limbs extended caudally. The cranial landmark is three rib spaces cranial to the xiphoid, and the caudal landmark is the greater trochanter of the femur. Position the patient so that the sternum and vertebrae are superimposed in a plane perpendicular to the table. Measure at the highest point for the kVp setting. Make the exposure during peak expiration (Figures 10-88 and 10-89).

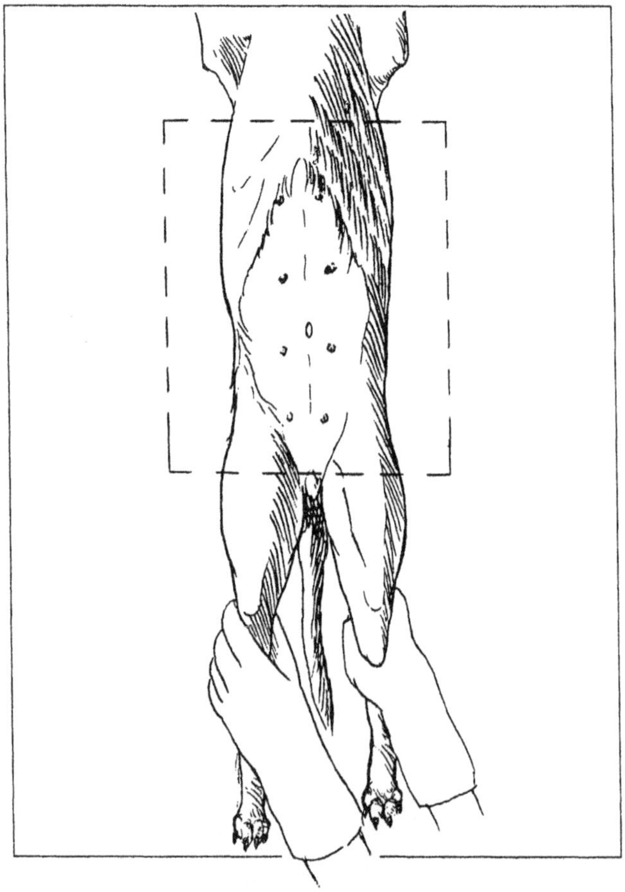

FIG. 10-88 Positioning for a ventrodorsal projection of the abdomen.

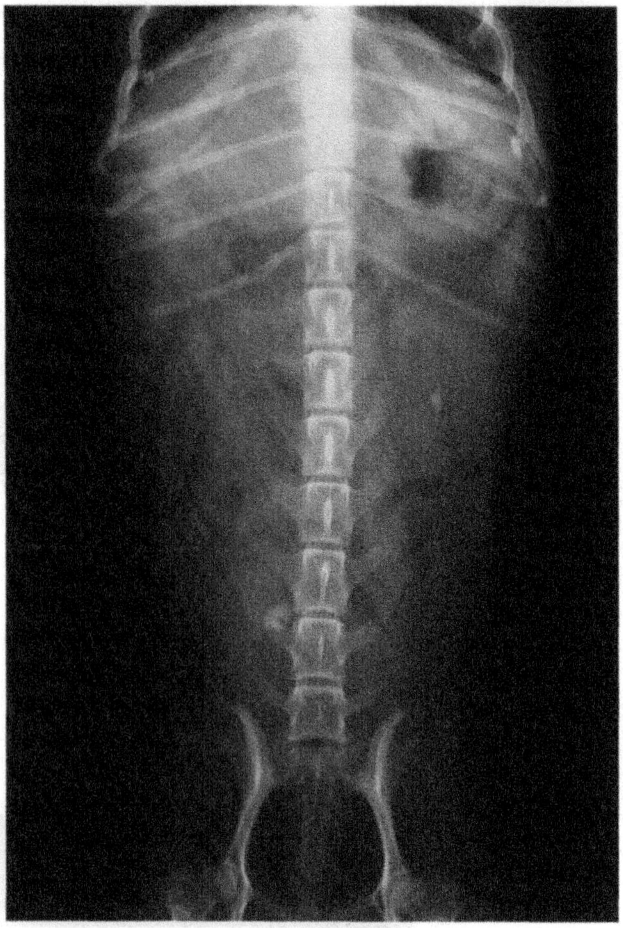

FIG. 10-89 Ventrodorsal projection of the abdomen.

Pelvis

Lateral Position

Place the patient in lateral recumbency with the wings of the ilium superimposed on each other, perpendicular to the table. Position the right limb slightly cranial and the left limb slightly caudal to separate the femoral heads. The cranial landmark is the wings of the ilium, and the caudal landmark is the caudal border of the ischium. Measure at the thickest point for the kVp setting. Sometimes the kVp needs to be increased because of the thick subject density (Figures 10-90 and 10-91).

When radiographing a pelvis in the lateral projection, increase 6 to 8 kVp, depending on the animal's muscle tone.

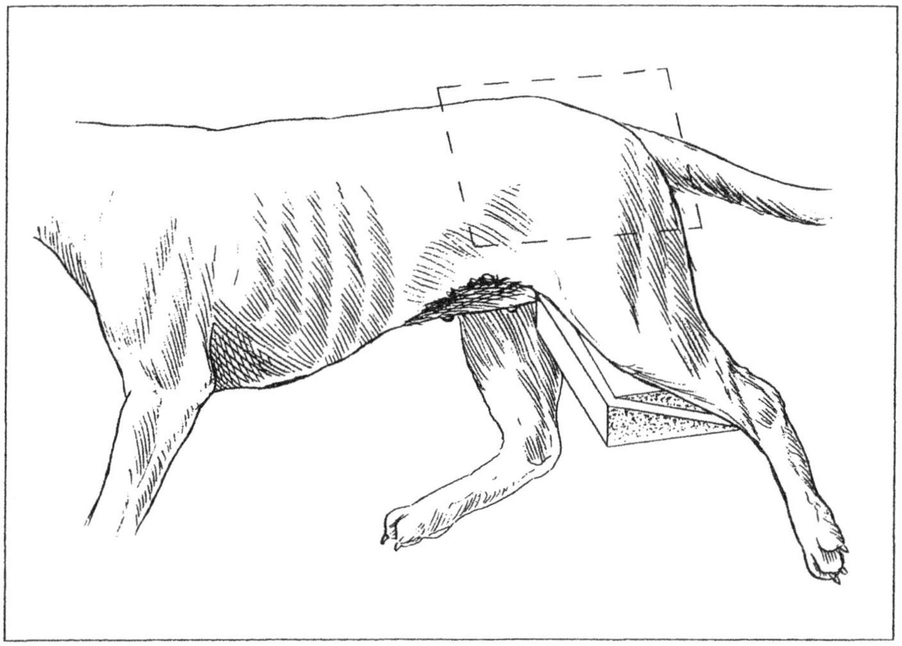

FIG. 10-90 Positioning for a lateral projection of the pelvis.

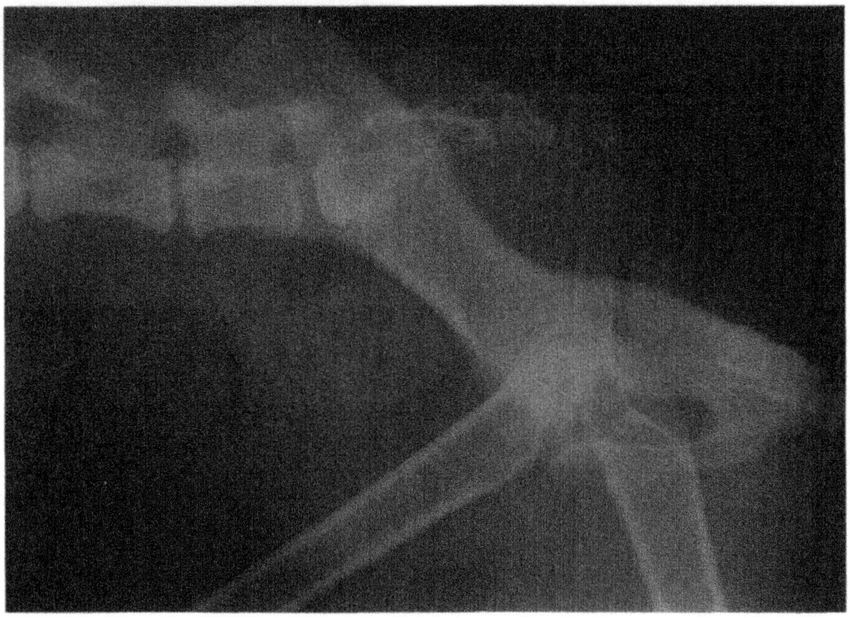

FIG. 10-91 Lateral projection of the pelvis.

Ventrodorsal Flexed Position

Place the patient in ventrodorsal position with the front limbs extended cranially. Position the patient so the wings of the ilium are in a plane parallel to the table and the stifles are pushed cranially. The cranial landmark is the wings of the ilium, and the caudal landmark is the caudal border of the ischium. Measure at the thickest point for the kVp setting. Identify the right or left side (Figures 10-92 and 10-93).

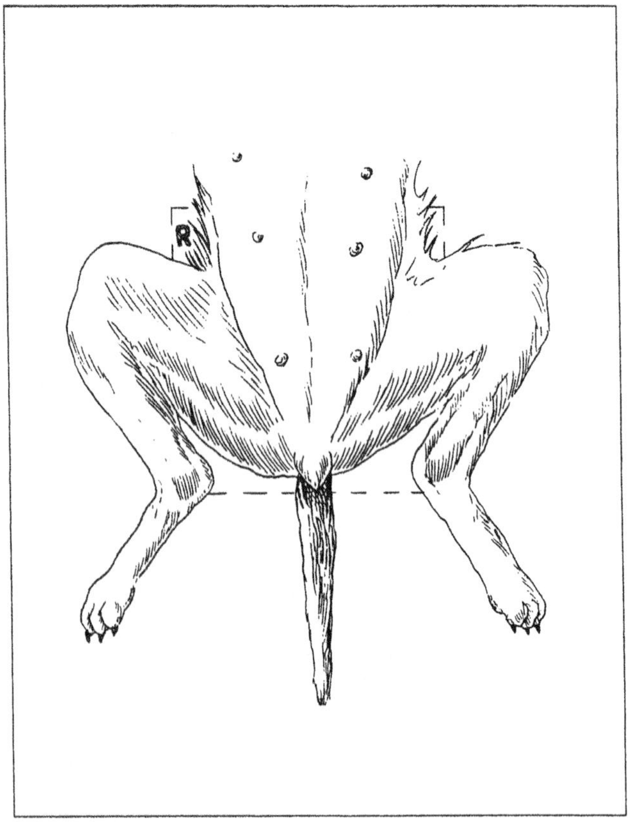

FIG. 10-92 Positioning for a ventrodorsal projection of the pelvis in the flexed position.

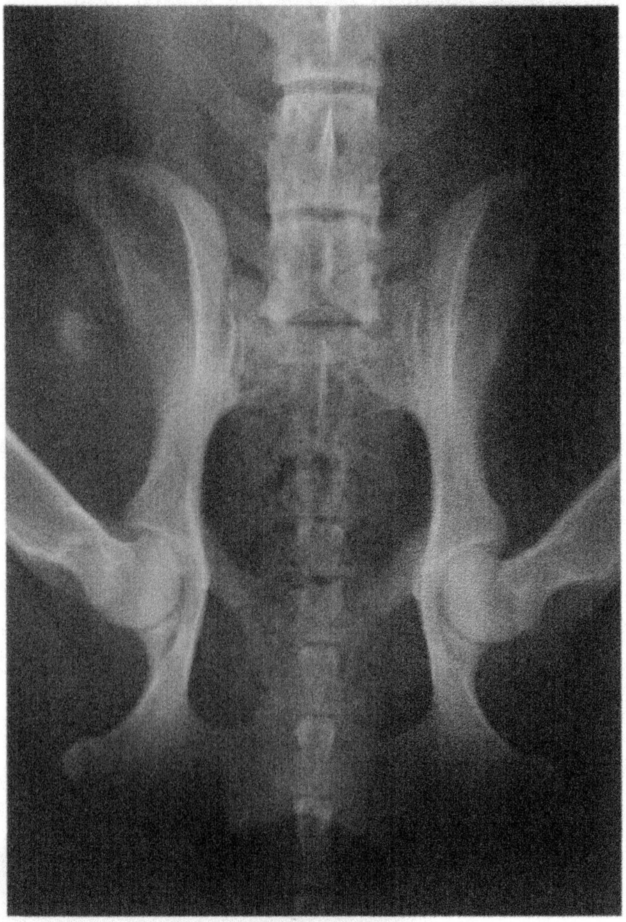

FIG. 10-93 Ventrodorsal projection of the pelvis in the flexed position.

Ventrodorsal Extended Position

General anesthesia may be necessary to achieve complete muscle relaxation and facilitate accurate positioning. Place the patient in ventrodorsal position with the front limbs extended cranially. Position the patient so that the wings of the ilium are in a plane parallel to the table. The cranial landmark is the wings of the ilium, and the caudal landmark is the stifle joint. While holding the limbs at the tarsi, pull both limbs caudally, rotating the stifle joints inward. The femora should be parallel to the table and to each another. Measure from the table to the stifle when the limbs are fully extended for the kVp setting. Identify the right or left side (Figures 10-94 and 10-95).

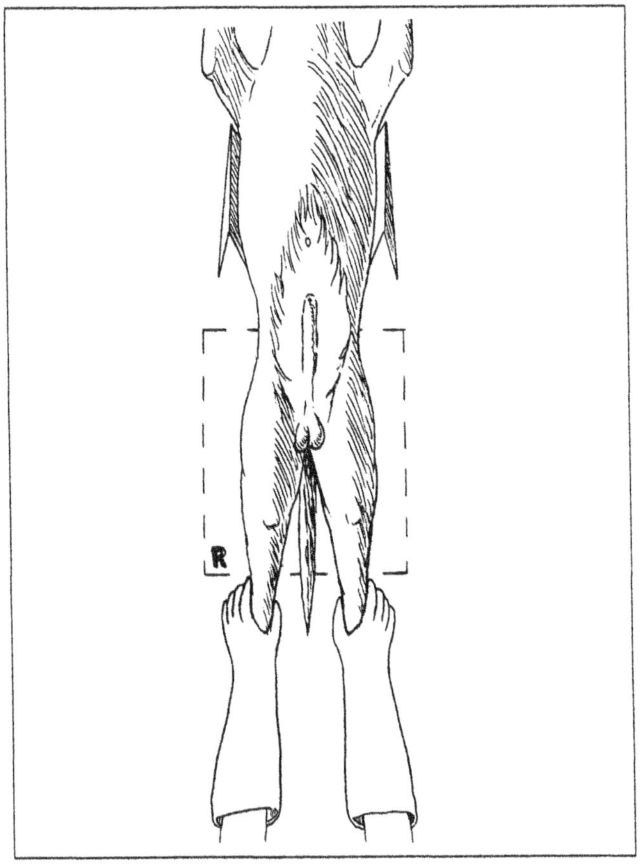

FIG. 10-94 Positioning for a ventrodorsal projection of the pelvis in the extended position.

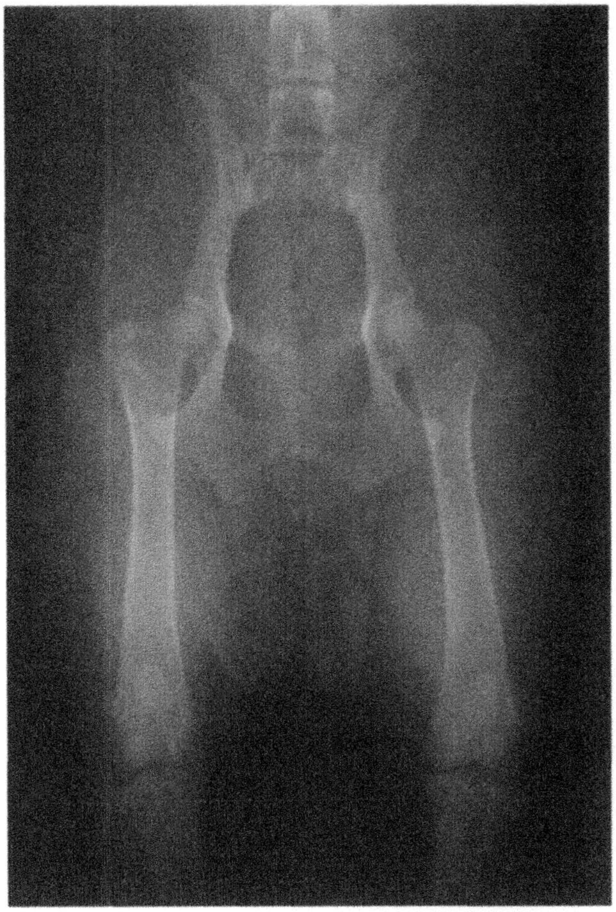

FIG. 10-95 Ventrodorsal projection of the pelvis in the extended position.

Femur

Mediolateral Position

Place the patient in lateral recumbency with the limb of interest closest to the table. Abduct the unaffected limb out of the way. Center the primary beam on the femoral shaft and collimate to include the coxofemoral and stifle joints. Measure at the thickest point for the kVp setting. Place a right or left marker on the cranial side of the limb (Figures 10-96 and 10-97).

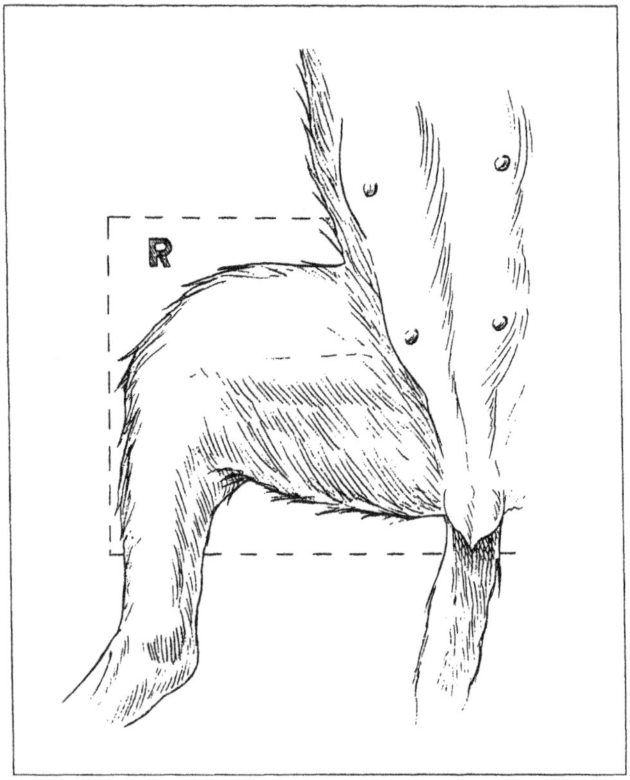

FIG. 10-96 Positioning for a mediolateral projection of the femur.

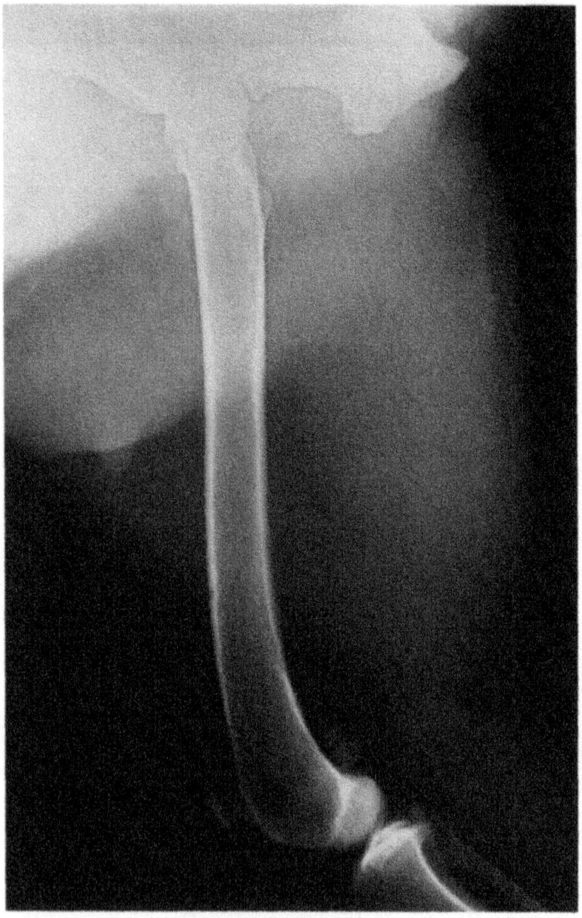

FIG. 10-97 Mediolateral projection of the femur.

Craniocaudal Position

Because of the structure of the femur, it is sometimes difficult to position it parallel to the table. This causes foreshortening of the limb, altering the true length and shape of the bone. Two methods are available for positioning a femur in craniocaudal projection. The *cross-table projection* involves positioning the patient in lateral recumbency with the limb to be imaged nondependent (Figure 10-98). Place the cassette caudal to the limb and perpendicular to the table. Keep the cassette as close to the limb as possible and parallel with the femur. Slightly abduct the limb by rotating the stifle joint. Bring the tube head down toward the table, and angle the primary beam perpendicular to the femur. Center the primary beam on the femoral shaft and collimate to include the coxofemoral and stifle joints. The *ventrodorsal extended projection* may require some sedation to achieve proper extension of the femur (Figure 10-99). Place the patient in ventrodorsal position. Extend the limb caudally so that the femur is parallel to the table. With this method, the increase in OFD causes magnification and a decrease in detail. For both methods, measure over the thickest point for the kVp setting. Place a right or left marker on the lateral side of the limb (Figure 10-100).

When imaging long bones, always include the joint above and the joint below.

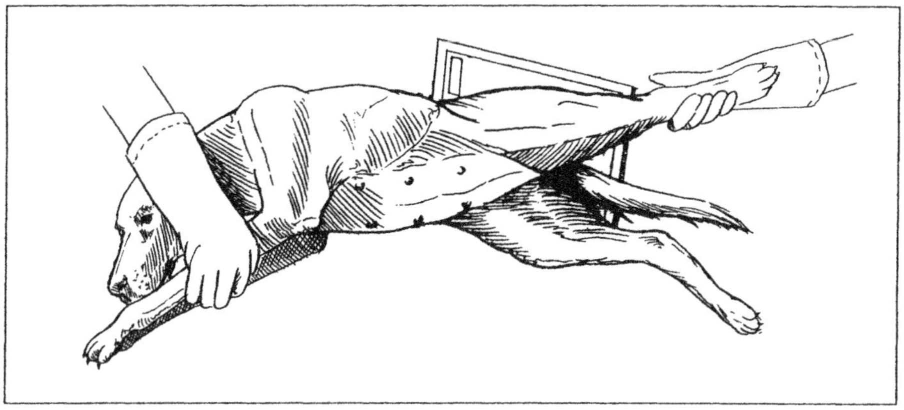

FIG. 10-98 Positioning for a cross-table craniocaudal projection of the femur.

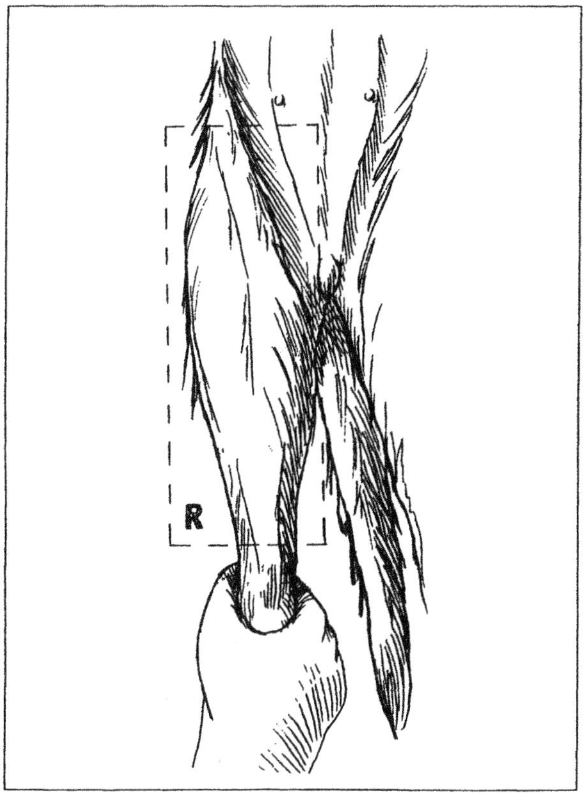

FIG. 10-99 Positioning for a craniocaudal projection of the femur using ventrodorsal extended projection.

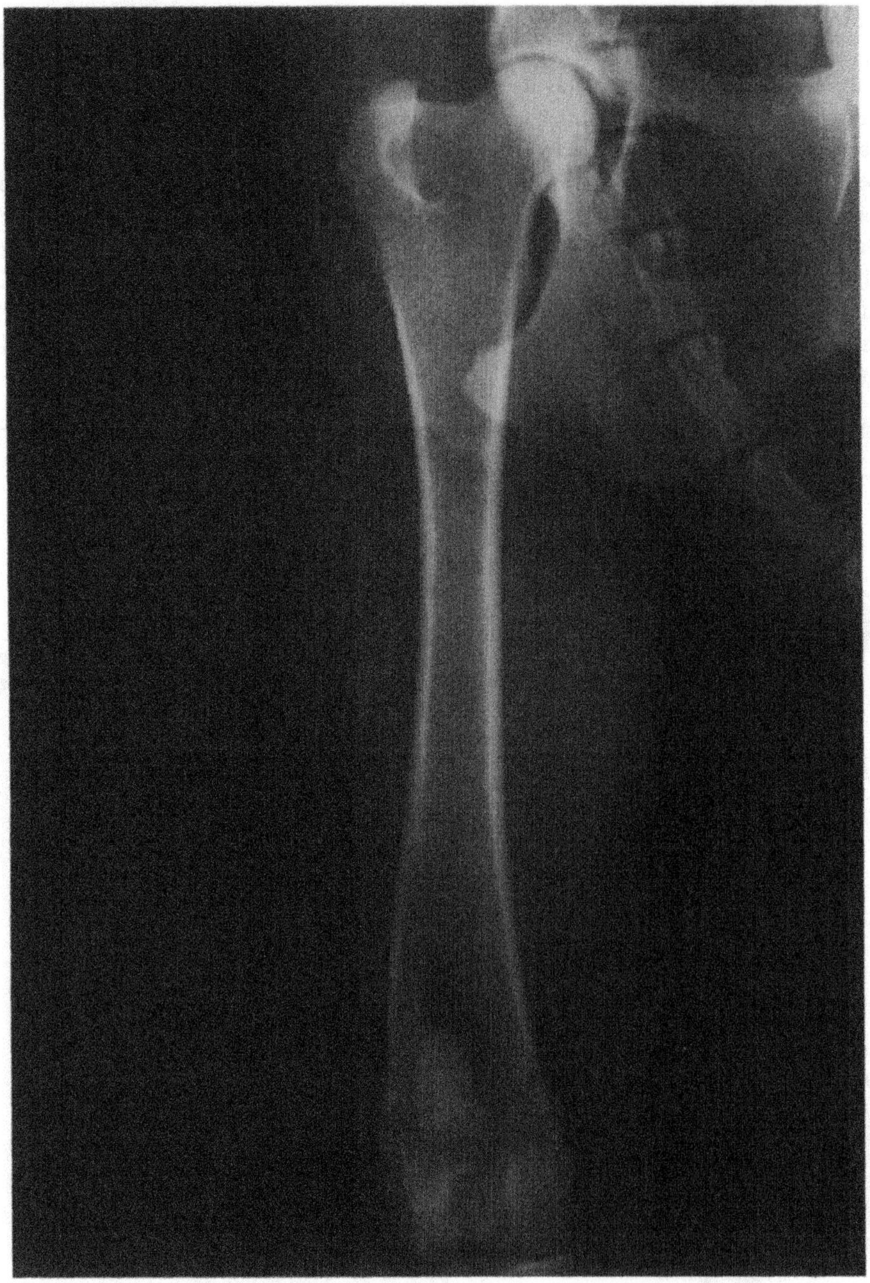

FIG. 10-100 Craniocaudal projection of the femur.

Stifle Joint

Mediolateral Position

Place the patient in lateral recumbency with the limb to be imaged closest to the table. Place padding under the pelvis and abduct the unaffected limb out of the way. With the stifle to be imaged in extension, place a small amount of cotton under the tarsus to bring the tibia parallel to the table. Center the primary beam on the stifle joint and collimate to include only the joint. Measure over the thickest point for the kVp setting. Place a right or left marker on the cranial side of the limb (Figures 10-101 and 10-102).

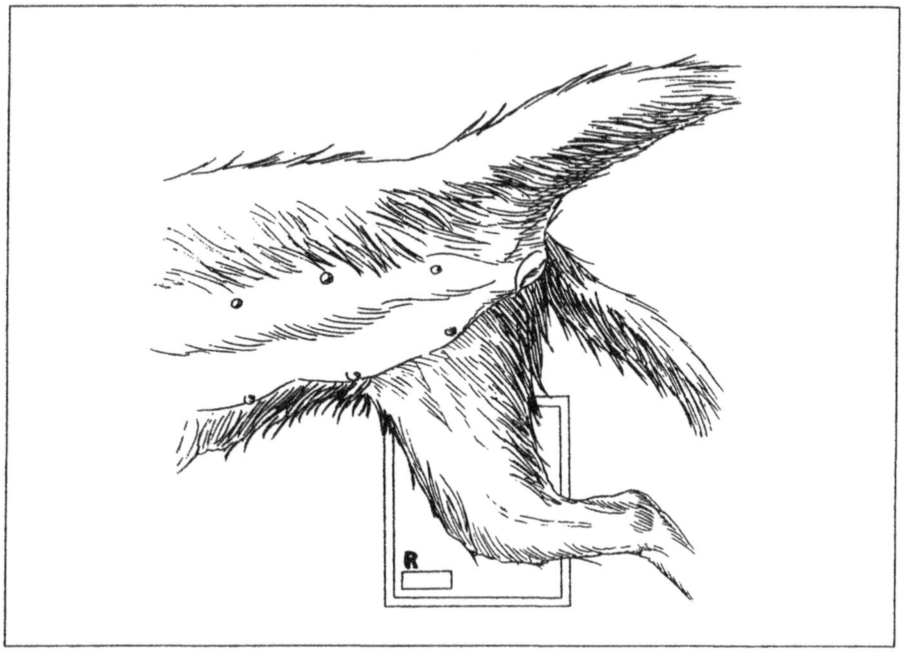

FIG. 10-101 Positioning for a mediolateral projection of the stifle joint.

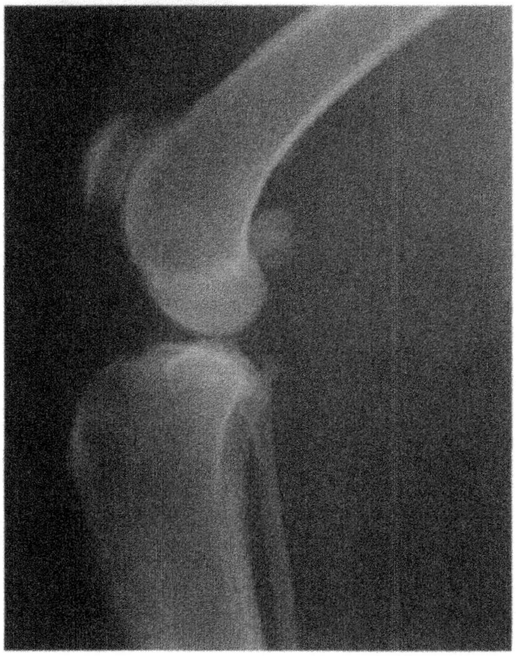

FIG. 10-102 Mediolateral projection of the stifle joint.

Caudocranial Position

Place the patient in sternal recumbency with two or three foam wedges under the flexed unaffected limb. The limb of interest is extended caudally. Palpating the tibial tuberosity aids in determining the amount of rotation necessary for an exact caudocranial projection. Center the primary beam on the stifle joint and collimate the beam to include only the joint. Measure over the distal femur for the kVp setting. Place a right or left marker on the lateral side of the limb (Figures 10-103 and 10-104).

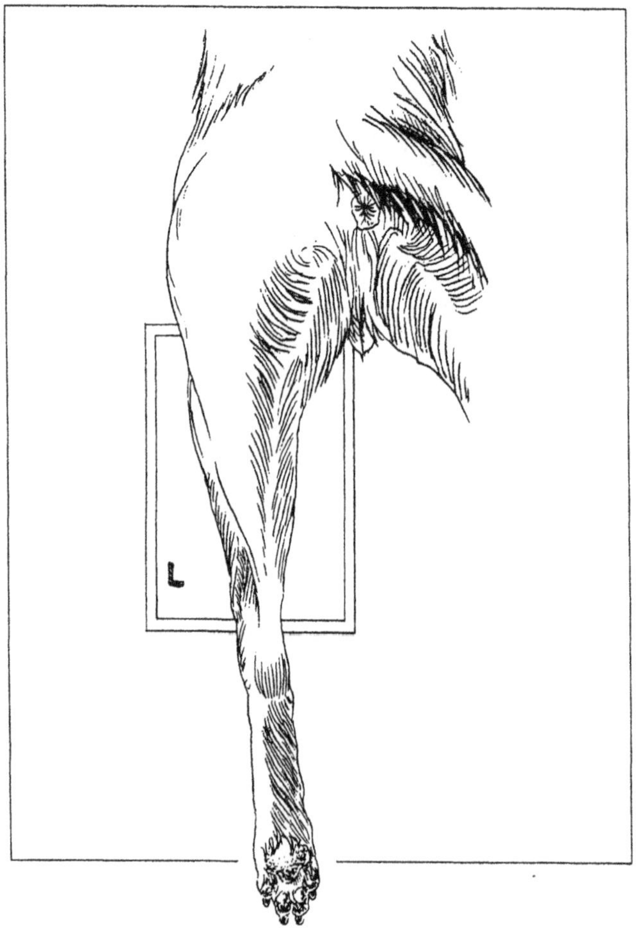

FIG. 10-103 Positioning for a caudocranial projection of the stifle joint.

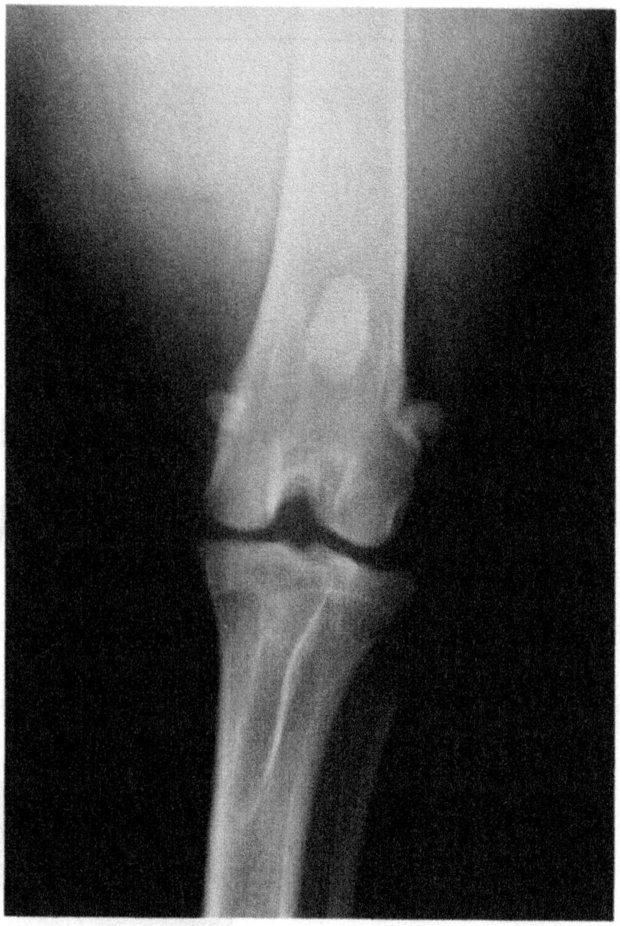

FIG. 10-104 Caudocranial projection of the stifle joint.

Tibia

Mediolateral Position

Place the patient in lateral recumbency with the limb of interest closest to the table. Abduct the unaffected limb out of the way. Place a small amount of cotton under the tarsus to bring the tibia parallel to the table. Center the primary beam on the tibia and collimate to include the stifle and tarsal joints. Measure over the thickest area for the kVp setting. Place a right or left marker on the cranial side of the limb (Figures 10-105 and 10-106).

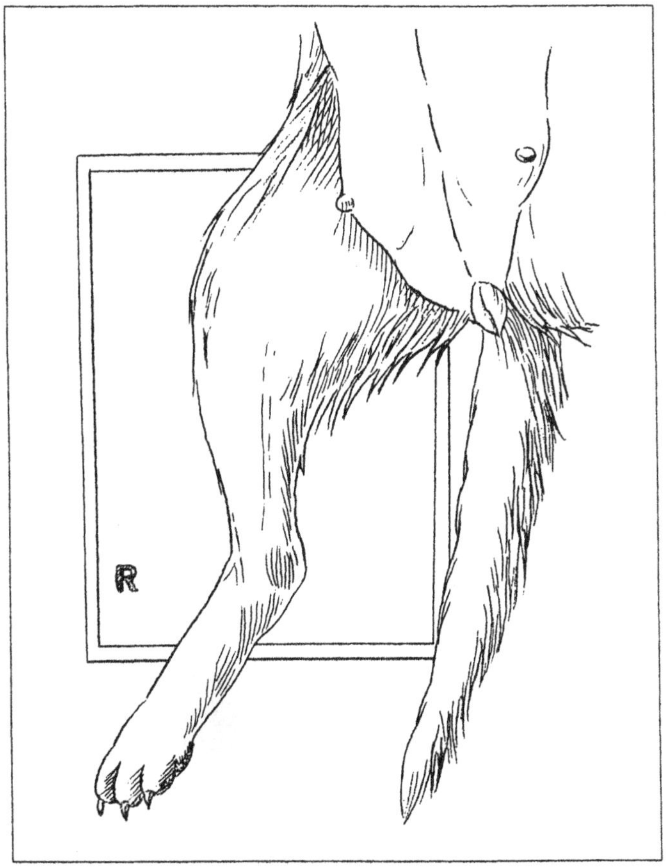

FIG. 10-105 Positioning for a mediolateral projection of the tibia.

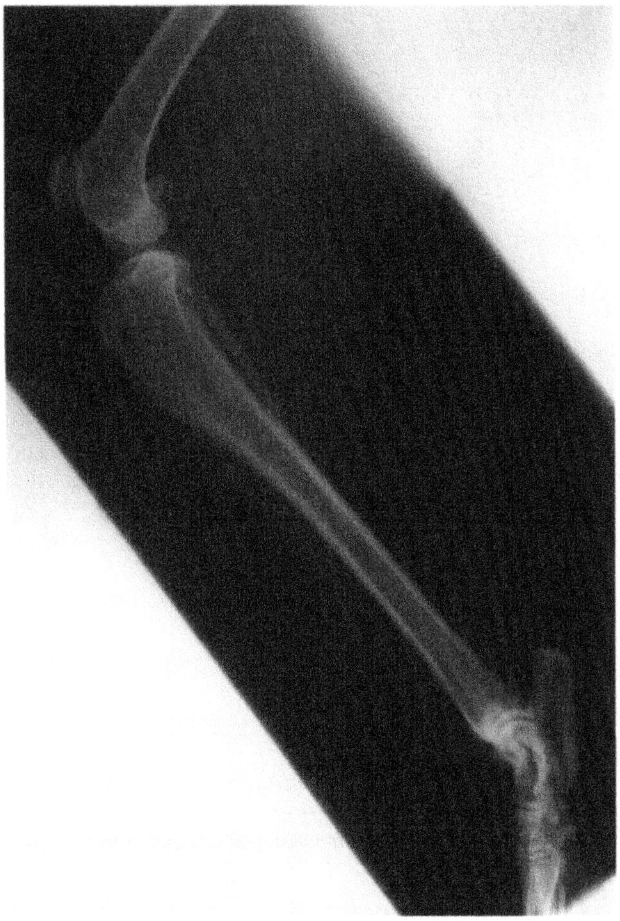

FIG. 10-106 Mediolateral projection of the tibia.

Caudocranial Position

Place the patient in sternal recumbency with two or three foam wedges under the flexed unaffected limb. The limb of interest is extended caudally. Palpating the tibial tuberosity aids in determining the amount of rotation necessary for an exact caudocranial position. Center the primary beam on the tibia and collimate to include the stifle and tarsal joints. Measure over the stifle joint for the kVp setting. Place a right or left marker on the lateral side of the limb (Figures 10-107 and 10-108).

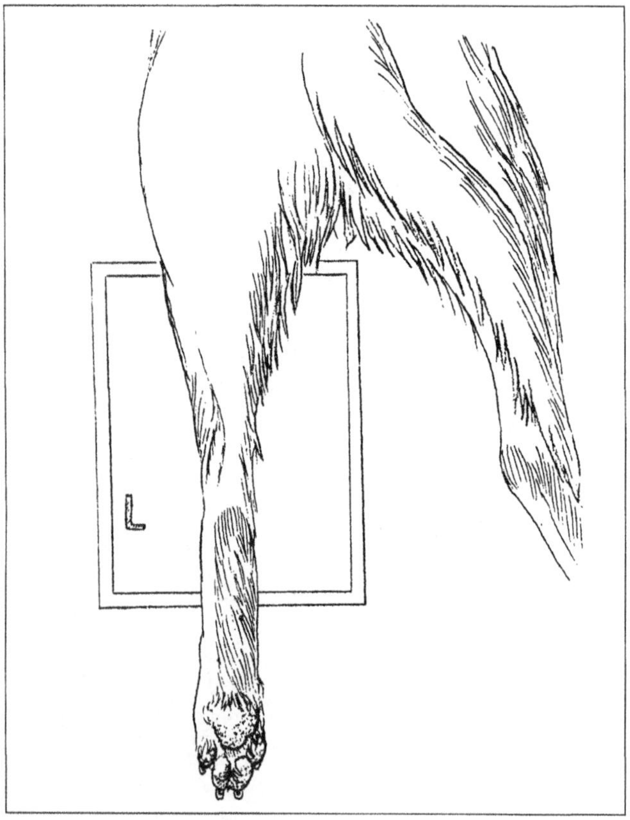

FIG. 10-107 Positioning for a caudocranial projection of the tibia.

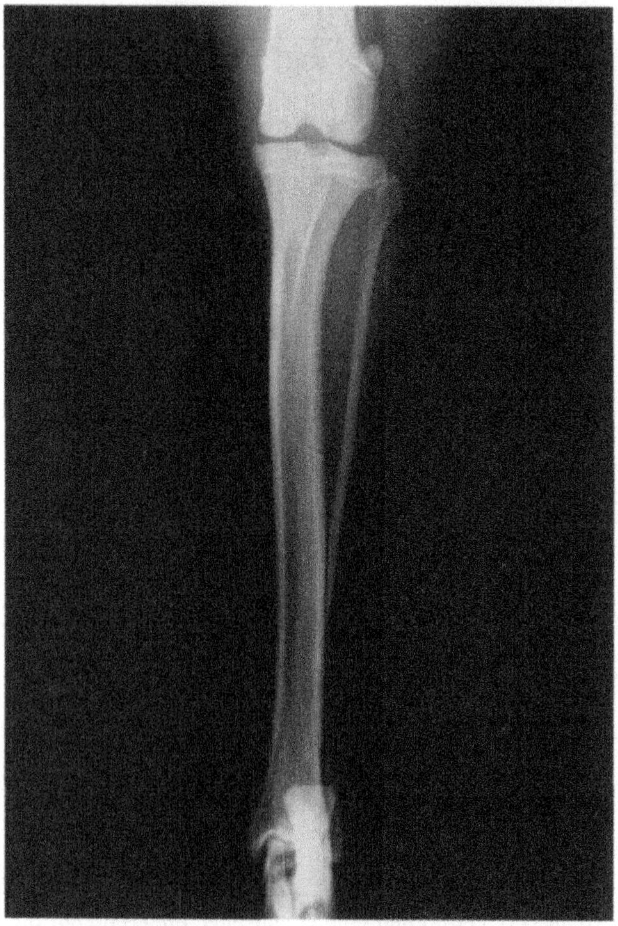

FIG. 10-108 Caudocranial projection of the tibia.

Tarsus

Mediolateral Position

Place the patient in lateral recumbency with the limb of interest closest to the table. Abduct the unaffected limb out of the way. Center the primary beam on the tarsal joint and collimate to include only the joint. Some padding may be necessary under the talus to achieve an exact mediolateral position. Measure at the thickest point for the kVp setting. Place a right or left marker on the dorsal side of the limb (Figures 10-109 and 10-110).

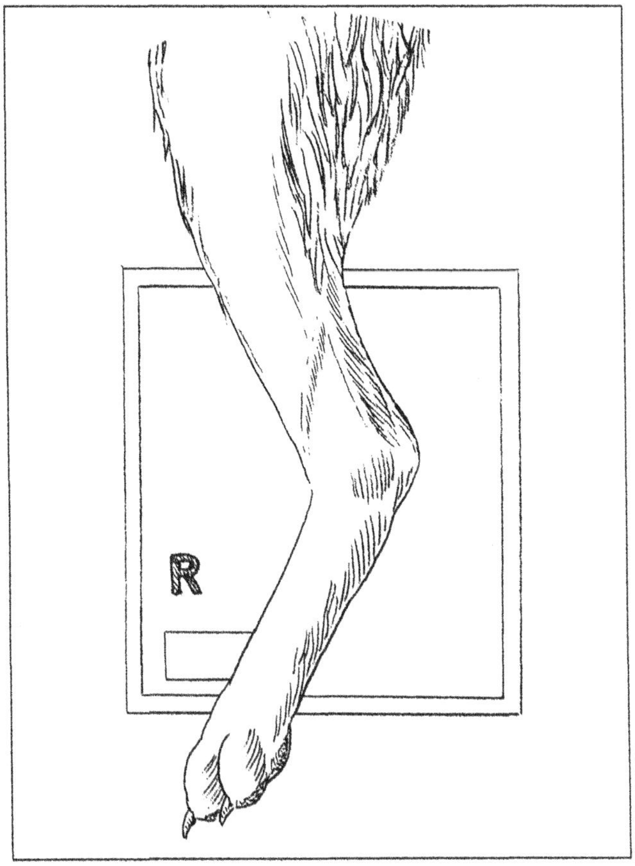

FIG. 10-109 Positioning for a mediolateral projection of the tarsal joint.

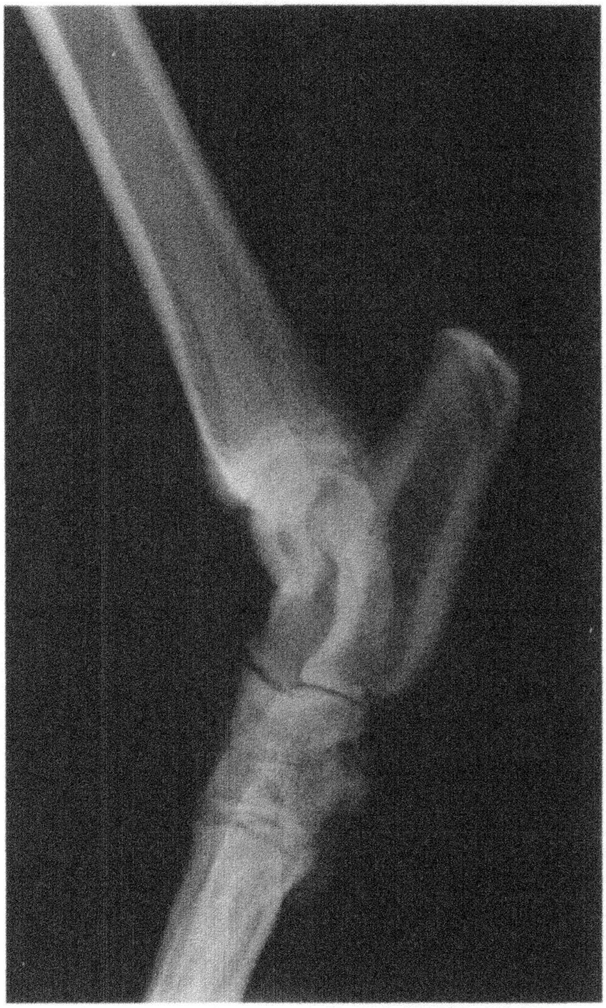

FIG. 10-110 Mediolateral projection of the tarsal joint.

Plantarodorsal Position

Place the patient in sternal recumbency with two or three foam wedges under the flexed unaffected limb. Extend the limb of interest caudally. Center the primary beam on the tarsal joint and collimate to include only the joint. Measure at the thickest point for the kVp setting. Place a right or left marker on the lateral side of the limb (Figures 10-111 and 10-112).

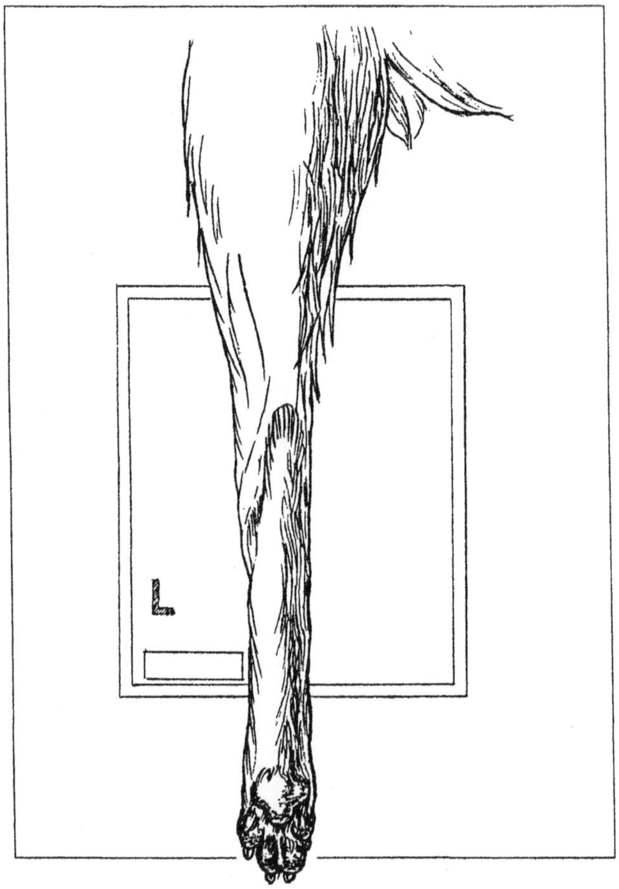

FIG. 10-111 Positioning for the plantarodorsal projection of the tarsal joint.

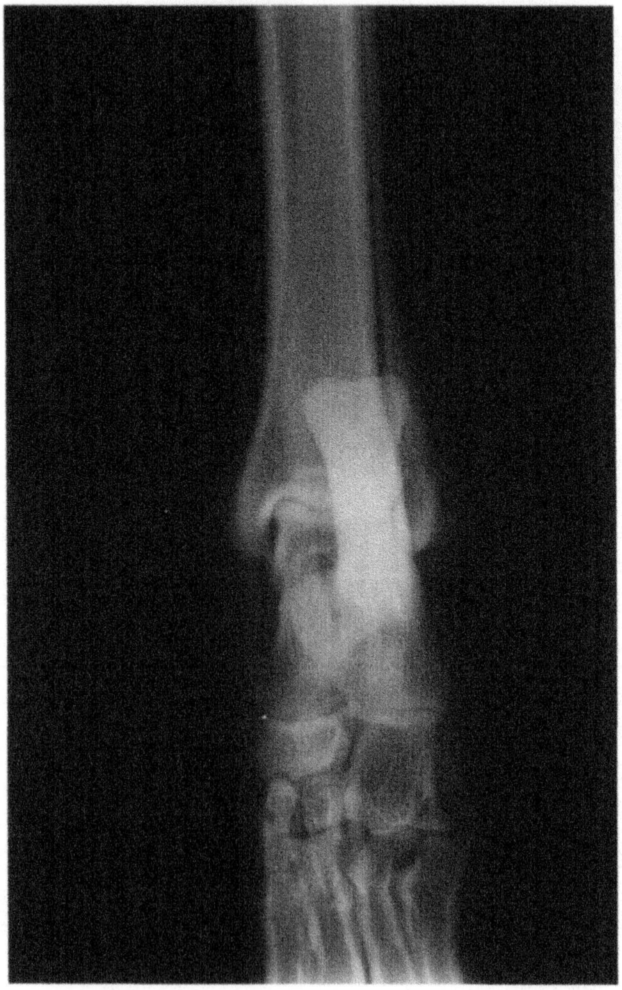

FIG. 10-112 Plantarodorsal projection of the tarsal joint.

Metatarsus and Digits

Mediolateral Position

Place the patient in lateral recumbency with the limb of interest closest to the table. Extend the unaffected limb caudally and out of the way. Center the primary beam on the metatarsus and collimate to include the tarsal joint and digits. Sometimes the usefulness of a lateral projection is limited because of the superimposition of the digits. To open a space between each metatarsal bone, position the limb slightly oblique. To image only the digits, tape each digit so that it is not superimposed over the others. Measure at the thickest point for the kVp setting. Place a right or left marker on the dorsal side of the limb (Figures 10-113 and 10-114).

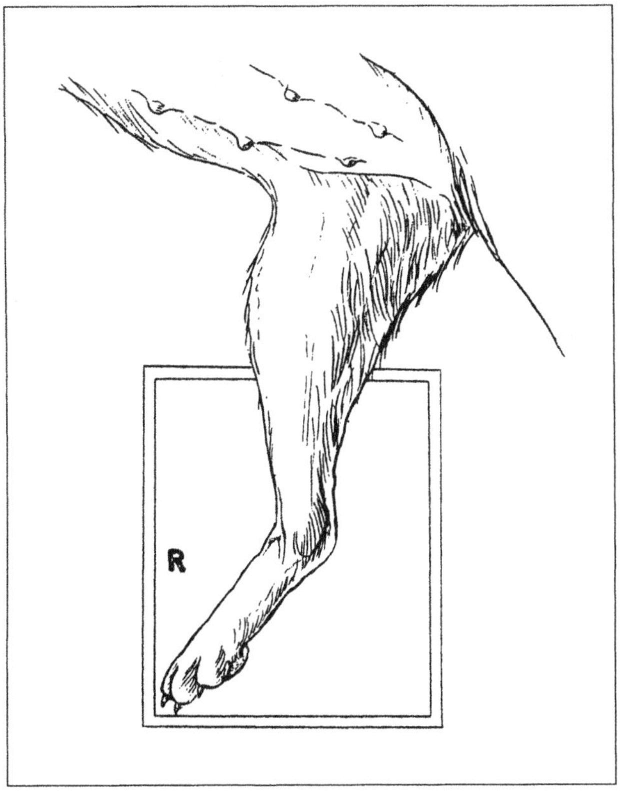

FIG. 10-113 Positioning for a mediolateral projection of the metatarsus and digits. Lateral oblique projections of the metatarsus are positioned similarly to that of the metacarpus.

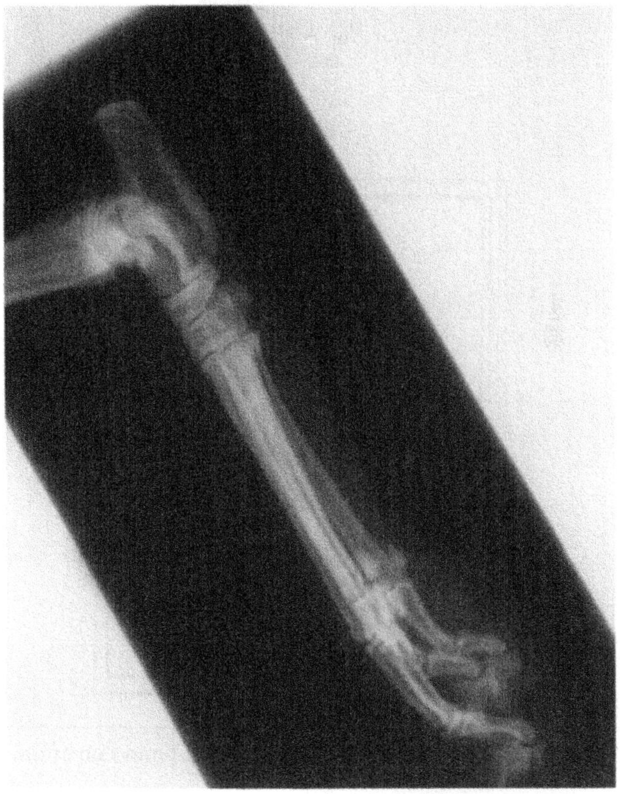

FIG. 10-114 Mediolateral projection of the metatarsus and digits.

Plantarodorsal Position

Place the patient in sternal recumbency with two or three foam wedges under the flexed unaffected limb. Extend the limb of interest caudally. Center the primary beam on the metatarsus and collimate to include the metatarsus and digits. Measure the thickest point for the kVp setting. Place a right or left marker on the lateral side of the limb (Figures 10-115 and 10-116).

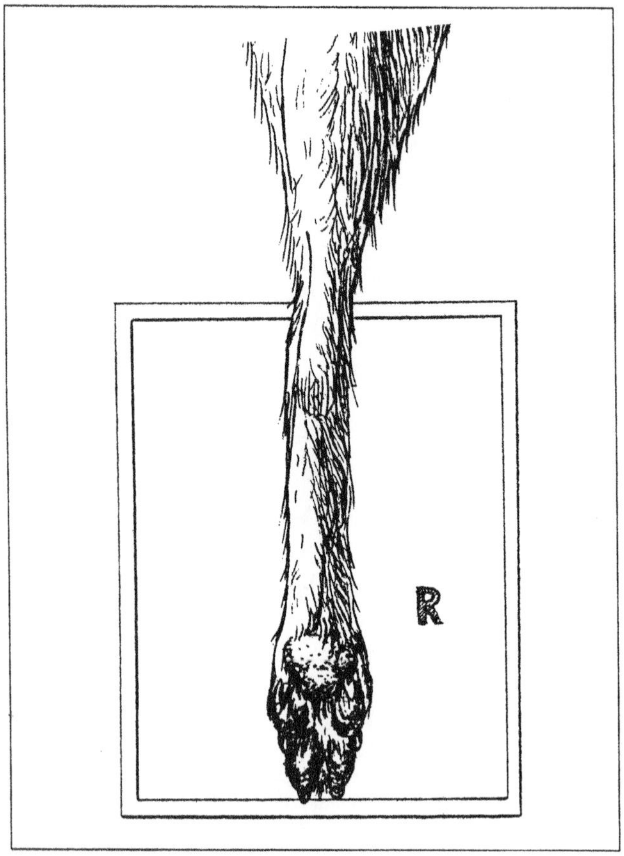

FIG. 10-115 Positioning for a plantarodorsal projection of the metatarsus and digits.

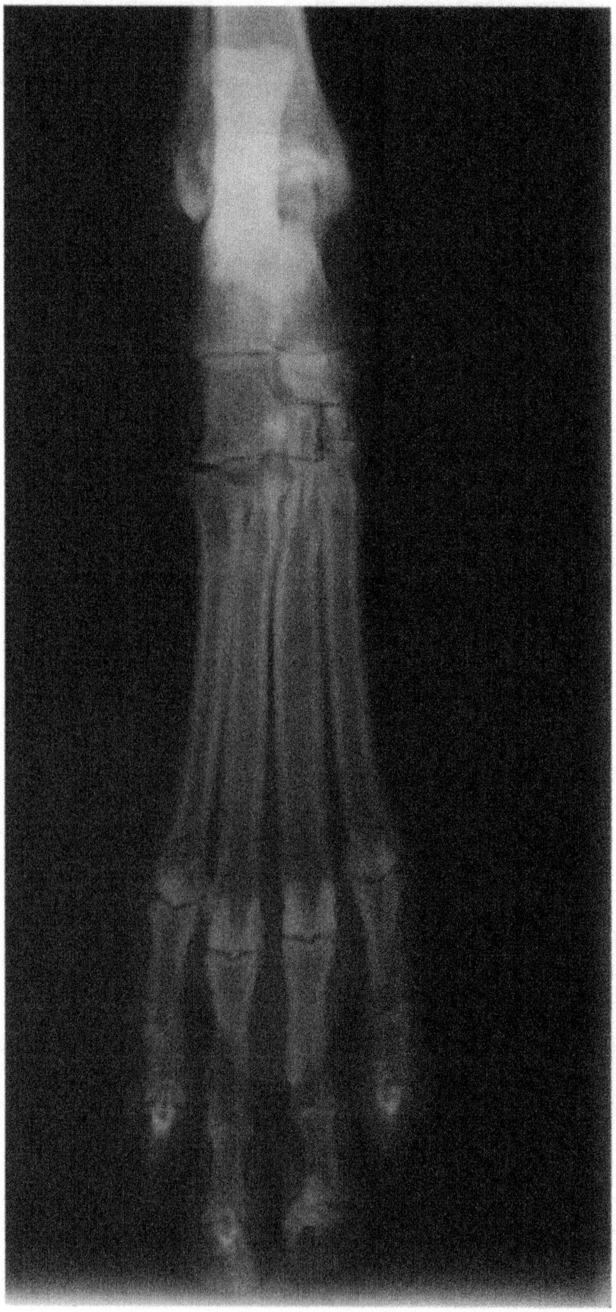

FIG. 10-116 Plantarodorsal projection of the metatarsus and digits.

Recommended Reading

Douglas SW et al: *Principles of veterinary radiography*, ed 4, London, 1987, Bailliere Tindall.

Kealy JK: *Diagnostic radiology of the dog and cat*, ed 2, Philadelphia, 1987, Saunders.

Morgan JP, Silverman S: *Techniques of veterinary radiography*, ed 5, Davis, Calif, 1993, Veterinary Radiology Associates.

Schebitz H, Wilkens H: *Atlas of radiographic anatomy of the dog and cat*, ed 4, Philadelphia, 1986, Saunders.

Smallwood JE et al: A standardized nomenclature for radiographic projections used in veterinary medicine, *Vet Radiol* 26(1):2, 1985.

Ticer JW: *Radiographic technique in veterinary practice*, ed 2, Philadelphia, 1984, Saunders.

11

Basic Small Animal Dental Radiography

CONNIE HAN

CHAPTER OBJECTIVES

- List the types of x-ray equipment used for veterinary dentistry.
- Explain the use of extraoral films in dental radiography.
- Discuss the dental applications of intraoral x-ray films.
- Describe the basic exposure techniques used in dental radiography.
- Define the parallel positioning technique and when it is used.
- Define the bisecting-angle positioning technique and when it is used.

Dental radiography is one of the most important diagnostic tools used in veterinary dentistry. It is used to determine the status of not only the crown but also the tooth root. Nearly two thirds of the tooth is located below the gingiva. Radiographs can help determine the degree of disease in areas that cannot be inspected visually.

Equipment

Most standard x-ray equipment found in veterinary practices can be used for dental radiographs. The tube head is more cumbersome to position than a dedicated dental x-ray unit. The only requirements are that the tube head can be angled along the axis of the table and that the focal-film distance (FFD) can be changed. Portable x-ray units used for ambulatory large animal radiography can also be used. As with any other radiographic procedure, portable units should not be handheld but placed on a tripod where the height can be adjusted. If the caseload warrants, human dental x-ray machines may be purchased, which quickly pay for themselves (Figure 11-1).

> Almost any x-ray machine can be used for dental radiography.

The type of film used in dental radiography can vary. Any combination of regular cassettes, standard nonscreen film, and intraoral film may be used. Regular cassettes or standard nonscreen films are used when a survey of the dental arcade is needed. Cases in which fractures are suspected or areas in which oral pathology or neoplasia exist call for survey views. These films generally have some superimposition of other oral structures, decreasing the fine detail.

Intraoral films are useful for individual teeth. These films are small and flexible, which allows for easier positioning (Figure 11-2). It is best to have at least two sizes of intraoral film to accommodate the many sizes of patients. Intraoral films provide excellent detail without superimposition of other oral structures.

> It is best to have at least two sizes of intraoral x-ray film.

As with any other radiographic procedure, film processing is important. Errors in the darkroom can rapidly make a radiograph nondiagnostic. The regular cassettes and the standard nonscreen film can be processed normally. The intraoral films can also be processed using standard manual tanks or automatic processors. Intraoral films take the same amount of time to process as the larger films.

An intraoral film can be run through an automatic processor by either of two methods. The first method involves taping the small film to a larger leader film, then running it as usual through the processor. The major problem with this method is that the intraoral film can become detached from the leader film and lost in the processor. The second method involves placing the film in special developing mounts that carry the intraoral film through the processor.

As the number of intraoral dental radiographs increases, however, the speed of processing needs to increase. One option is rapid developer and fixer solutions used in individual containers (Figure 11-3). The containers can be used in the darkroom (Figure 11-4) or in chairside darkroom units in the dental area (Figure 11-5). With the rapid-developing solutions, depending on the temperature of the chemicals, the film can be developed in 15 to 30 seconds. When multiple films are made, processing speed is important. For high-volume practices, special automatic processors for small dental film can be purchased.

Exposure

As with any new radiographic procedure, a technique for dental radiography needs to be established. Intraoral films

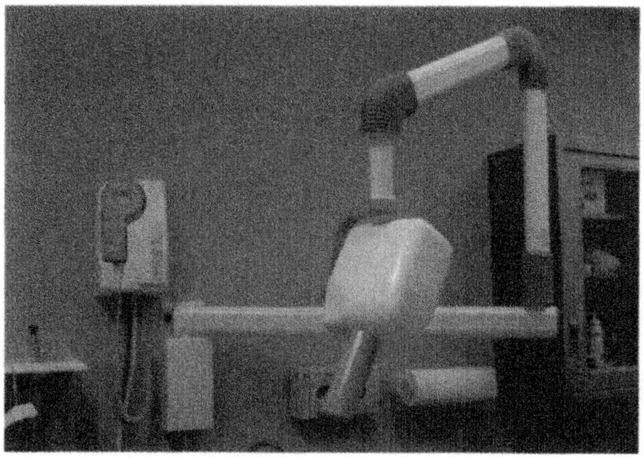

FIG. 11-1 Image-Vet 70 Plus AFP Imaging dedicated dental x-ray machine.

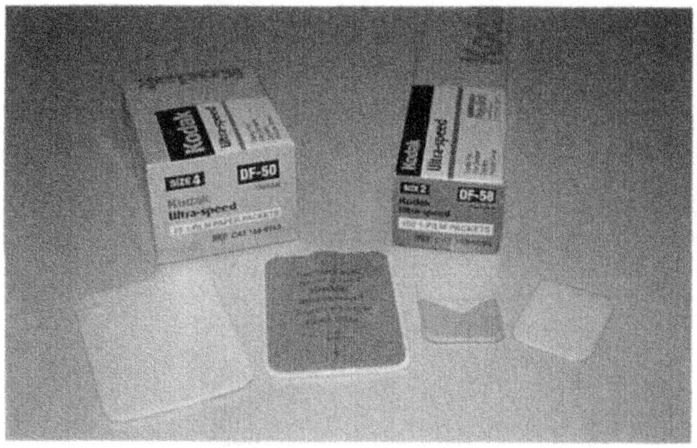

FIG. 11-2 Two sizes of Kodak ultra-speed intraoral dental x-ray film. It is beneficial to have at least two sizes of intraoral film available.

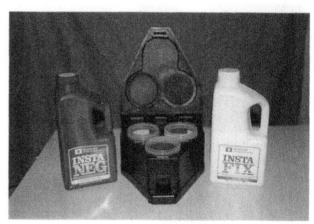

FIG. 11-3 Insta-Neg and Insta-Fix (Microcopy) rapid-processing chemicals for darkroom and chairside dental processors.

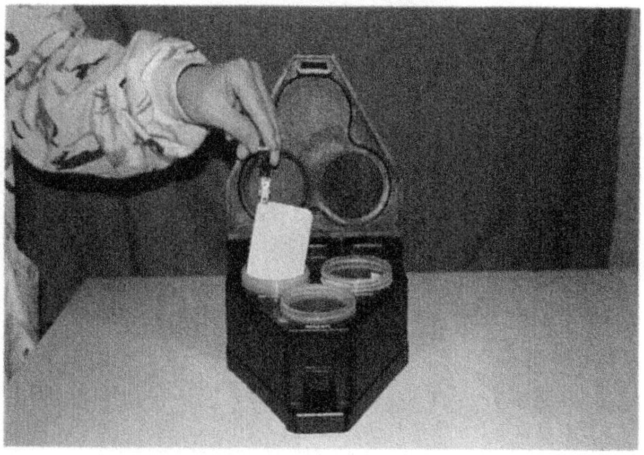

FIG. 11-4 Tabletop dental film processor used in the darkroom.

can be made with stationary tubes that have a fixed FFD of 36 to 40 inches. An exposure of approximately 40 mAs is needed. If the tube head can be lowered, an FFD of 12 to 15 inches is ideal. At this FFD, approximately 10 mAs can be used. Some x-ray machines have the capability of using either a small or a large focal spot. When using intraoral film at a decreased FFD, an mA station that uses a small focal spot is beneficial. This counteracts the penumbra created from the shortened FFD, thereby increasing the detail on the radiograph.

Use an mA station with a small focal spot whenever possible.

The kilovoltage peak (kVp) for either FFD varies from 65 to 80 kVp, depending on the size of the animal. A small-breed dog or cat may require 65 kVp for the primary beam to penetrate the area properly. However, a large-breed dog may need as high as 80 kVp for the x-ray beam to penetrate. Some variation in kVp may exist between an intraoral film of the incisors and the molars. Compared with the molars, a slightly lower kVp for the incisors is often needed.

Positioning

The most difficult part of dental radiography involves the positioning of the patient. If the animal is not correctly positioned, a distorted image of the tooth root will result.

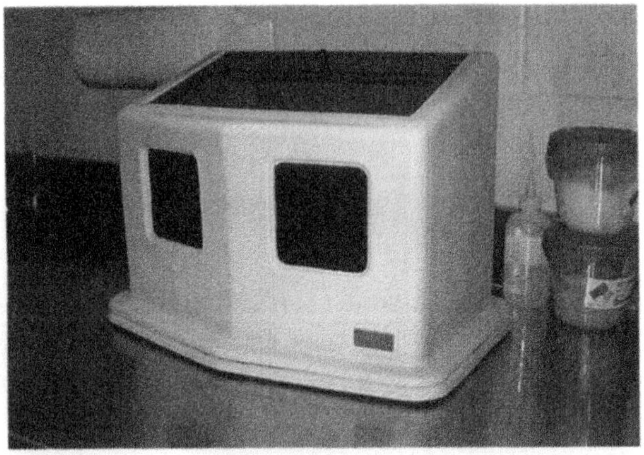

FIG. 11-5 Chairside processor that can be used in the dental area.

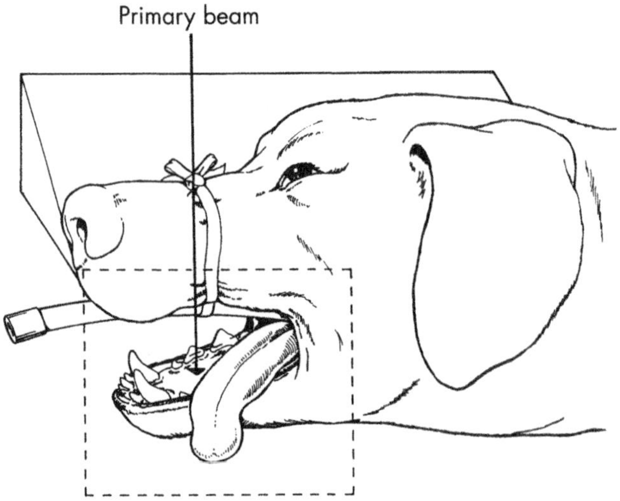

FIG. 11-6 Positioning for a survey of the mandibular dental arcade.

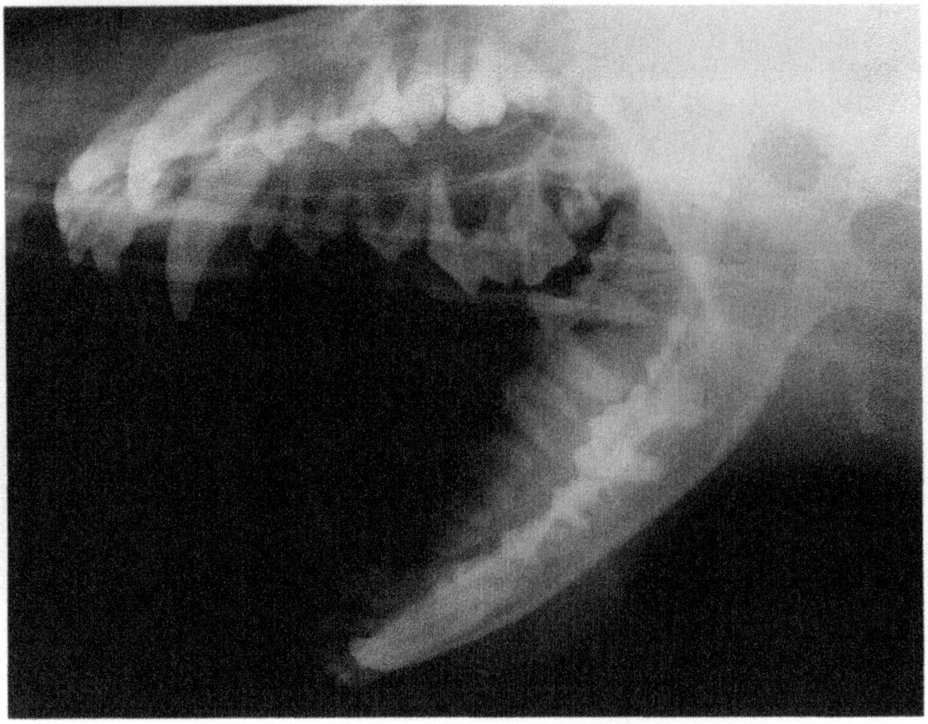

FIG. 11-7 Survey radiograph of the mandibular dental arcade.

Extraoral radiographs using a standard cassette or 8 × 10–inch sheet of nonscreen film are used to survey the mandibular or maxillary arcade. The cassette is placed in the grid, whereas the nonscreen film is placed on the tabletop. A mouth gag is positioned to prop open the mouth. For a *mandibular survey*, roll the head slightly in the dorsoventral position (Figures 11-6 and 11-7). The amount of obliquity depends on the degree of superimposition over the area of interest, but it usually averages 30 degrees. Place a small amount of cotton under the neck to keep the mandible parallel to the film. For a *maxillary survey*, roll the head slightly in the ventrodorsal position (Figures 11-8 and 11-9). Again, the amount of obliquity depends on the amount of superimposition over the area of interest.

Parallel technique is used for mandibular premolars and molars.

Positioning for intraoral films can be challenging. Basically, two techniques are used: the parallel technique and the bisecting-angle technique. The *parallel technique* is used only with mandibular premolars and molars. The film is pressed into the lingual vestibule parallel to the teeth. The primary beam is positioned perpendicular to the film (Figure 11-10). However, the anatomy surrounding the other teeth does not allow for a parallel technique. The film cannot physically be positioned parallel to the tooth root.

For the areas that do not allow parallel technique, a *bisecting-angle technique* is used. If the primary beam is positioned perpendicular to the tooth, the image appears longer

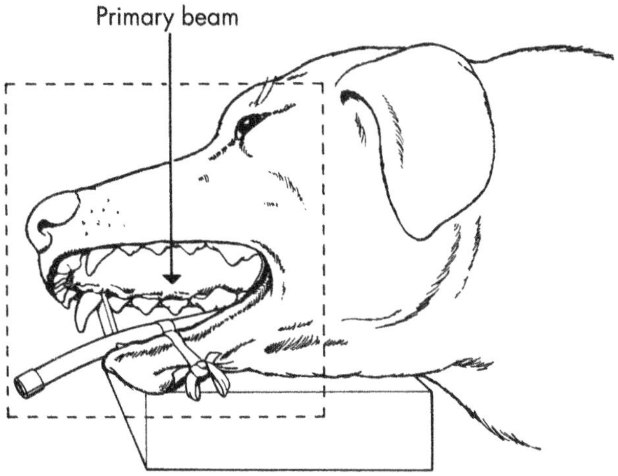

FIG. 11-8 Positioning for a survey of the maxillary dental arcade.

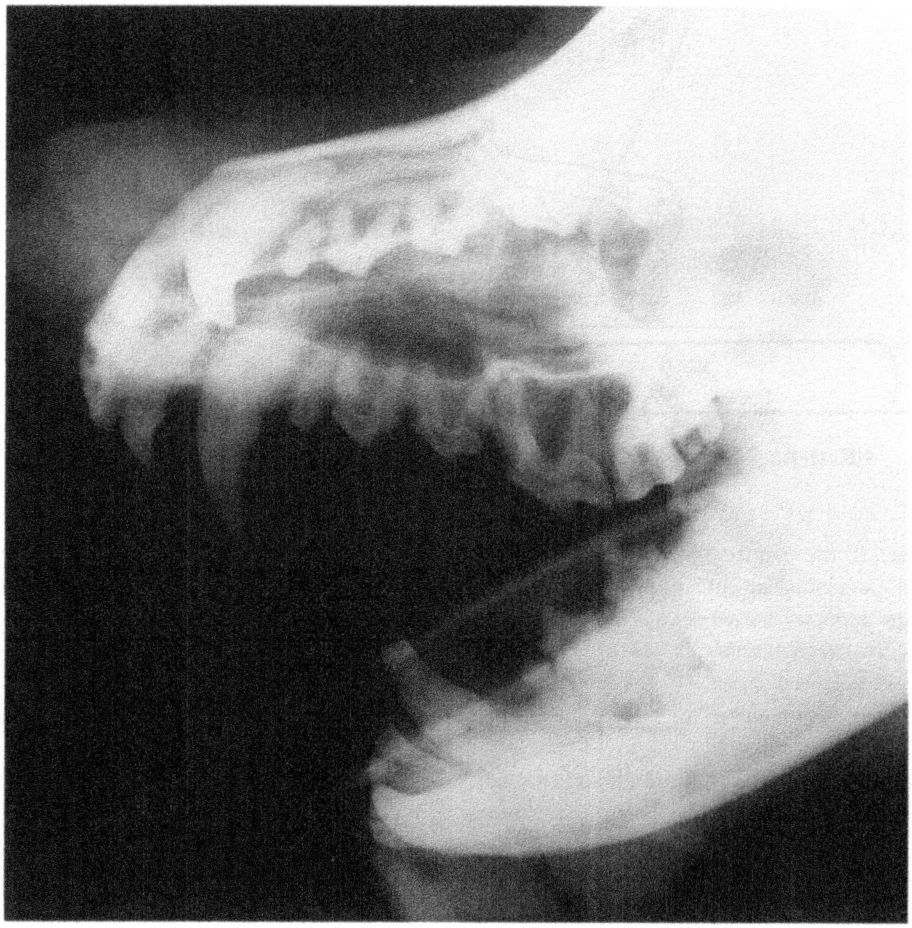

FIG. 11-9 Survey radiograph of the maxillary dental arcade.

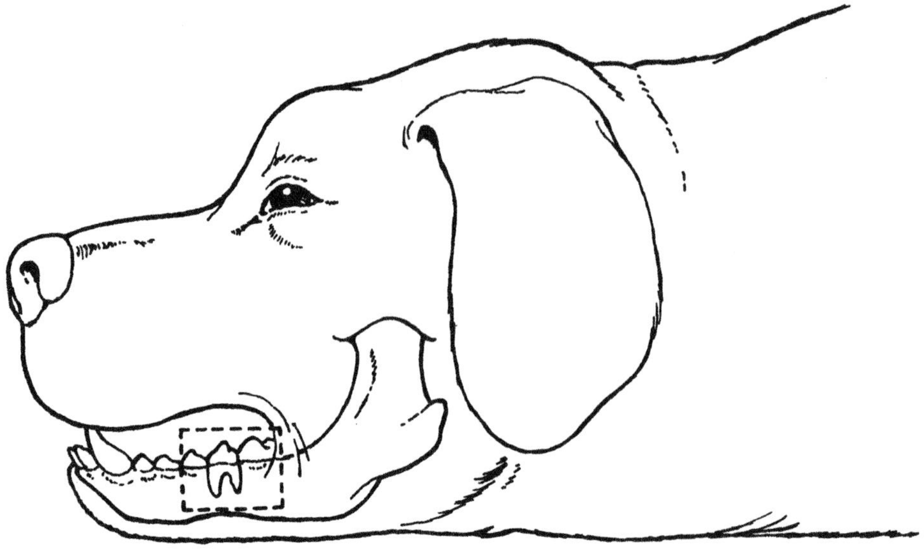

FIG. 11-10. Parallel technique, used to radiograph the mandibular premolars and molars.

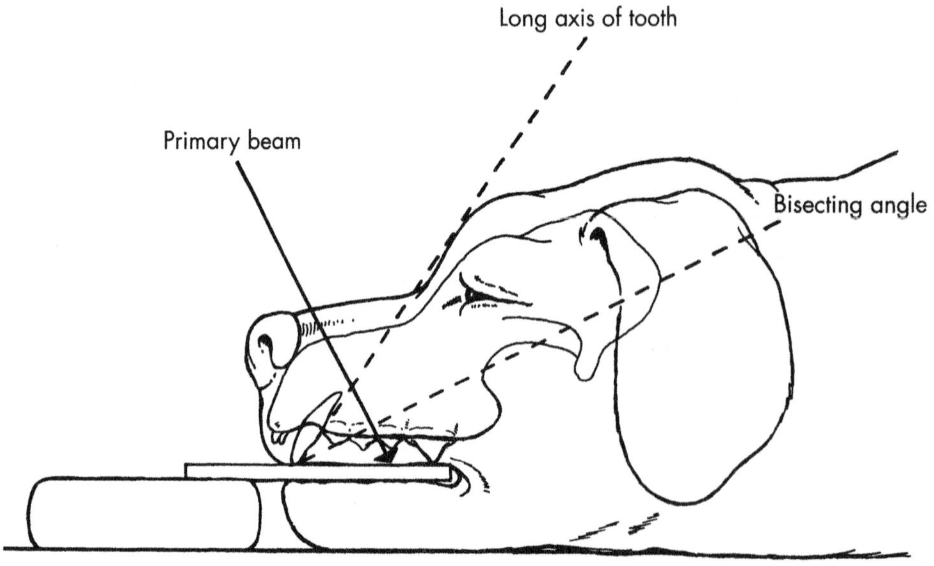

FIG. 11-11 Bisecting-angle technique, used to prevent distortion of the tooth image.

than the actual size. If the primary beam is positioned perpendicular to the film, the image appears shorter than the actual size. By using a bisecting angle, the tooth is portrayed closer to its actual size. When positioning a tooth for bisecting-angle technique, draw an imaginary line along the axis of the tooth and another along the axis of the film. Where these two lines join, forming an angle, position the primary beam perpendicular to a line that bisects that angle (Figure 11-11). This technique is used for all the maxillary teeth and the mandibular incisors.

Bisecting-angle technique is used when the film cannot be positioned parallel to the tooth.

Dental radiography can be a challenging procedure. Once mastered, it becomes a beneficial addition to any veterinary practice.

Recommended Reading

Harvey CE, Emily PP: *Small animal dentistry*, St Louis, 1993, Mosby.

Pratt P: *Principles and practice of veterinary technology*, St Louis, 1998, Mosby.

Shipp AD, Fahrenkrug P: *Practitioner's guide to veterinary dentistry*, Beverly Hills, Calif, 1992, Shipp's Laboratories.

Wiggs RB, Lobprise HB: *Veterinary dentistry: principles and practice*, Philadelphia, 1997, Lippincott.

12

Contrast Studies

CHERYL HURD

CHAPTER OBJECTIVES

- State the importance of making survey radiographs before administration of the contrast medium.
- List the types of contrast media, and state which type is used for each contrast study.
- Describe the contraindications for each type of contrast media.
- State the importance of proper patient preparation before the administration of contrast medium.
- Explain the difference between positive and negative contrast media and how they appear on the radiograph.

The purpose of a contrast radiographic study is to delineate an organ or organ system from the surrounding soft tissues. Such a study is useful in determining the size, shape, position, location, and function of an organ. The information obtained from a contrast study complements or confirms the information from the survey (plain) radiographs. A contrast study should never be used in place of survey radiographs.

In contrast studies, areas of interest appear either radiopaque or radiolucent on the finished radiograph. *Radiopaque* areas appear white; positive-contrast agents appear radiopaque (white) on a radiograph. *Radiolucent* areas on the finished radiograph appear black; negative-contrast agents produce radiolucencies (black areas) on a radiograph.

> Radiopaque appears white on the radiograph.

> Radiolucent appears black on the radiograph.

Survey radiographs made before a contrast study establish proper exposure technique and patient preparation. In addition, a diagnosis may be achieved from the survey radiographs, eliminating the need for the contrast study. Because most contrast studies require multiple images, it is important to label each film with the time and sequence. Always record the amount, type, and route of administration of the contrast medium.

> Always make survey radiographs before administering contrast media.

Positive-Contrast Media

Positive-contrast media contain elements with a high atomic number (high density). Elements with a high atomic number absorb more x-rays. Thus, fewer x-rays penetrate the patient and expose the film, making a white area on the radiograph.

Two common types of positive-contrast agents are barium sulfate and water-soluble organic iodides (Table 12-1).

Barium Sulfate

Barium sulfate is commonly used for positive-contrast studies of the gastrointestinal (GI) tract. It is insoluble and is not affected by gastric secretions. Therefore it provides good mucosal detail on radiographs. Barium sulfate preparations are relatively inexpensive and are manufactured in the form of powders, colloid suspensions, and pastes. One disadvantage of using barium sulfate is that it can take 3 or more hours to travel from the stomach to the colon. It can also be harmful to the peritoneum, so it should never be used when GI perforations are suspected. Barium sulfate is insoluble and the body cannot eliminate it, resulting in granulomatous reactions. When administering barium sulfate orally (per os, by mouth), care must be taken to prevent the patient from aspirating. Aspiration of large amounts of barium into the lungs can be fatal. Barium sulfate may also aggravate an already obstructed bowel by causing further impaction.

> **Never administer barium sulfate to an animal when perforation is suspected.**

Organic Iodides

Water-soluble organic iodides in ionic or nonionic forms are also used for positive-contrast procedures. Different forms of the water-soluble organic iodides can be administered intravenously, orally, into a hollow viscous, or into the subarachnoid space. Being water soluble, these iodides are absorbed into the bloodstream and excreted by the kidneys. Another advantage is that organic iodides are well tolerated by the body and provide excellent contrast.

Ionic iodides

A common oral form of ionic water-soluble organic iodide is a solution of meglumine diatrizoate and sodium diatrizoate. It is used for contrast studies of the GI tract when perforation is suspected. When this iodide is administered orally, transit through the GI system is rapid, usually within 45 to 60 minutes. However, it is a hypertonic solution that draws fluid into the bowel lumen. Thus the contrast medium is diluted, decreasing the quality of the resultant films. Fluid loss may further complicate hypovolemia in a dehydrated animal. Water-soluble organic iodides should never be used in place of barium sulfate, and they are used only when perforations are suspected.

Ionic water-soluble organic iodides for intravenous (IV) injection are prepared in various combinations of meglumine and sodium diatrizoate. Diatrizoates can also be infused into hollow organs such as the urinary bladder or into fistulous tracts. Sodium diatrizoate is often used for excretory urography because it provides better opacification of the kidneys. Nausea, vomiting, and decreased blood pressure can occur after rapid administration of a large IV bolus of contrast medium. Ionic water-soluble organic iodides cannot be used for myelography because they are irritating to the brain and spinal cord.

> **Ionic iodides can be infused into hollow organs or injected intravenously.**

Nonionic iodides

Nonionic water-soluble organic iodides are used for myelography. Because of their low osmolarity and chemical nature, fewer adverse effects occur when nonionic iodides are infused in the subarachnoid space. Three common media are iohexol, iopamidol, and iodixanol (see Table 12-1).

> **Nonionic iodides are used for myelography.**

Nonionic water-soluble organic iodides are suitable for myelography but also can be used intravenously. However, they are approximately 10 times more expensive than ionic media.

Negative-Contrast Media

Negative-contrast agents include air, oxygen, and carbon dioxide, all of which have a low atomic number (low density) and appear radiolucent on the finished radiograph. Oxygen and carbon dioxide are more soluble than water. Care must be taken not to overinflate the organs, such as the bladder, with these gases. Air embolism can occur when ulcerative lesions cause organ rupture, leading to cardiac arrest.

> **Overinflation of organs such as the urinary bladder with negative-contrast agents can lead to air embolism or rupture.**

Double-Contrast Procedures

Double-contrast procedures use both positive-contrast and negative-contrast media to image an organ or organ system. The most common organs imaged with double-contrast studies are the urinary bladder, stomach, and colon. In most cases the negative-contrast medium is added first, then the positive-contrast medium. Adding negative-contrast medium to positive-contrast medium can cause air bubbles to form, which might be misinterpreted as lesions.

TABLE 12-1
COMMONLY USED CONTRAST AGENTS

TRADE NAME	GENERIC NAME	IODINE (MG/ML)	MANUFACTURER
Barium Liquid E-X Paque	Barium sulfate suspension 60%	—	E-Z-EM, Inc.
Novopaque	Barium sulfate suspension 60%	—	Lafayette
Gastrografin	Sodium diatrizoate and meglumine diatrizoate	367	Fort Dodge
IONIC WATER-SOLUBLE ORGANIC IODIDES			
Hypaque sodium 50%	Sodium diatrizoate 50%	300	Amersham Medical
Hypaque meglumine 60%	Meglumine diatrizoate 60%	282	Amersham Medical
Renografin 60	Sodium diatrizoate 8% and meglumine diatrizoate 52%	292	Squibb
Renografin 76	Sodium diatrizoate 10% and meglumine diatrizoate 66%	370	Squibb
Conray 60	Meglumine iothalamate 60%	282	Shering-Plough
Conray 325	Sodium iothalamate 66.8%	235	Shering-Plough
NONIONIC WATER-SOLUBLE ORGANIC IODIDES			
Isovue-M 200	Iopamidol	200	Squibb
Omnipaque 240	Iohexol	240	Amersham Medical
Omnipaque 180	Iohexol	180	Amersham Medical
Visipaque 320	Iodixanol	320	Amersham Medical
Visipaque 270	Iodixanol	270	Amersham Medical

Gastrointestinal Tract Studies

Esophagography

Esophagography (or esophagraphy) is used to evaluate functional and structural alterations of the esophagus. Because it is a dynamic study, esophagography should ideally be performed with fluoroscopy. If fluoroscopic equipment is not available, conventional radiography may be used successfully (Figure 12-1).

Indications

Dysphagia, regurgitation, foreign body, mass, suspected rupture, stricture, megaesophagus, tracheo-esophageal fistula, esophageal dysfunction.

Precautions

Water-soluble organic iodides should be used in cases of suspected perforation or rupture.

Contrast agents

MEDIA	DOSAGE
Barium sulfate paste 60%	1 ml/lb
Barium sulfate liquid 60%	3 ml/lb
Barium sulfate mixed with canned food	½ to 1 can food (add enough liquid barium to coat food thoroughly)
Water-soluble organic iodide	1 ml/lb

Equipment

- ◆ Large-dose syringe
- ◆ Canned food

Survey

Lateral and ventrodorsal views of thoracic and cervical areas, including the total length of the esophagus.

Patient preparation

If ingesta are seen in the esophagus on survey radiographs, fast the animal for 12 hours and repeat the survey radiographs.

Procedure

Administer the contrast medium via the buccal pouch using a large-dose syringe. Make lateral and ventrodorsal views of the cervical and thoracic esophagus immediately after administration. If the contrast medium alone passes, repeat the procedure with the barium sulfate mixed with canned food.

Comments

Administer the contrast medium slowly to avoid aspiration. Use a slightly oblique ventrodorsal projection to avoid superimposition of the spine on the esophagus.

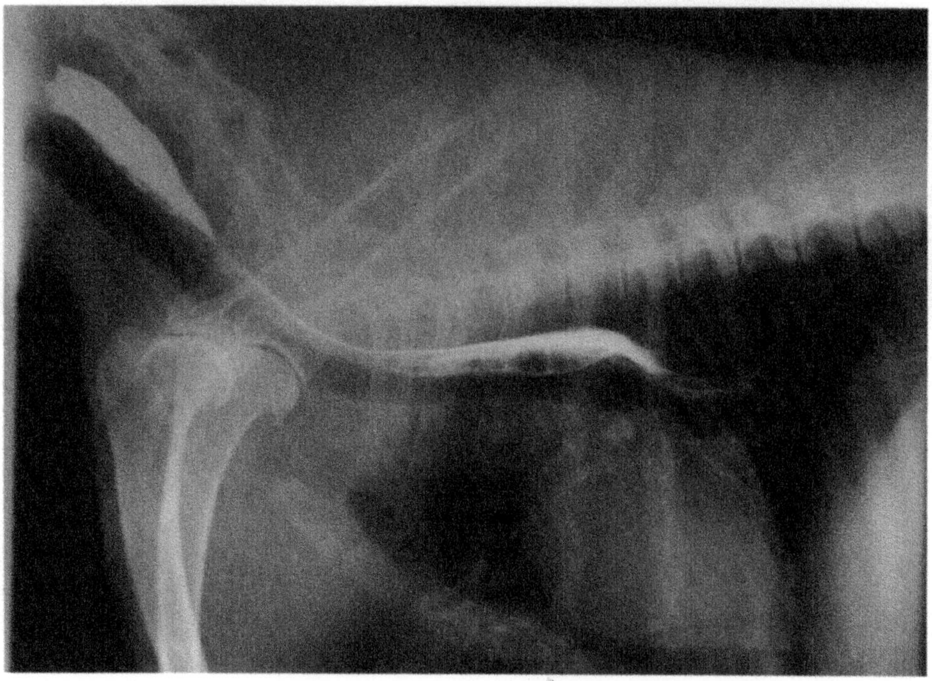

FIG. 12-1 Lateral projection of a normal canine esophagogram.

Upper Gastrointestinal Series

Upper GI studies are dynamic and can be imaged with fluoroscopy, although studies are usually recorded with multiple radiographs. Contrast medium is administered orally, and films are made during transit of contrast through the stomach and small bowel into the colon (Figure 12-2).

Indications

Vomiting, small bowel diarrhea, melena, obstruction, wall distortions (dilation, stenosis), wall lesions (ulcers, neoplasia), abdominal organ displacement, observation of GI function.

Precautions

In cases of suspected perforation or rupture, water-soluble organic iodides should be used rather than barium. Water-soluble organic iodides should be avoided in dehydrated patients.

> Water-soluble iodides are contraindicated in a dehydrated animal because of their hypertonic properties.

Contrast agents

MEDIA	**DOSAGE**
Barium sulfate liquid 60%	3-5 ml/lb
Water-soluble organic iodide	1 ml/lb

Equipment

- Large-dose syringe
- Stomach tubes
- Towels

Survey

Ventrodorsal and lateral views of abdomen before enemas.

Patient preparation

Animal should be free of ingesta. If not, fast the animal 24 hours before the study. Give enemas the previous night, as well as 3 hours and 1 hour before the study.

Procedure

Make lateral and ventrodorsal views of the abdomen before administering the contrast medium. Administer the medium into the buccal pouch or by a stomach tube. Immediately after administration, make lateral and ventrodorsal views of the abdomen. Then, lateral and ventrodorsal abdominal views are taken at 15, 30, and 60 minutes postadministration. Repeat the abdominal views hourly until the contrast medium has reached the colon.

Comments

If tranquilization is necessary, acetylpromazine for dogs and ketamine for cats are the drugs of choice. Give enough contrast medium to fully distend the stomach. If stomach or bowel perforation is suspected, use a water-soluble organic iodide. All films should be marked with the time after administration.

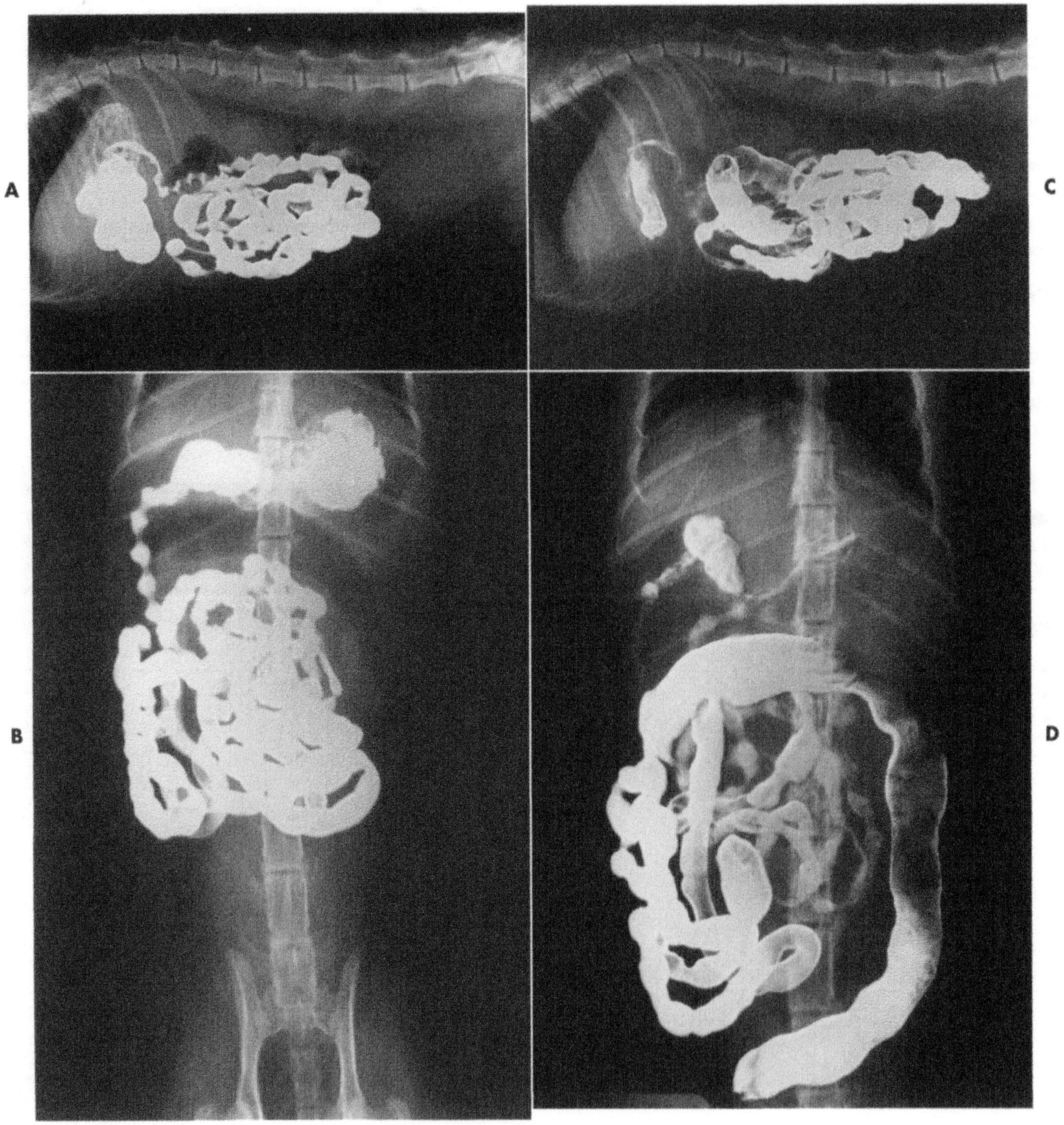

FIG. 12-2 Normal feline upper gastrointestinal series. **A,** Lateral view made 15 minutes after barium administration. **B,** Ventrodorsal view made 15 minutes after barium administration. **C** and **D,** Lateral and ventrodorsal views made 3 hours after barium administration. The study is complete at this point because the barium has reached the colon.

Gastrography

Pneumogastrograms are helpful in determining the position of the stomach. Double-contrast gastrograms best demonstrate the gastric mucosa for ulcerations and mass lesions (Figure 12-3).

Indications

Suspected gastric masses, radiolucent foreign bodies, outflow obstruction.

Precautions

Contraindicated if fluid, ingestus, or diarrhea is present. Double-contrast gastrography preceded by glucagon is contraindicated in patients with diabetes mellitus or pheochromocytoma.

Contrast agents

MEDIA	DOSAGE
NEGATIVE-CONTRAST GASTROGRAPHY OR IN CONJUNCTION WITH UPPER GI SERIES	
Air	3-5 ml/lb
Carbonated beverages	30-60 ml
Effervescent granules or tablets	Enough to produce 3-5 ml gas/lb
POSITIVE-CONTRAST GASTROGRAPHY	
Barium sulfate suspension 60%	3-5 ml/lb
Water-soluble organic iodide solution (cannot be used with double-contrast gastrography)	3-5 ml/lb
DOUBLE-CONTRAST GASTROGRAPHY WITHOUT UPPER GI SERIES	
Barium sulfate suspension	
<17 lb body weight	1.5 ml/lb
17-88 lb body weight	1 ml/lb
>88 lb body weight	0.7 ml/lb
Air	10 ml/lb
GLUCAGON HYDROCHLORIDE (LILLY)	
<17 lb body weight	0.05 ml/lb IV
17-44 lb body weight	0.09 ml/lb IV
44-88 lb body weight	0.12 ml/lb IV
>88 lb body weight	0.16 ml/lb IV

Equipment

- ◆ Stomach tube
- ◆ Three-way valve
- ◆ Mouth gag
- ◆ Large syringe

Survey

Ventrodorsal and lateral views of the abdomen.

Patient preparation

Fast the animal for 12 to 24 hours.

Procedure

NEGATIVE-CONTRAST GASTROGRAPHY, PNEUMOGASTROGRAPHY. Place stomach tube to administer air. If using effervescent granules, administer them in the buccal pouch via a dose syringe. This prevents the loss of foam before it reaches the stomach. After the introduction of negative-contrast medium into the stomach, remove the tube. Make right lateral, left lateral, ventrodorsal, and dorsoventral views of the cranial abdomen.

POSITIVE-CONTRAST GASTROGRAPHY. Place a stomach tube and administer either barium sulfate suspension or water-soluble organic iodide solution. Withdraw the stomach tube. Make right lateral, left lateral, ventrodorsal, and dorsoventral views of the cranial abdomen.

DOUBLE-CONTRAST GASTROGRAPHY WITH UPPER GI SERIES. When most of the barium sulfate has emptied from the stomach, place a stomach tube and administer the negative-contrast medium. Remove the tube and roll the patient from side to side to coat the gastric mucosa adequately. Make right lateral, left lateral, ventrodorsal, and dorsoventral views of the cranial abdomen.

DOUBLE-CONTRAST GASTROGRAPHY WITHOUT UPPER GI SERIES. Paralyze the stomach with glucagon. Place the stomach tube and administer positive-contrast medium. With the tube still in place, administer the negative-contrast medium. Remove the tube and roll the patient from side to side to coat the gastric mucosa adequately. Make right lateral, left lateral, ventrodorsal, and dorsoventral views of the cranial abdomen.

Comments

Since glucagon is a protein, hypersensitivity is a possibility.

A

B

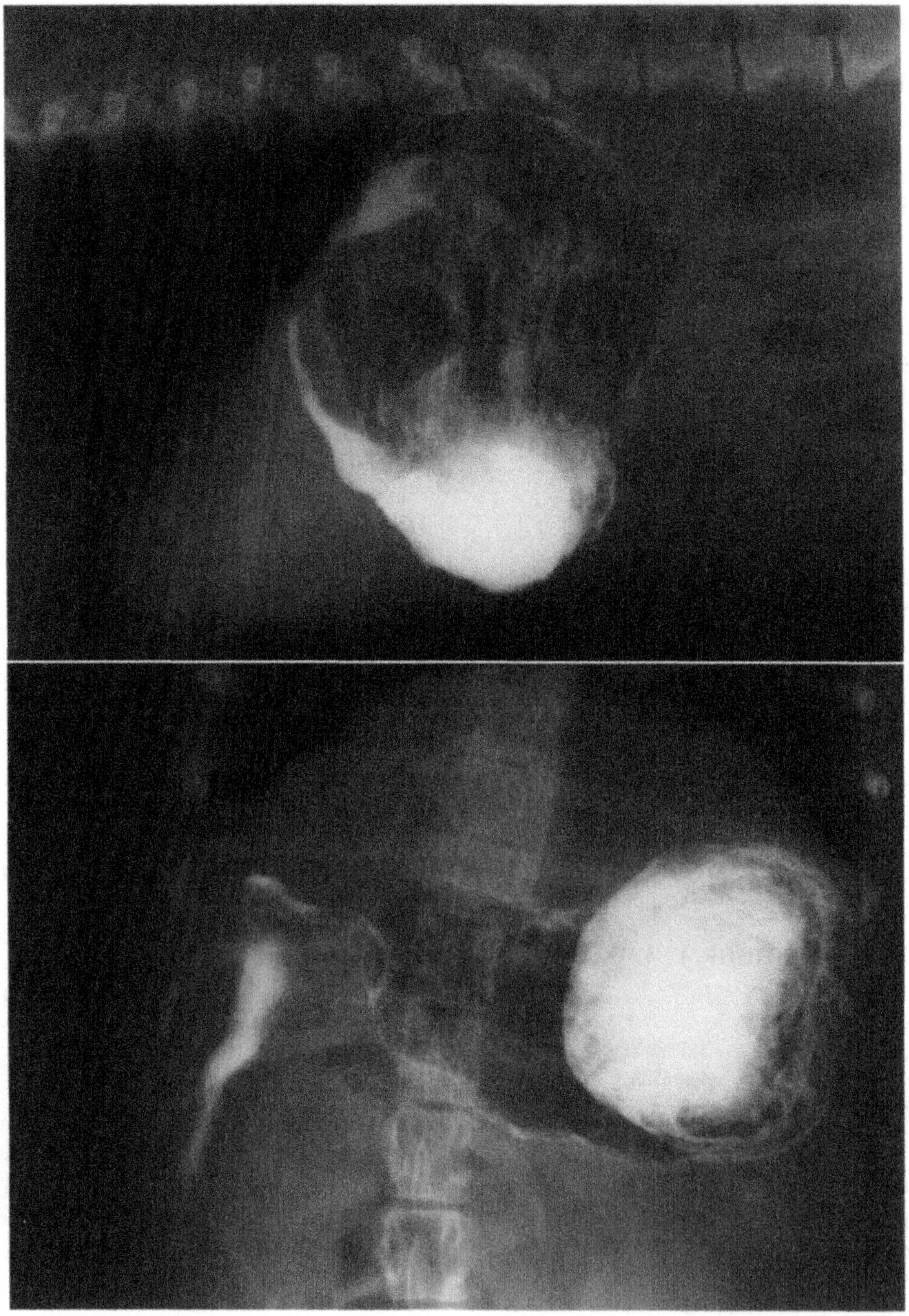

FIG. 12-3 Normal canine double-contrast gastrogram. **A,** Lateral projection. **B,** Ventrodorsal projection.

Barium Enema

The barium enema procedure is used to study the position and contour of the colon. Do not attempt to study the colon using an upper GI series (Figure 12-4).

Indications

Large bowel diarrhea, tenesmus, fresh blood in the feces, colonic or rectal neoplasia, colitis, mucosal disease, ileocolic intussusception.

Precautions

Barium should not be used if GI perforation is suspected. Barium enemas are not recommended for patients that have had proctoscopy within 12 hours or cleansing enemas within 4 hours before the study.

Contrast agents

MEDIA	DOSAGE
Barium sulfate 20%	5-7 ml/lb
Air	Volume equal to amount of contrast material removed

Equipment

- ◆ Enema catheter or Foley catheter
- ◆ Syringe
- ◆ Enema can and adapter with 3-way valve

Survey

Ventrodorsal and lateral views of the abdomen before enemas.

Patient preparation

The colon should be free of fecal material. Animal should be fasted for 24 hours. Give enemas the night before. General anesthesia is required.

Procedure

Make lateral and ventrodorsal views of the abdomen before administration of the contrast medium. Place the catheter in the rectum and inflate the cuff to prevent leakage. Administer three quarters of the calculated dose. Radiograph the animal in ventrodorsal position to check the amount of bowel distention. If the colon is not fully distended, add 5 ml of contrast medium and repeat the radiograph. Continue until proper distention is achieved. With proper distention, make a lateral view of the abdomen. With the catheter still in place, remove the contrast medium and replace it with negative-contrast medium. Make lateral and ventrodorsal views of the abdomen. Remove as much of the contrast medium as possible before removing the catheter.

Comments

Air may be used as the medium for negative-contrast study. Avoid overdistention of the colon. Use higher kVp values for positive-contrast studies. Saline should be used to dilute contrast medium to a 20% solution.

A

B

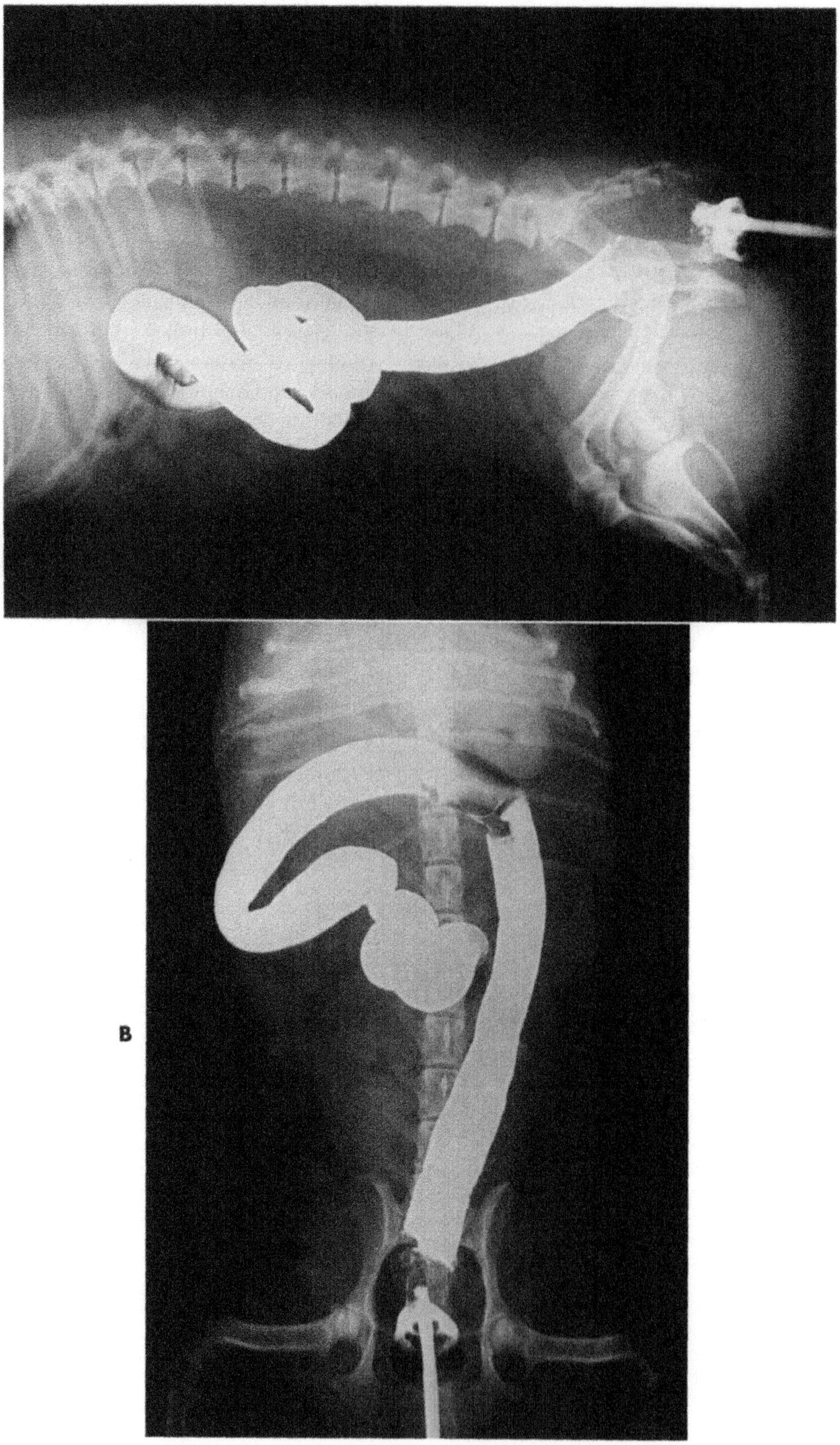

FIG. 12-4 Normal canine barium enema. **A,** Lateral projection. **B,** Ventrodorsal projection. After imaging with the positive-contrast medium in the colon, remove as much contrast agent as possible. Replace the removed positive-contrast agent with an equal amount of negative-contrast agent. Repeat the lateral and ventrodorsal projections.

Urinary Tract Studies

Cystography

Cystography involves the use of positive-contrast and negative-contrast agents to evaluate the bladder.

Indications

Hematuria, polyuria, dysuria, trauma to caudal abdomen, calculus, neoplasia, mural lesions, congenital anomalies, diverticulum, functional abnormalities, determining location of urinary bladder.

Contrast agents

MEDIA	DOSAGE
Water-soluble organic iodides	3-5 ml/lb
Air	3-5 ml/lb

Equipment

- Urethral catheter
- Lubricating jelly
- Syringe and catheter adapter
- Three-way stopcock

Survey

Ventrodorsal and lateral views of the abdomen, including the entire urinary tract, made after the colon is free of fecal material.

Patient preparation

Give one to two enemas to eliminate fecal material. Tranquilization or general anesthesia may be necessary to inflate the bladder fully.

Procedure

PNEUMOCYSTOGRAM. Before the contrast study, make lateral and ventrodorsal views centered over the bladder. Place a urinary catheter securely in the bladder. Withdraw all the urine. Inject the negative-contrast medium slowly while palpating the bladder. Terminate the injection if much resistance is met. Make lateral and ventrodorsal views centered over the bladder after the contrast medium has been administered (Figure 12-5).

DOUBLE-CONTRAST CYSTOGRAM. Make lateral and ventrodorsal views centered over the bladder before the contrast study. Place a urinary catheter securely in the bladder. Withdraw all the urine. Inject the negative-contrast medium slowly while palpating the bladder. Terminate the injection if much resistance is met. Make lateral and ventrodorsal views centered over the bladder after the contrast medium has been administered. After the radiographs for the pneumocystogram have been made, slowly inject 3 to 10 ml of the positive-contrast medium into the bladder. Roll the animal from side to side to coat the bladder walls. Make lateral and ventrodorsal views centered over the bladder. Sometimes it is necessary to make the opposite lateral and a dorsoventral projection to pool the contrast medium in all parts of the bladder (Figure 12-6).

> When performing a double-contrast cystogram, always infuse the negative-contrast agent first.

POSITIVE-CONTRAST CYSTOGRAM. Make lateral and ventrodorsal views centered over the bladder before the contrast study. Place a urinary catheter securely in the bladder. Withdraw all the urine. Inject the positive-contrast medium, which should be diluted 50% with saline, slowly while palpating the bladder. Terminate the injection if resistance is met. Make lateral and ventrodorsal views centered over the bladder after the contrast has been administered (Figure 12-7).

Comments

If a rupture or perforation is suspected, inject only a small quantity of contrast medium and then observe radiographically. A severely diseased urinary bladder could rupture with excessive intraluminal pressure. The dose of contrast varies according to the patient's size and the ability of the urinary bladder to distend, so always palpate the bladder when distending it with contrast medium. However, it is important to distend the bladder properly. Positive-contrast studies may be performed using contrast medium diluted 50% with saline. Obtain all urine samples for bacteriologic studies before injection of the contrast medium.

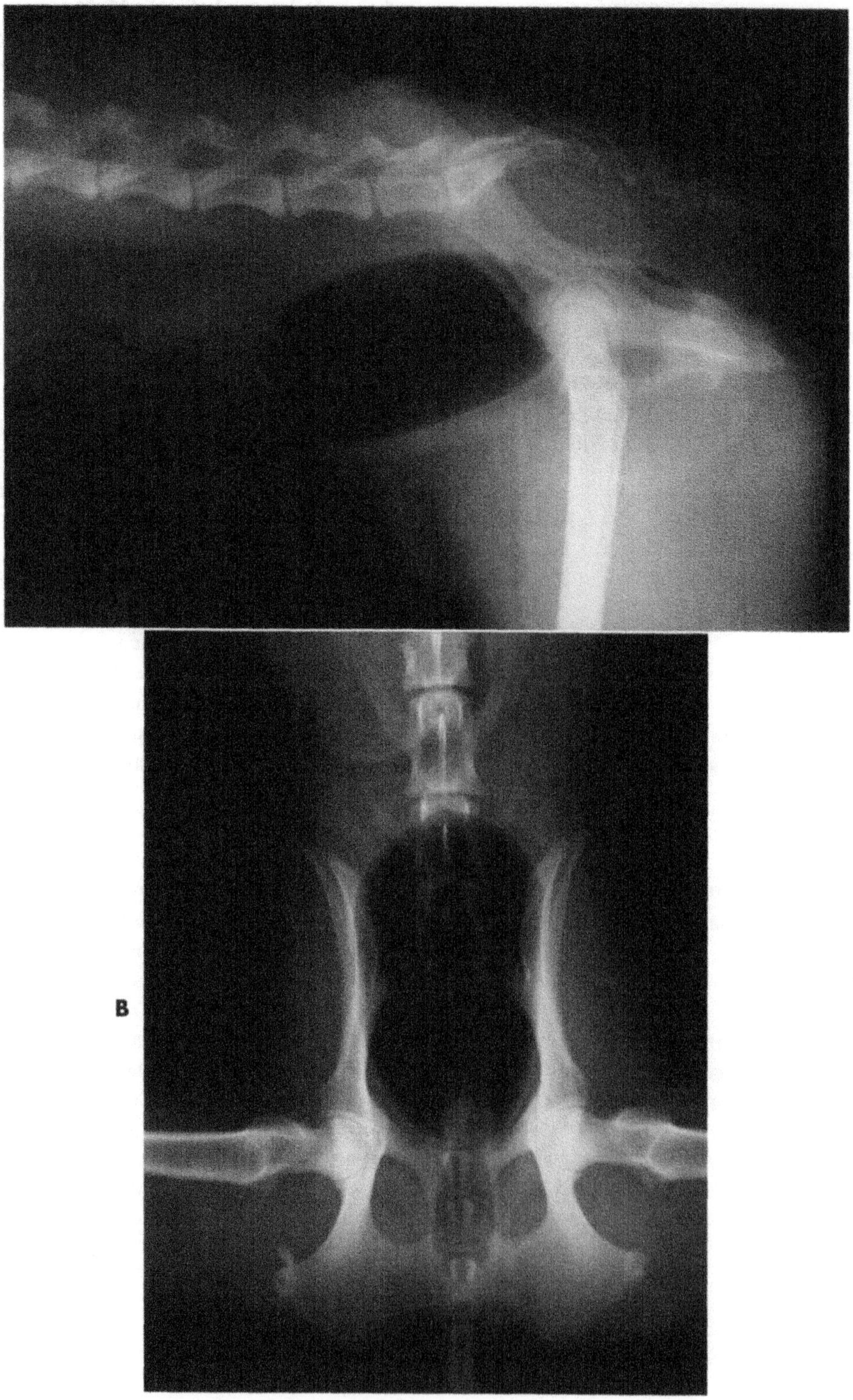

FIG. 12-5 Normal canine pneumocystogram. **A,** Lateral projection. **B,** Ventrodorsal projection. Note the complete distention of the urinary bladder.

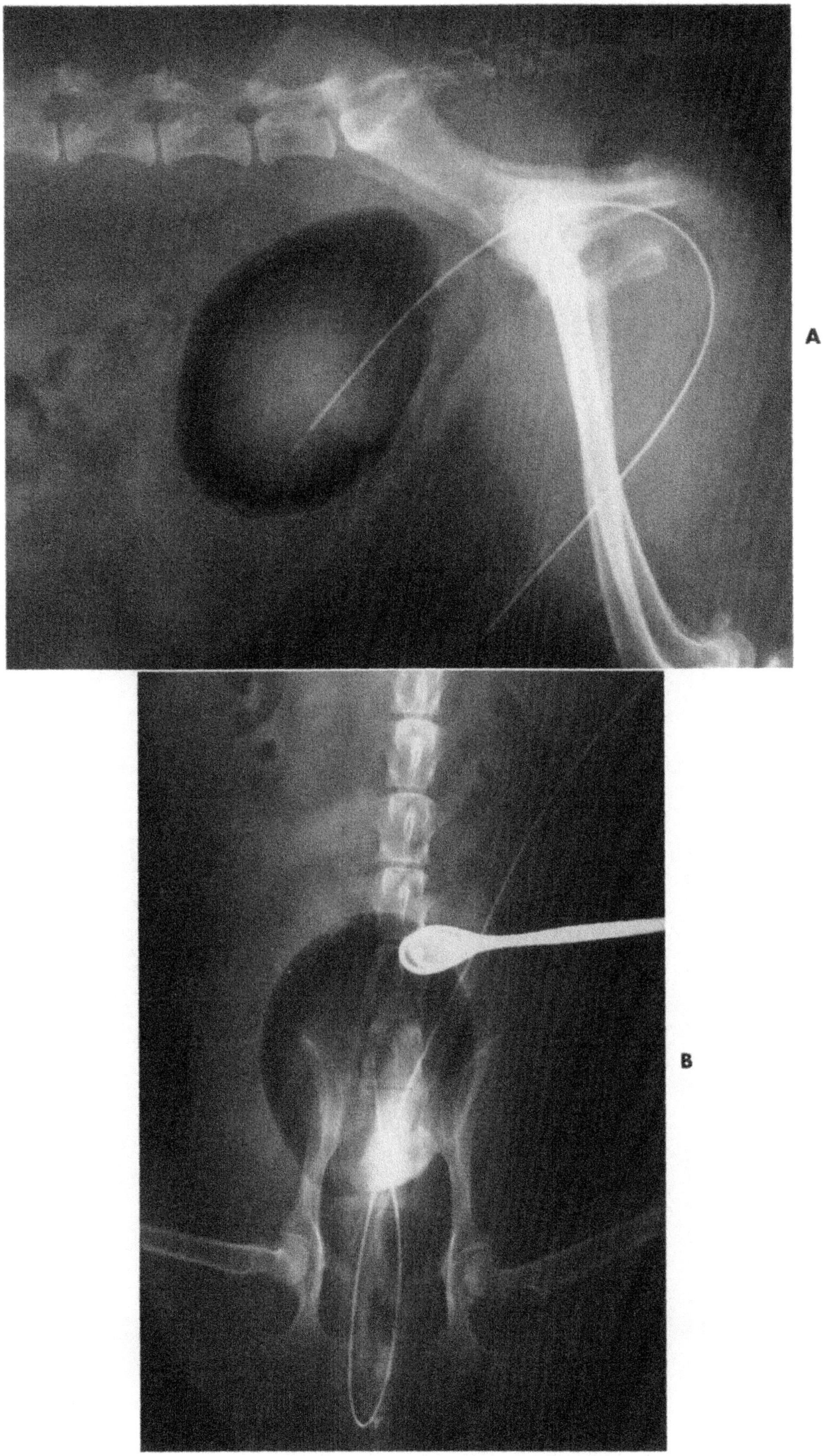

FIG. 12-6 Canine double-contrast cystogram with transitional cell carcinoma of the bladder wall. **A,** Lateral projection; a lesion is outlined in the vertex and trigone of the bladder. **B,** Ventrodorsal projection; a tongue forceps is placed on the prepuce to prevent leakage of the air from the bladder.

A

B

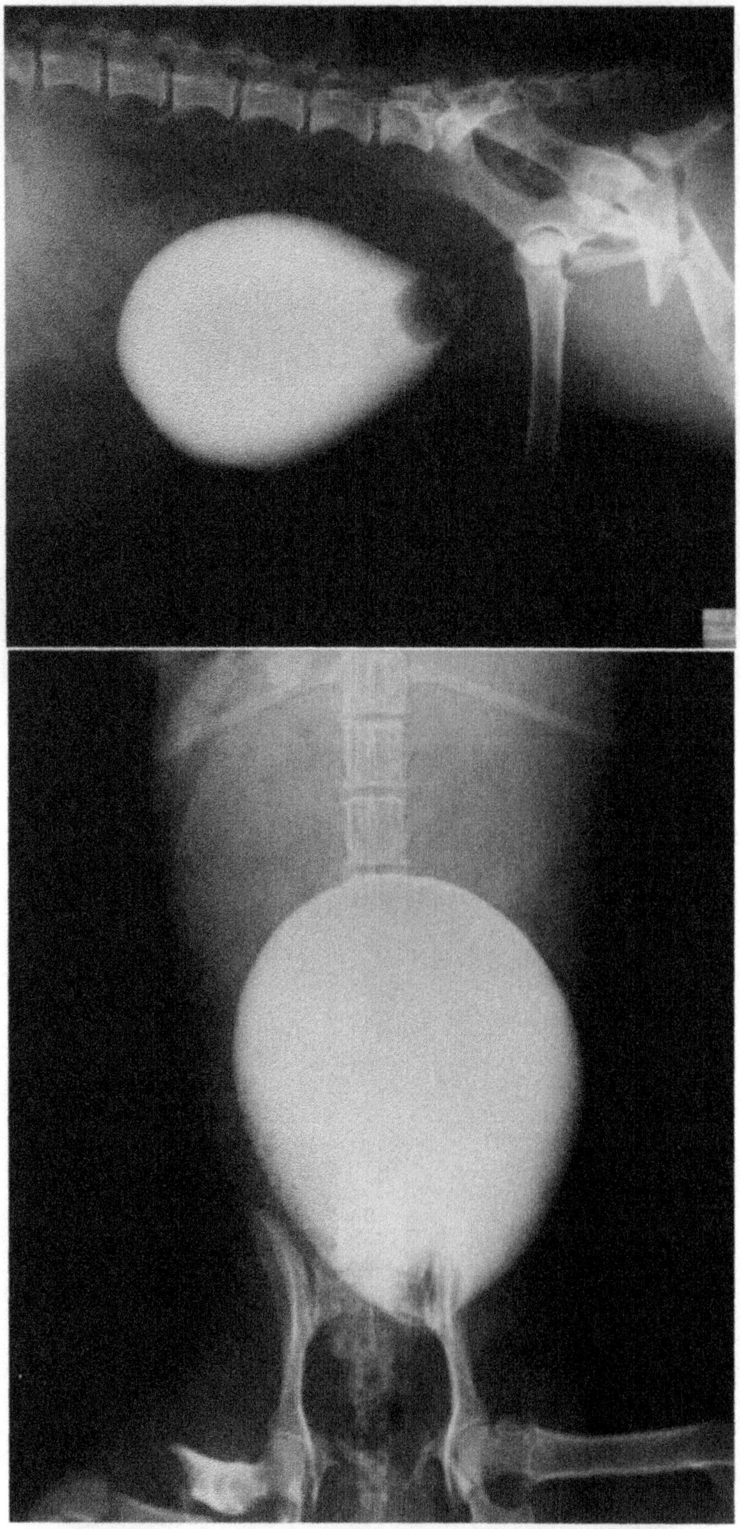

FIG. 12-7 Canine positive-contrast cystogram. **A,** Lateral projection. **B,** Ventrodorsal projection. This animal had been hit by a car, sustaining pelvic and femoral fractures. With a suspected rupture of urinary bladder, this was an emergency procedure without the normal patient preparation.

Urethrography

Urethrography is used to evaluate the urethra. The urethrogram can be made using a retrograde or voiding method (Figure 12-8).

Indications

Dysuria, pelvic fractures, urinary incontinence, hematuria, mucosal defects, displacement or deviation of urethra, calculus, obstruction, evaluation of prostate gland.

Contrast agents

MEDIA	DOSAGE
Water-soluble organic iodides	3-5 ml/lb

Equipment

- ◆ Urethral catheter
- ◆ Lubricating jelly
- ◆ Syringe
- ◆ Stopcock

Survey

Lateral and ventrodorsal views of the caudal abdomen after enemas.

Patient preparation

The colon should be free of fecal material. Tranquilization or anesthesia is required.

Procedure

VOIDING URETHROGRAPHY. Make lateral and ventrodorsal views of the caudal abdomen before the contrast study. Place a urinary catheter securely in the bladder. Inflate the bladder with diluted positive-contrast medium. With the animal in lateral recumbency, cassette in place, and machine ready, apply external pressure to the bladder. Make an exposure when urine is seen flowing from the urethra.

> Wooden spoons can be used to apply pressure to the urinary bladder, which still keeps the hands out of the primary beam.

RETROGRADE URETHROGRAPHY. Make lateral and ventrodorsal views of the caudal abdomen before the contrast study. Place a urinary catheter securely in the bladder. Inflate the bladder with diluted positive-contrast medium. With the animal in lateral recumbency, cassette in place, and machine ready, attach a syringe with an adequate amount of positive-contrast medium to the urinary catheter. Slowly begin to inject the contrast medium. As the contrast medium is injected, slowly withdraw the catheter. When the catheter tip reaches distal urethra, inject a bolus of contrast while the exposure is being made.

Comments

Lateral views are usually adequate.

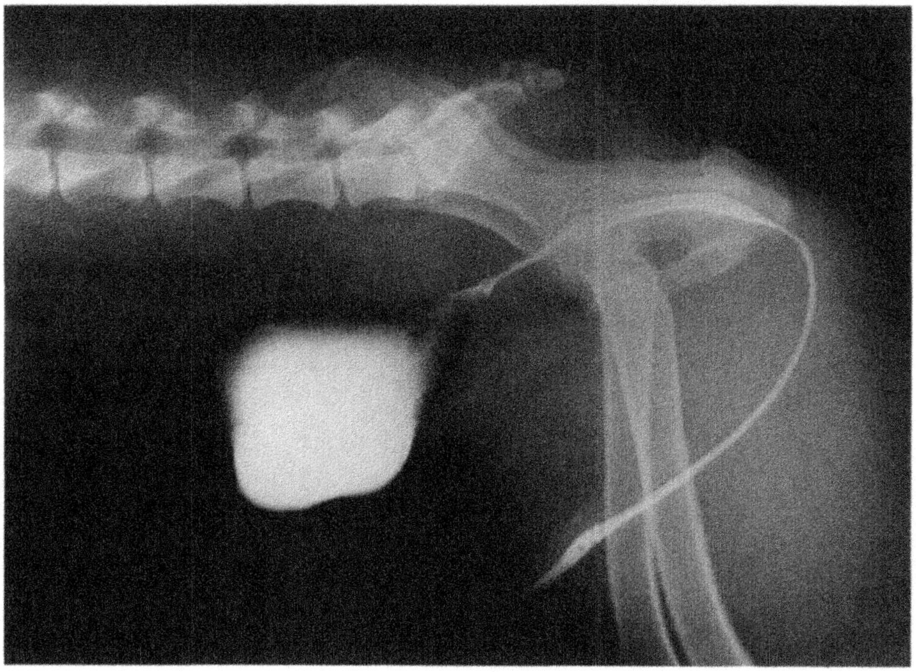

FIG. 12-8 Normal canine retrograde urethrogram, lateral projection.

Excretory Urography

An excretory urogram, formerly an intravenous pyelogram (IVP), provides information relative to renal function and the structure of the kidneys and ureters. The basis for the study is the kidney's capacity to concentrate and excrete circulating organic iodinated contrast media. Excretory urography contrasts the kidneys, ureters, and urinary bladder (Figure 12-9).

Indications

Identifying size, shape, location, and margination of kidneys and ureters; detection of suspected hydronephrosis, obstruction, renal calculus, congenital anomalies, and ureteral rupture; providing crude estimate of renal function.

Contrast agents

MEDIA	DOSAGE
Water-soluble organic iodide	1 ml/lb or 200-400 mg iodide/lb

Equipment

- IV catheter
- Extension set
- Syringe with heparinized saline
- Syringe with contrast

Survey

Lateral and ventrodorsal views of abdomen after enemas.

Patient preparation

The GI tract should be free of ingesta. Fast the animal 24 hours before study. Give enemas the previous night and 3 hours and 1 hour before the study. A patent cephalic catheter should be securely in place. Provide tranquilization or anesthesia as needed.

Procedure

Flush cephalic catheter with heparinized saline. With the animal in ventrodorsal position and the machine ready, start injection of contrast medium. Inject the contrast medium as rapidly as possible. Make an exposure 10 to 20 seconds from the start of the injection, even if the entire dose has not been given. Flush the catheter with heparinized saline after the contrast injection has been completed. Immediately make ventrodorsal and lateral views of the abdomen. Repeat radiographs (lateral and ventrodorsal) 5, 15, and 30 minutes postinjection.

Comments

If ectopic ureters are suspected, make oblique views 30 minutes postinjection. Inject the contrast medium as quickly as possible. Place time markers to label every view. The urinary bladder cannot be completely evaluated from an excretory urogram alone because proper distention cannot be achieved.

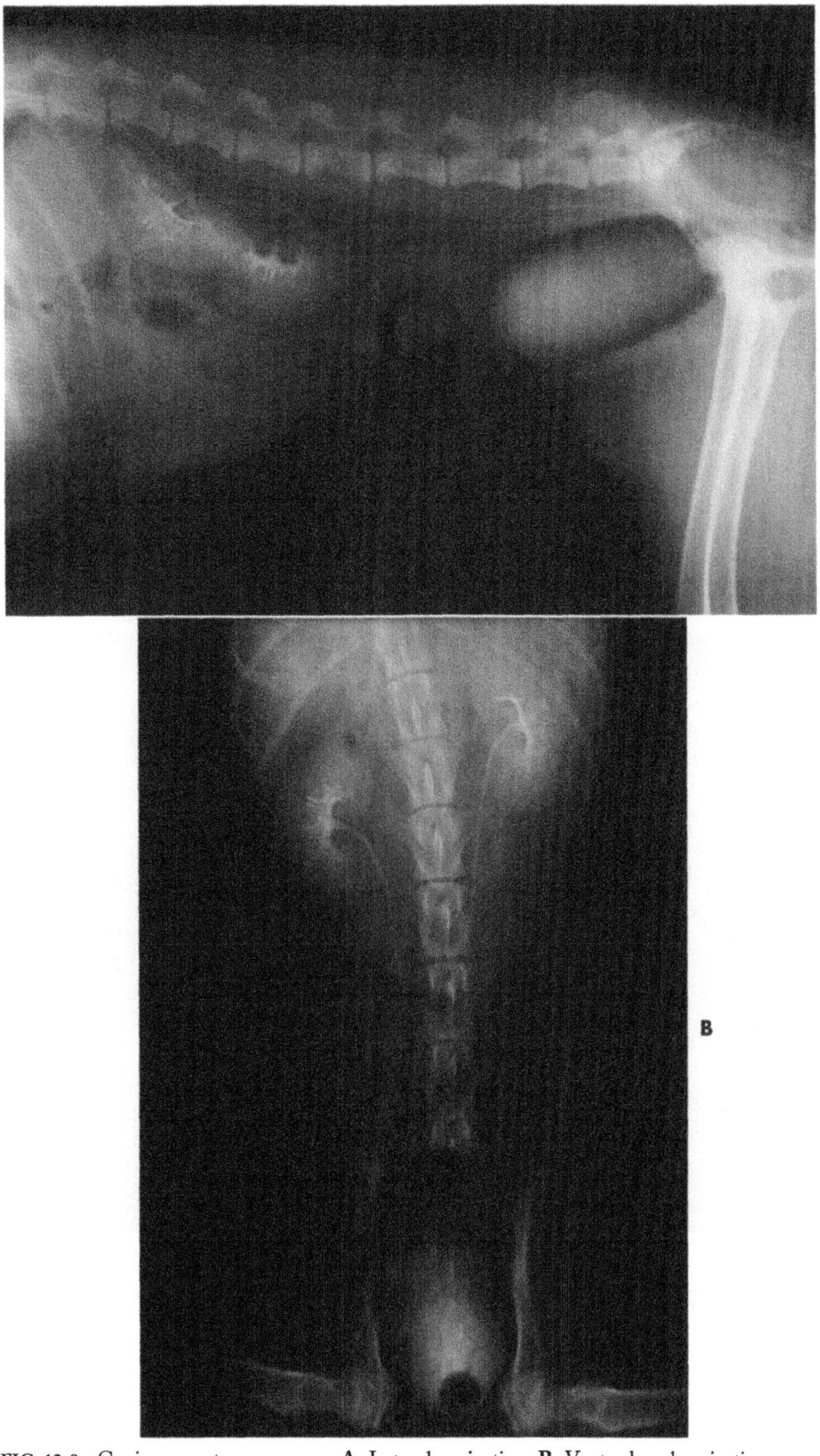

A

B

FIG. 12-9 Canine excretory urogram. **A,** Lateral projection. **B,** Ventrodorsal projection. These views were taken 5 minutes after IV injection of positive-contrast medium.

Vaginography

Vaginography involves the administration of contrast medium into the vagina to evaluate vaginal masses, strictures, and urethral problems. If it is impossible to catheterize the bladder, sometimes the vaginogram can be used to introduce contrast medium into the bladder (Figure 12-10).

Indications

Ectopic ureter, vaginal masses, urethral tumor, obstruction.

Contrast agents

MEDIA	DOSAGE
Water-soluble organic iodides	0.5 ml/lb

Equipment

- Foley catheter
- Syringe
- Stopcock
- Tongue forceps

Survey

Lateral view of the caudal abdomen centered over the bladder, including the pelvis.

Patient preparation

Anesthesia may be required, depending on temperament of animal.

Procedure

Distend the urinary bladder with a 50% dilution of saline and contrast medium. Place a Foley catheter in the vulva. Inflate the bulb with water or air so the catheter is taut when pulled back. Clamp tongue forceps onto the lips of the vulva to help prevent the catheter from slipping. Inject the contrast medium slowly. With the animal in lateral recumbency, make an exposure centered over the bladder at the end of the injection.

Comments

Vaginal rupture can occur if excessive pressure is used.

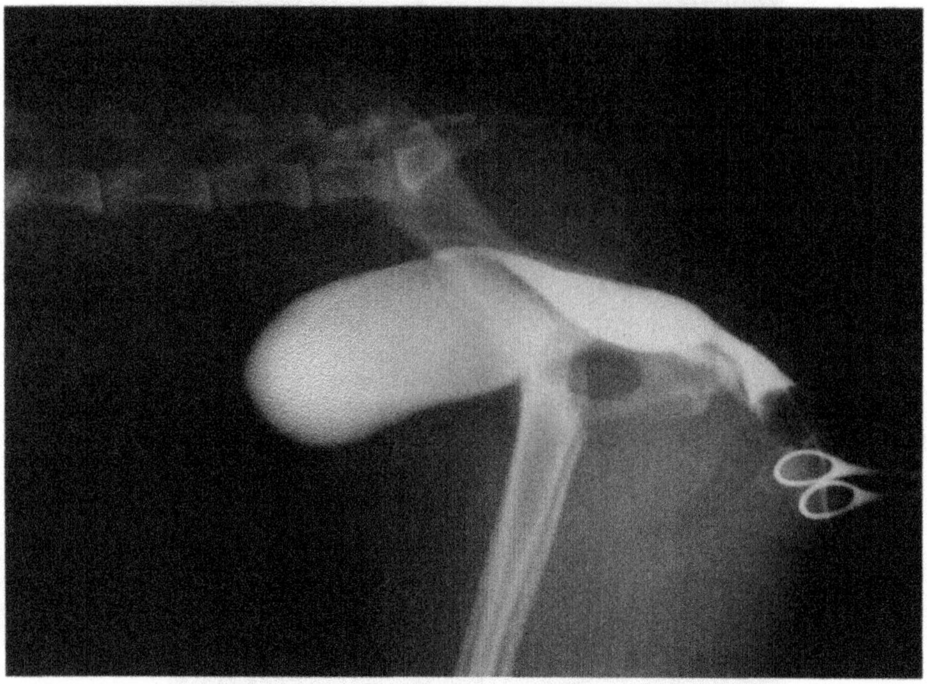

FIG. 12-10 Canine vaginogram, lateral projection.

Miscellaneous Studies

Celiography

Celiography is useful for evaluating the abdominal cavity and the integrity of the diaphragm (Figure 12-11).

Indications

Diaphragmatic hernia.

Contrast agents

MEDIA	DOSAGE
Water-soluble organic iodide	1 ml/lb

Equipment

- 20- to 22-gauge, 1-inch needle
- Syringe

Survey

Lateral and ventrodorsal views of the abdomen.

Patient preparation

Clip and surgically prep an 8 × 8–cm area, slightly right of midline, caudal to the umbilicus. Provide tranquilization or anesthesia as needed.

Procedure

With the animal in ventrodorsal recumbency and the site prepped, elevate the abdominal wall and advance the needle cranially into the abdomen, keeping the needle parallel with the abdominal wall. Aspirate to make sure the needle is not in a venous structure. Inject the contrast medium while the needle is being removed. Roll the animal to disperse the contrast medium throughout the abdomen. Make lateral and ventrodorsal views of the abdomen.

A
B
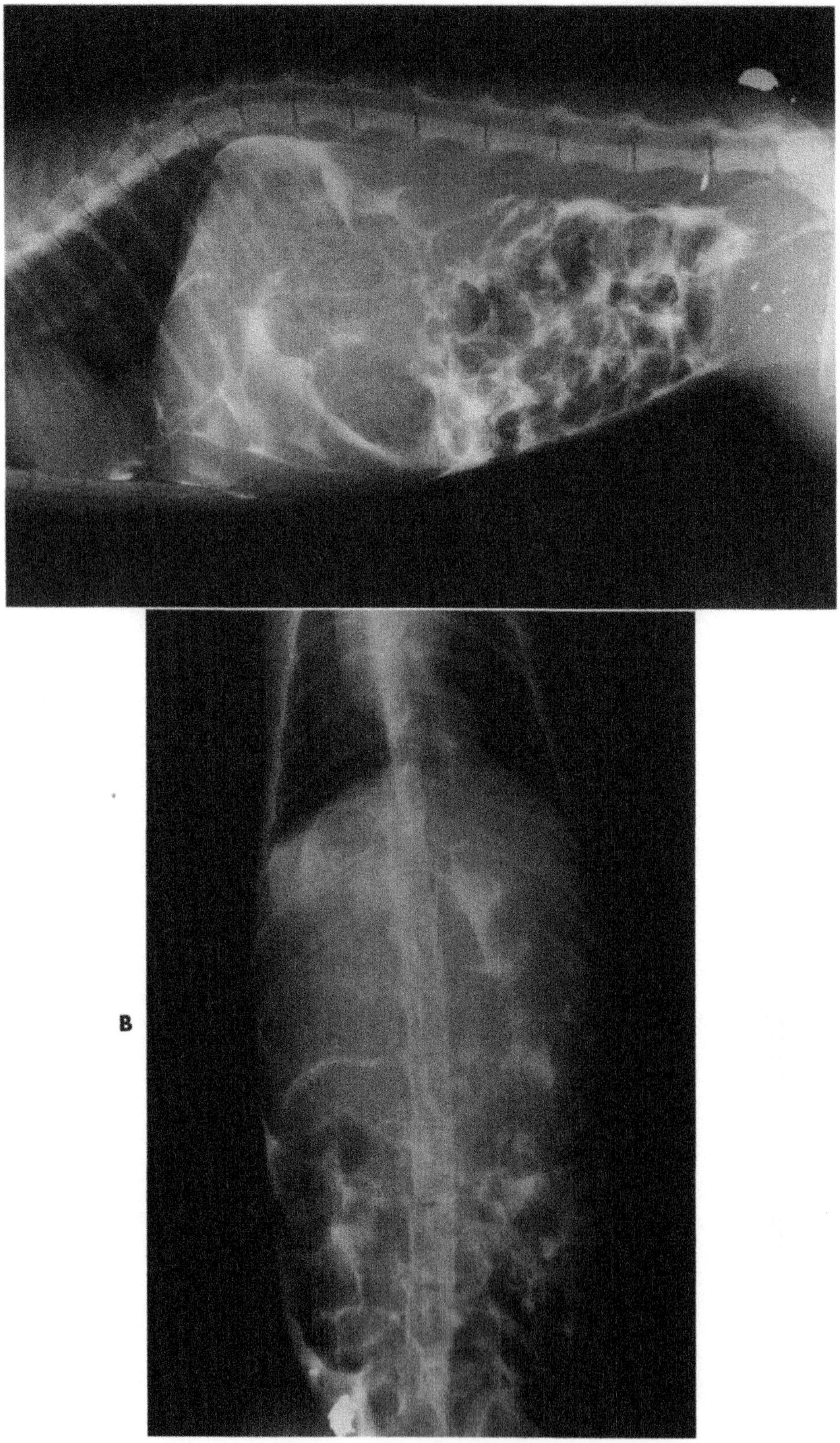

FIG. 12-11 Feline celiogram. **A,** Lateral projection. **B,** Ventrodorsal projection. This cat sustained a traumatic diaphragmatic hernia. Note the contrast medium in the thoracic cavity on both projections.

Fistulography

With fistulography, the extent and origin of fistulous tracts can be determined by injecting positive-contrast medium into the draining wounds and radiographically documenting the path of the tract (Figure 12-12).

Indications

Evaluating fistulous tracts of unknown origin or extent; detection of radiolucent foreign bodies.

Precautions

Possible dissemination of infection.

Contrast agents

MEDIA	DOSAGE
Water-soluble organic iodide	Enough to fill the tract

Equipment

- Appropriately sized catheter
- Syringe
- 4 × 4–inch gauze sponges

Survey

Make two views of the area at right angles to each other before injecting the contrast medium.

Patient preparation

The area of interest should be clean and dry.

Procedure

Insert a catheter filled with contrast medium into the tract as far as possible. Pack the skin around the wound with 4 × 4–inch gauze sponges. Inject part of the contrast medium, then slowly withdraw the catheter while injecting the rest of the contrast medium. Inject enough so contrast medium fills the entire tract. Massage the area to work the contrast medium into deeper tracts. Wipe any contrast medium from the skin. Make at least two radiographic views of the area at right angles to each other.

A

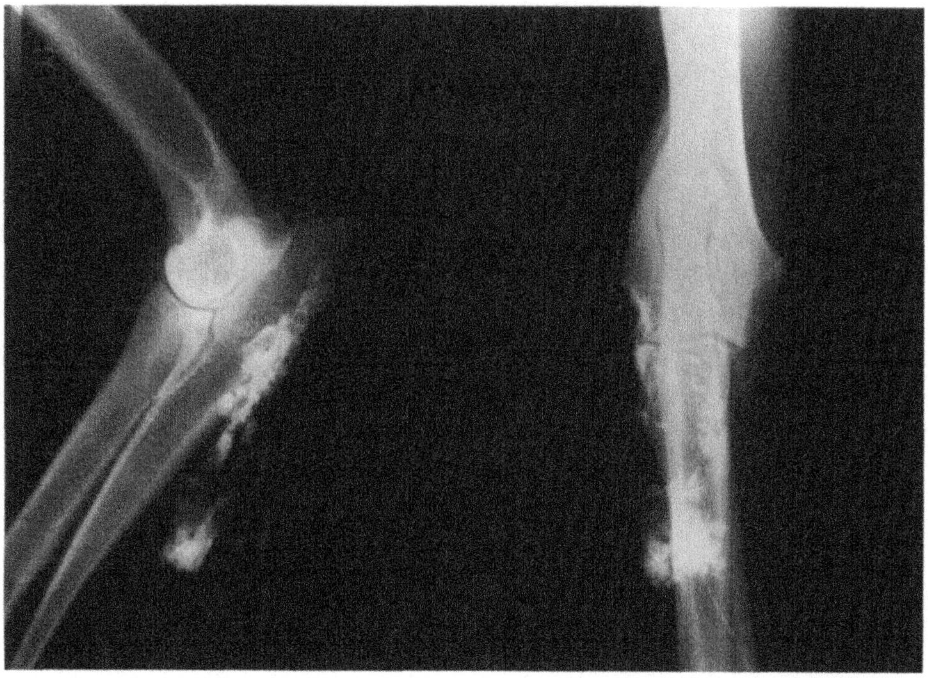

B

FIG. 12-12 Fistulogram of canine elbow area. **A,** Lateral projection. **B,** Craniocaudal projection.

Myelography

Myelography is done to evaluate the location and nature of lesions of the spinal cord. The myelogram is performed by injection of contrast medium into the subarachnoid space.

Indications

Suspected intervertebral disc disease, neoplasms, vertebral instability, malformations, fractures.

Precautions

Evidence of infection in the cerebrospinal fluid.

Contrast agents

MEDIA	DOSAGE
NOTE: Dosage is the same for all contrast agents.	
Iohexol	0.7 ml/lb for cervical areas only
Iopamidol	0.7 ml/lb for lumbar areas only
Visipaque	1 ml/lb for whole spine dosage

Equipment

- ◆ Drape
- ◆ Sterile gloves
- ◆ 0.22-µ millipore filter (Millex–GS, Millipore Products Division, Bedford, Massachusetts)
- ◆ 1½- to 3½-inch spinal needle (depends on size of animal)
- ◆ 18-gauge, 1-inch needle
- ◆ Syringe for contrast medium
- ◆ Extension set
- ◆ 3-ml syringe to collect cerebrospinal fluid
- ◆ Tubes for cerebrospinal fluid analysis

Survey

Lateral and ventrodorsal views centered and collimated over the area of interest; cervical, thoracic, thoracolumbar (T-L), or lumbar vertebrae.

Patient preparation

General anesthesia is required. Clip the hair over the cervical or lumbar area and do three surgical scrubs. For cervical injection, insert the needle in the atlantooccipital joint. For lumbar injection, insert the needle between the fifth and sixth lumbar vertebrae.

Procedure

CERVICAL MYELOGRAPHY. Depending on the preference of the myelographer, the patient is placed in either sternal or lateral recumbency with neck flexed. Clip and surgically prep an area over the atlantooccipital joint. Place a drape over the clipped site. The needle is then inserted into the cisterna magna. Once cerebrospinal fluid has been withdrawn, the contrast medium is slowly injected, and the needle is removed. The head should remain elevated for a few minutes to allow the contrast medium to flow caudally. The neck may also need to be massaged to aid flow of the contrast medium. Lateral and ventrodorsal views of the cervical spine are made (Figure 12-13).

LUMBAR MYELOGRAPHY. The patient is placed in lateral recumbency. If needed, the spine may be flexed to help open the vertebral spaces. This is done by bringing the rear limbs cranially between the front limbs and pulling the front limbs caudally. An area over the fifth and sixth lumbar vertebrae is clipped and surgically prepped. Place a drape over the prep site. Once the needle is in the subarachnoid space, the cerebrospinal fluid can be collected and the contrast medium slowly injected. With the needle in place, a lateral view is made. This prevents the contrast from leaking back into the needle tract and going epidural. Once the lateral projection has been made, the needle is removed, and a ventrodorsal view is quickly made (Figure 12-14).

Comments

Deliver the contrast medium slowly. Oblique, flexed, or extended views may be necessary. After cervical myelography, keep the head elevated to decrease the chance of seizures.

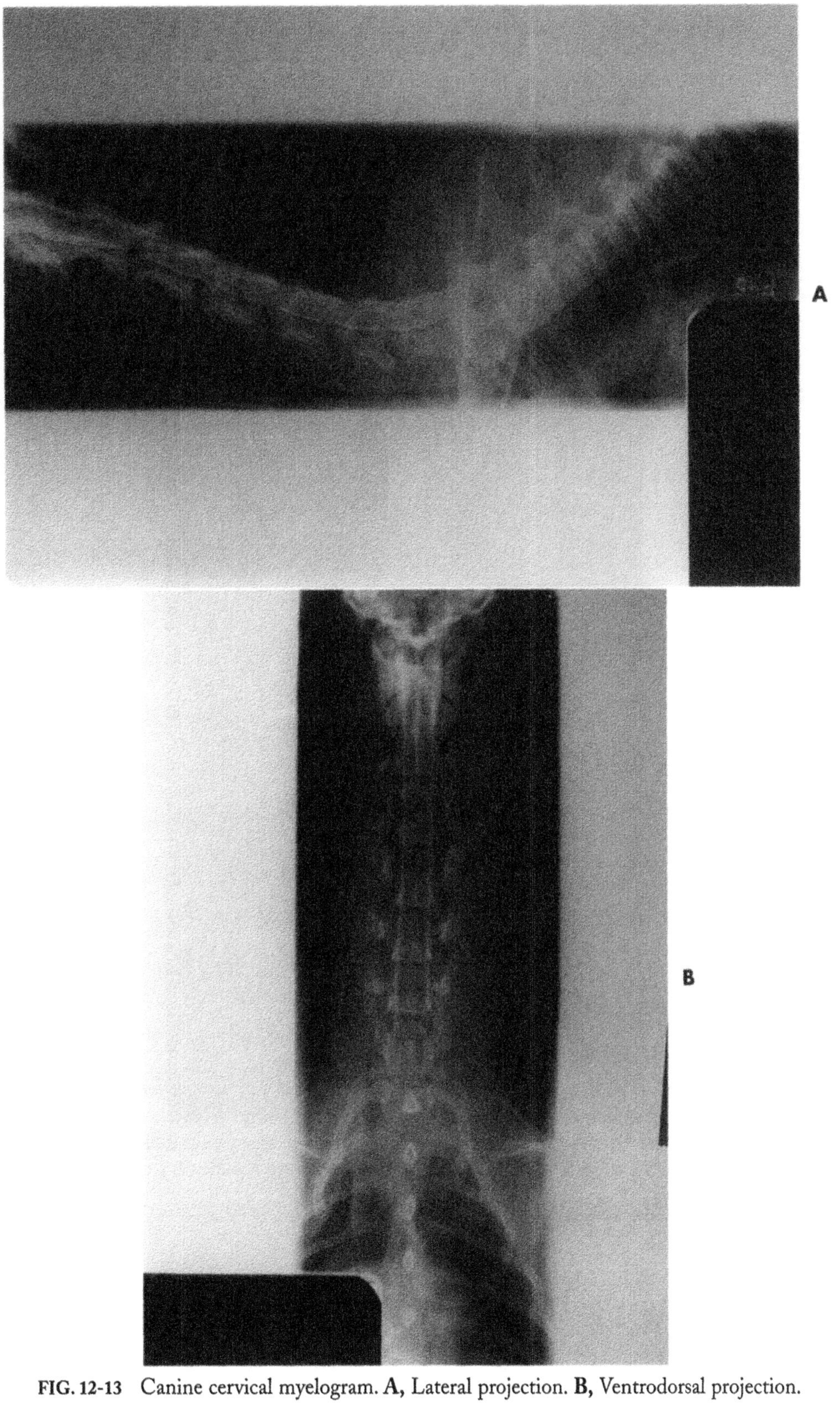

FIG. 12-13 Canine cervical myelogram. **A,** Lateral projection. **B,** Ventrodorsal projection.

A

B

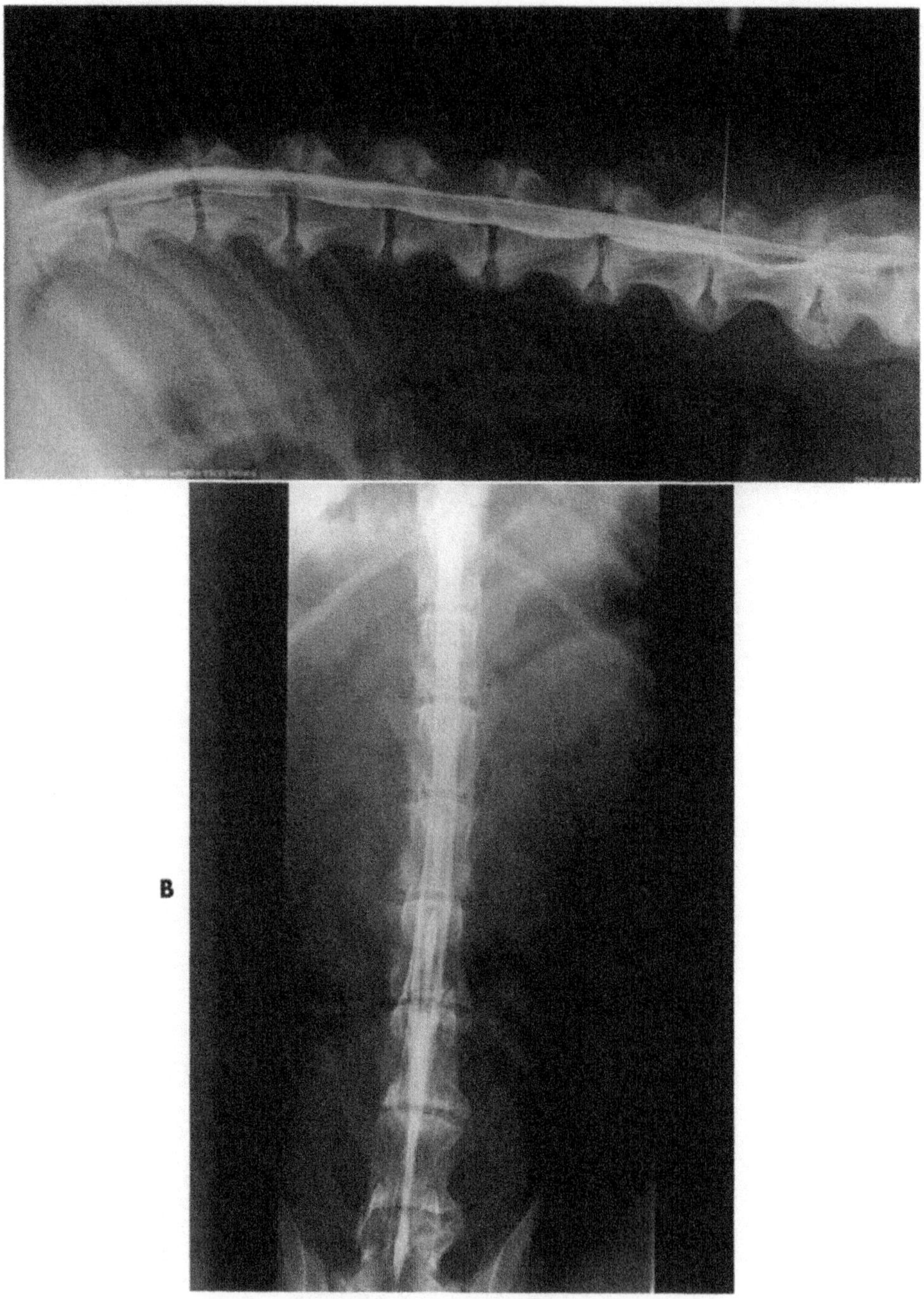

FIG. 12-14 Canine lumbar myelogram. **A,** Lateral projection. **B,** Ventrodorsal projection. Note that the needle remains in place for the lateral view but is removed for the ventrodorsal view.

Sialography

Sialography is performed to visualize the salivary ducts and glands (Figure 12-15).

Indications

Suspected salivary mucoceles.

Contrast agents

MEDIA	DOSAGE
Water-soluble organic iodide	0.5-1 ml

Equipment

- ◆ Blunt cannula (lacrimal) or blunted 22-, 25-, and 26-gauge needles
- ◆ Tissue forceps
- ◆ Syringe
- ◆ Mouth gag

Survey

Lateral and ventrodorsal views of the skull.

Patient preparation

General anesthesia is required.

Procedure

Four ducts, the parotid, zygomatic, mandibular, and sublingual, can be cannulated and injected with contrast medium. After the duct of interest has been identified, the cannula is then inserted into the duct up to the hub. The contrast medium is injected, then lateral and ventrodorsal views of the skull are made.

Comments

Much time, patience, and experience are required when performing sialograms.

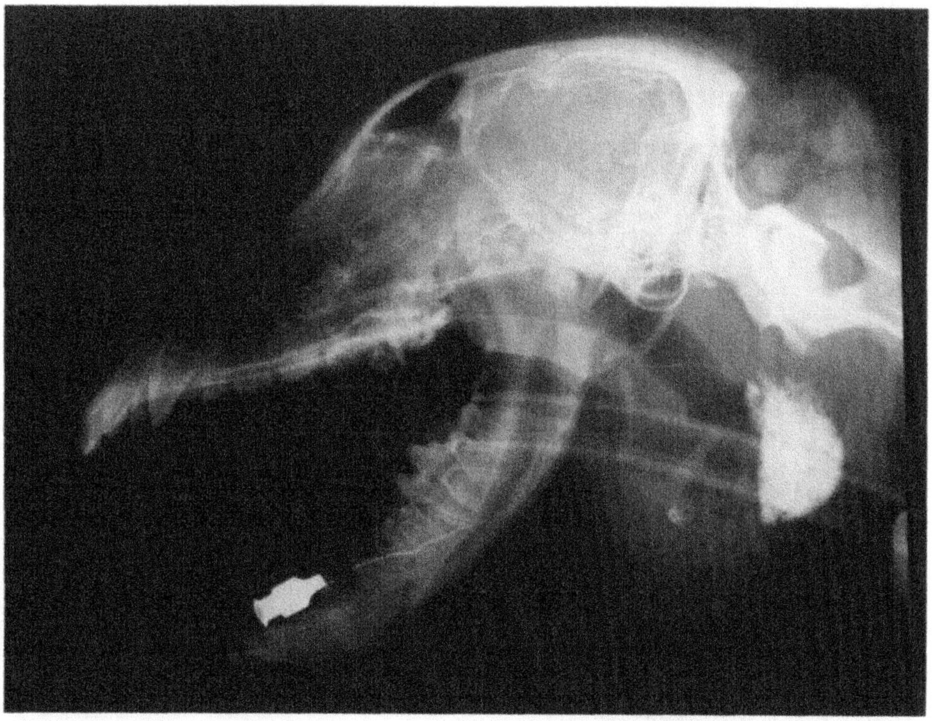

FIG. 12-15 Canine sialogram, lateral projection.

Arthrography

Arthrography involves introduction of contrast medium, either positive or negative, into the synovial fluid to contrast the articular surfaces and joint capsule (Figure 12-16).

Indications

Outlining articular cartilage defects and joint capsule abnormalities.

Contrast agents

MEDIA	DOSAGE
Water-soluble organic iodide	4-5 ml

Equipment

- 20-gauge, 1-inch needle
- Two 6-ml syringes

Survey

Two views, mediolateral and craniocaudal or caudocranial, are necessary before administration of the contrast medium.

Patient preparation

General anesthesia is required. An 8 × 8–cm area is clipped, surgically prepped, and draped.

Procedure

A 20-gauge needle with the syringe attached is inserted into the joint. Aspiration of synovial fluid confirms correct placement of the needle. The syringe is then removed and replaced with the second syringe filled with 4 to 5 ml of contrast medium. The contrast medium is injected with a slight amount of pressure, and the needle is withdrawn. The joint should then be flexed and extended to allow the contrast medium to mix with the synovial fluid. Two views, mediolateral and craniocaudal or caudocranial, of the joint are then made.

Comments

Radiographic views should be made within 1 minute after injection, because some of the contrast medium may be absorbed if an extended period has elapsed after injection. Arthrography may also be performed on horses and cattle, using a larger needle and more contrast medium.

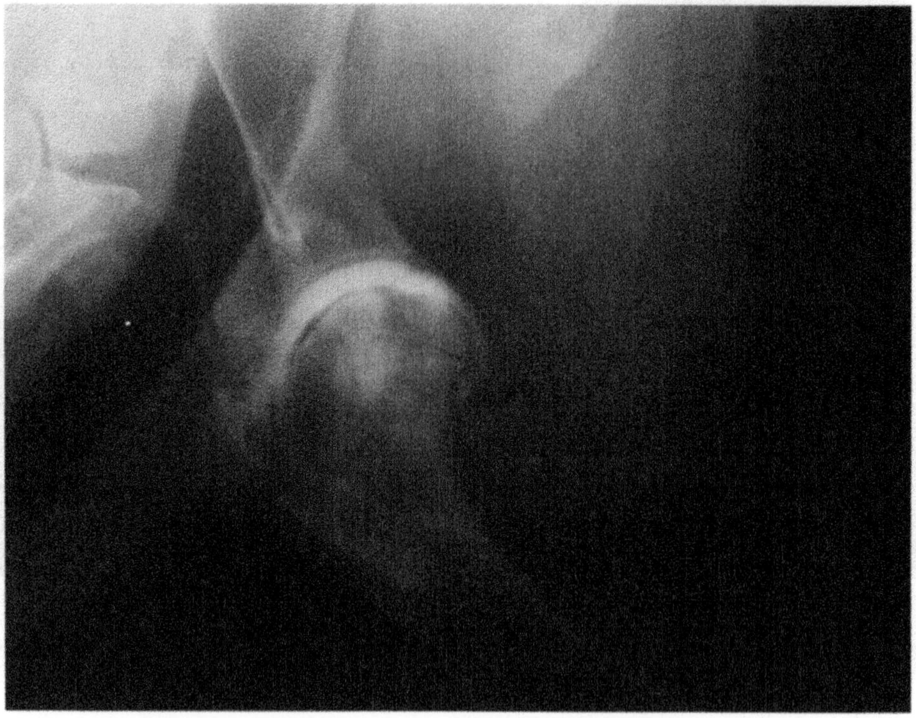

FIG. 12-16 Arthrogram of canine shoulder joint, lateral projection.

Nonselective Angiocardiography

Nonselective angiocardiography requires injection of contrast medium into a cephalic or jugular catheter to obtain information about cardiac abnormalities (Figure 12-17).

Indications

Detection of some congenital diseases (e.g., right-to-left shunts, pulmonic stenosis); cardiomyopathy in cats; right atrial or ventricular masses; pericardial disease.

Precautions

Problems could arise if the patient is allergic to the contrast medium.

Contrast agents

MEDIA	DOSAGE
Water-soluble organic iodide	1 ml/lb

Equipment

- Cephalic or jugular catheter
- Syringe

Patient preparation

Sedation or anesthesia is usually necessary to obtain adequate images. A cephalic or jugular catheter should be securely placed.

Procedure

Place the animal in lateral recumbency and set the technique on the machine. Have as many cassettes as possible ready for use. Administer a bolus injection of contrast medium. Make the first radiograph while the injection is being made. Make radiographs 1 second apart for 9 seconds.

Comments

Selective angiocardiography is rarely performed by veterinarians in practice because of the specialized equipment required.

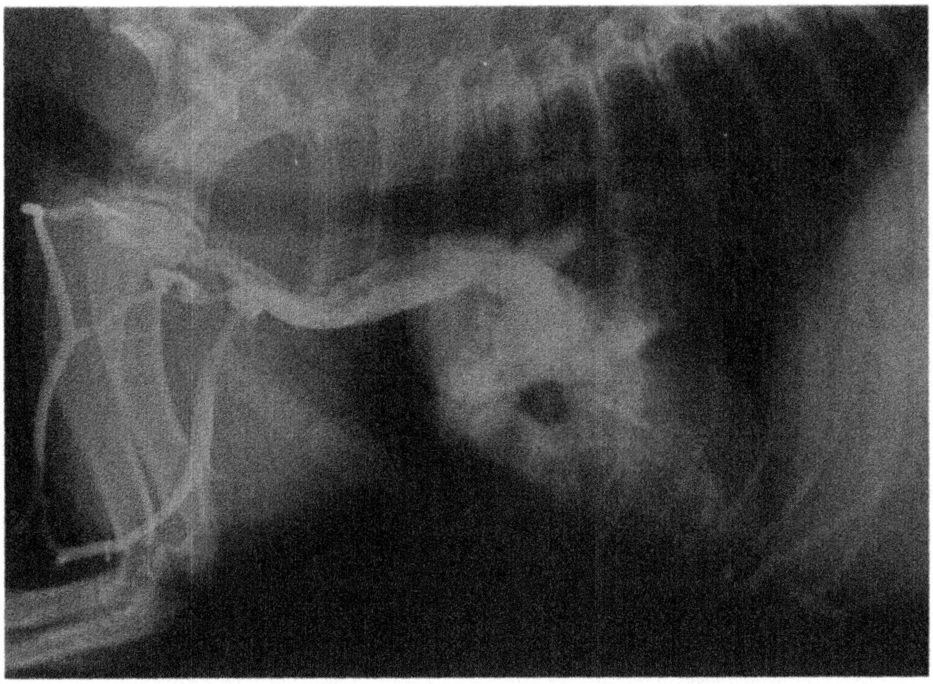

FIG. 12-17 Nonselective angiocardiogram, lateral projection.

Recommended Reading

Bettmann MA: Angiographic contrast agents: conventional and new media compared, *AJR Am J Roentgenol* 139:787, 1982.

Douglas SW et al: *Principles of veterinary radiography*, ed 4, London, 1987, Bailliere Tindall.

Fischer HW: Catalog of intravascular contrast media, *Radiology* 159:561, 1986.

Morgan JP, Silverman S: *Techniques of veterinary radiography*, ed 5, Davis, Calif, 1993, Veterinary Radiology Associates.

Ticer JW: *Radiographic technique in veterinary practice*, ed 2, Philadelphia, 1984, Saunders.

Widmer WR et al: Iohexol and iopamidol myelography in the dog: a clinical trial comparing adverse effects and myelographic quality, *Vet Radiol Ultrasound* 33(6):327, 1992.

13

Exotic Animal Radiography

KIM ZODY

CHAPTER OBJECTIVES

- Explain the three basic restraint methods preferred for exotic animal radiography.
- List the various restraint and positioning devices used for rodents and small mammals, for reptiles, and for birds.
- State when to use rapid cassettes, detail cassettes, and nonscreen film for all exotic animals.
- Explain how to determine appropriate mAs and kVp techniques for all exotic animals.
- List the views that are necessary for rodent and small mammal radiography, for reptile radiography, and for avian radiography.
- State the precautions that are necessary when radiographing rabbits and guinea pigs.
- Define the important positioning technique to remember when producing a lateral image of a lizard.
- List some important considerations to keep in mind when manually restraining birds.

With the increasing popularity and expense of exotic pets, owners expect to receive top-quality care, including the most advanced diagnostic radiography available. Most of the same principles, equipment, and positioning methods used to radiograph domestic animals can be used to radiograph exotic species.

A high-output x-ray machine capable of 200 or 300 mA is recommended so that faster exposure times can be used. Exposure times of $\frac{1}{40}$ second or less are needed to decrease the motion artifact that may occur on the finished radiograph. If a high-output machine is not available, the focal-film distance (FFD) may need to be decreased to compensate.

Magnification radiography is another option that may be useful when radiographing small areas. This requires an x-ray machine that allows the operator to choose a small focal spot. The object-film distance (OFD) is increased by either 20 or 30 inches, and the FFD is decreased to either 20 or 10 inches. Patient motion with blurring of the radiograph becomes more of a problem with this technique. Chemical restraint is recommended.

The unique challenges that exotic animal radiography present can intimidate even the most experienced staff. However, this does not have to be the case. High-quality, consistent radiographs can be produced with an understanding of a few special considerations and the application of good exposure techniques and consistent positioning methods.

Few exotic species, unless critically ill, can be safely restrained manually or even physically. *Chemical restraint* is

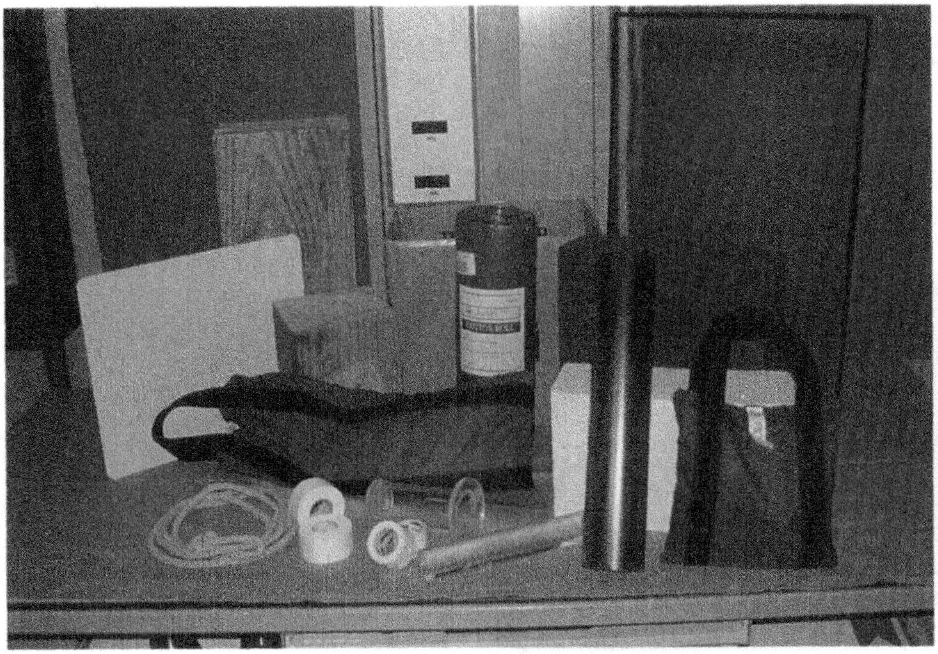

FIG. 13-1 Exotic animal positioning aids and restraint devices.

generally the preferred method. *Manual restraint* involves the assistance of gowned and gloved individuals holding the animal, whereas *physical restraint* is the use of devices such as adhesive cloth tape, ropes, sandbags, roll cotton, wooden blocks, foam wedges, Plexiglas radiolucent plates, and radiolucent tubes (Figure 13-1). Injectable sedation and gas anesthesia are the safest and most reliably consistent restraint methods. Ideally, a combination of physical and chemical restraint should be employed.

This chapter covers three main areas of exotic animal radiography: (1) rodent and small mammal, (2) reptile, and (3) avian.

Rodent and Small Mammal Radiography

Since manual restraint is virtually impossible with all but the most critically ill of rodent and small mammal patients, some form of chemical restraint is essential. The use of physical restraint devices such as tape, foam wedges, roll cotton, and radiolucent tubes are recommended (Figure 13-2).

Nonscreen film can be used because of the high degree of detail produced. In some cases, however, the probability of patient movement negates its use, since longer exposure times are necessary. Because of small patient size, a tabletop technique is preferred over grid techniques. Higher mA, shorter exposure time, and lower kVp, coupled with collimation, should be used to minimize scatter radiation and decrease the possibility of motion artifacts.

Rodents and small mammals must be chemically restrained when using nonscreen film.

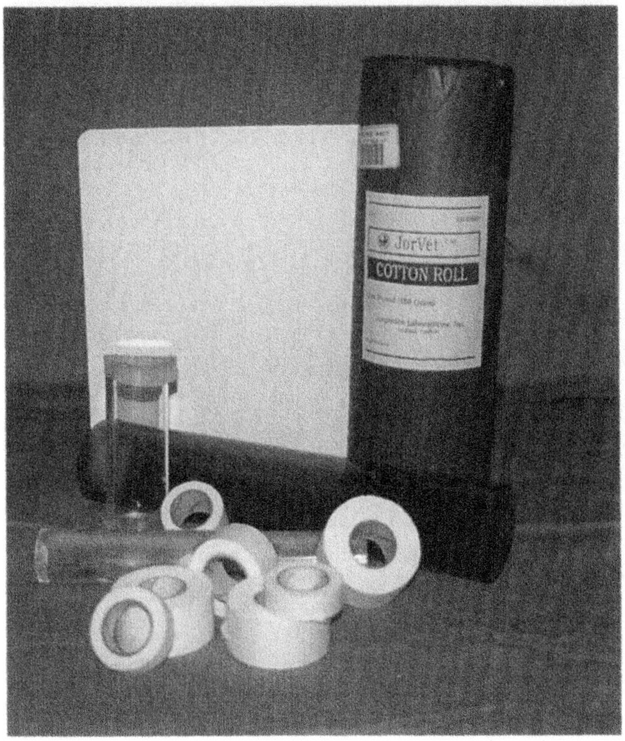

FIG. 13-2 Rodent and small mammal positioning aids and restraint devices.

Rodent Radiography

Entire body dorsoventral-ventrodorsal view

Place sedated or anesthetized animal directly on the cassette in sternal or dorsal recumbency. Tape the head to the cassette, placing adhesive tape across the base of the skull. Tape all four legs to the cassette, with front legs extended out cranially and rear legs extended back caudally. Center the primary beam on the thoracolumbar area and collimate to include the entire animal. Measure over the highest point on the patient's body (Figures 13-3 and 13-4).

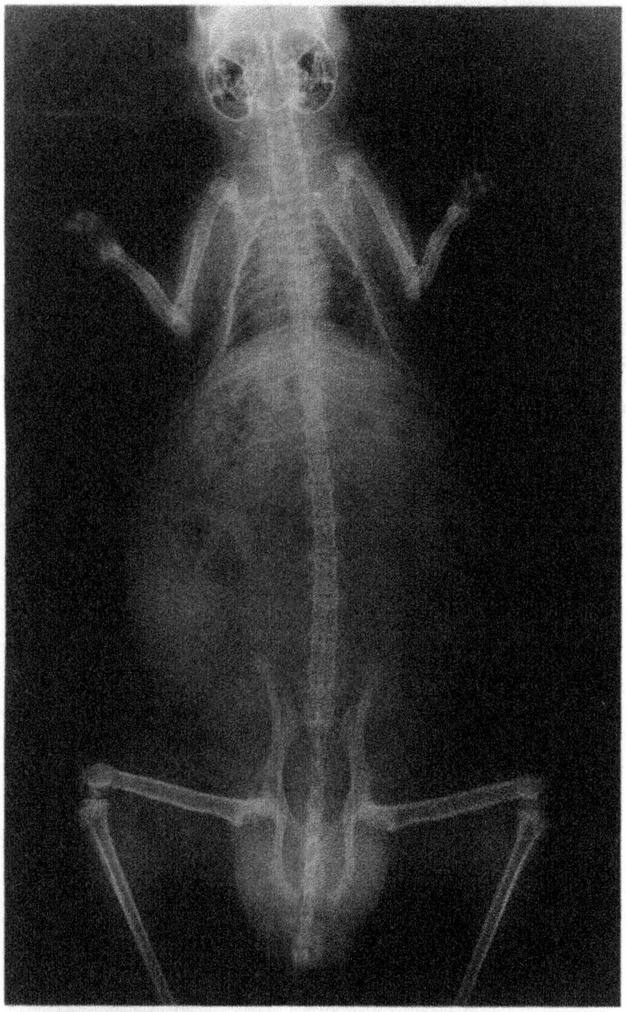

FIG. 13-3 Dorsoventral radiograph of chinchilla.

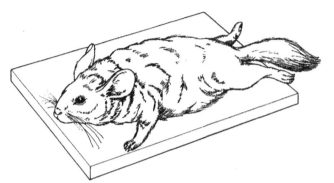

FIG. 13-4 Dorsoventral positioning of chinchilla.

Entire body lateral view

Place anesthetized or sedated patient directly on the cassette in right lateral recumbency. Tape across the head and neck just behind the base of the skull. Tape all four legs to the cassette, extending front limbs cranially and rear limbs caudally. If necessary, place a small amount of padding, either roll cotton or foam wedges, between the front and rear legs or under the body to prevent "obliquing." Center on the thoracolumbar junction and collimate to include the entire animal. Measure over the highest point on the patient's body (Figures 13-5, 13-6, 13-7, and 13-8).

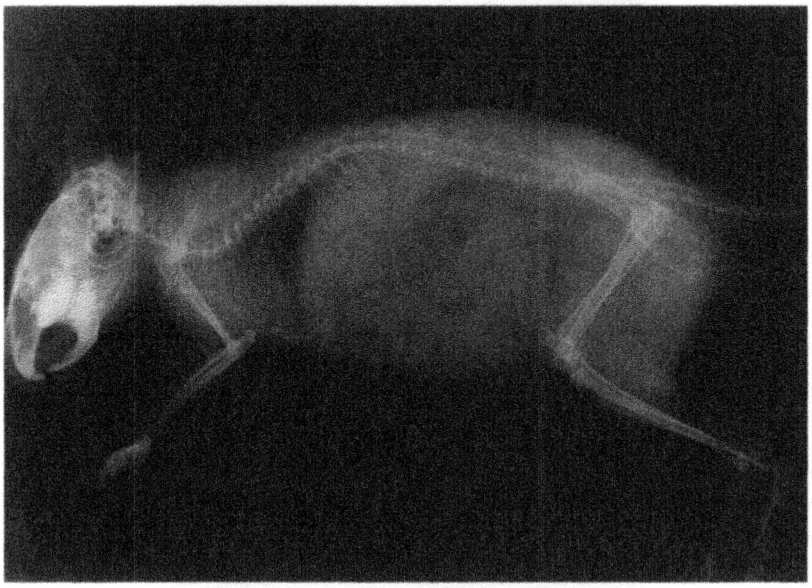

FIG. 13-5 Lateral radiograph of chinchilla.

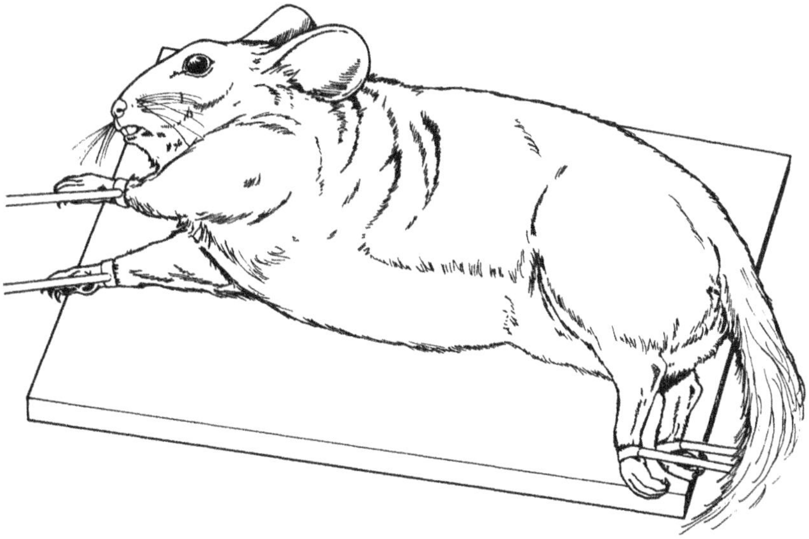

FIG. 13-6 Lateral positioning of chinchilla.

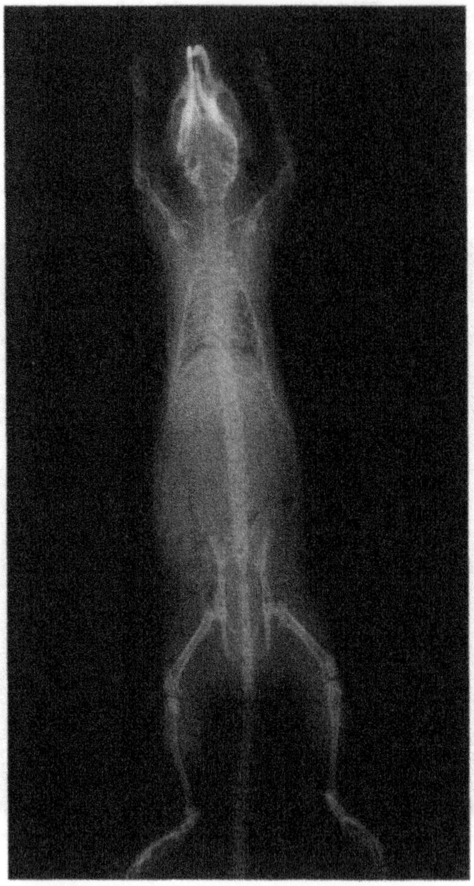

FIG. 13-7 Ventrodorsal radiograph of rat.

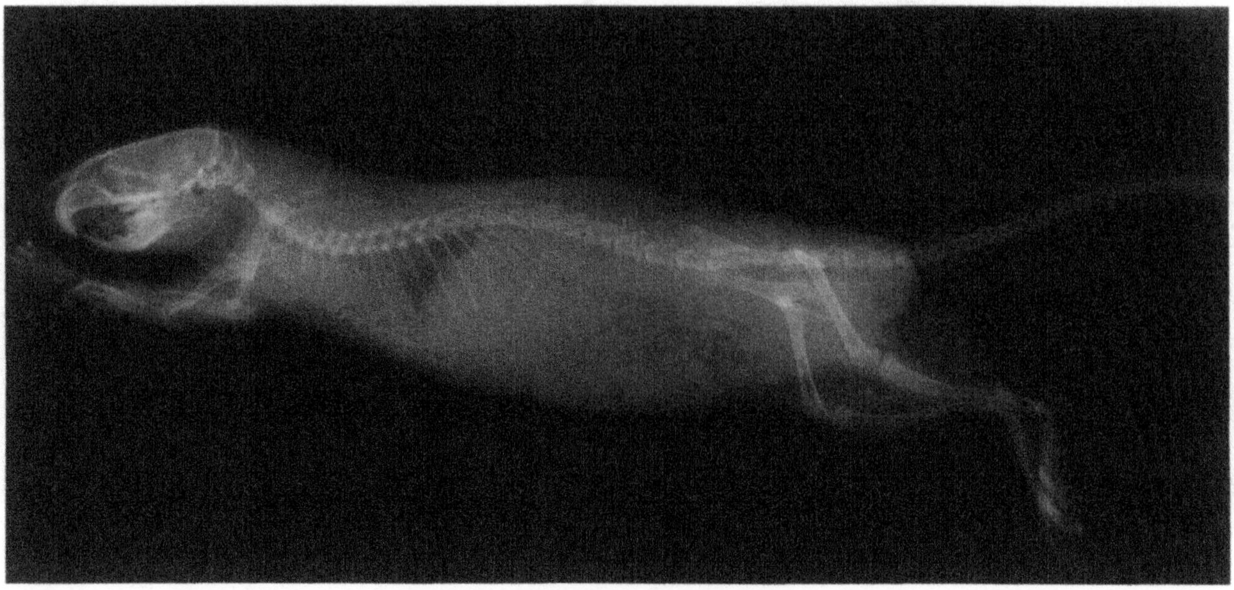

FIG. 13-8 Lateral radiograph of rat.

Entire body dorsoventral-ventrodorsal radiolucent tube view

A radiolucent Plexiglas tube can be advantageous since ventrodorsal-dorsoventral and lateral views can be obtained without patient manipulation (Figure 13-9). A major disadvantage to the use of a tube is that the patient's legs or tail may be superimposed over the thorax or abdomen as a result of less-than-optimum positioning (Figures 13-10, 13-11, and 13-12). If a radiolucent Plexiglas tube is not available, a piece of unexposed but developed film can be used. Cut the film to an appropriate width for the desired tube diameter. Roll the film into a tube without overlapping the edges, and secure with cellophane tape. Place the rodent in the film tube, and cover the ends with corks or pieces of cloth stretched over the openings.

> For rodent radiography, a piece of rolled film (unexposed but developed) can be used in place of a Plexiglas tube.

For ventrodorsal-dorsoventral view place the patient in the tube and cover both ends with corks or plastic caps. Lay the tube directly on the cassette. Adhesive tape can be used if it is necessary to prevent slight patient movement. Center on the thoracolumbar area and collimate to include the animal's entire body. Remember to add 2 to 4 kVp to the measurement to compensate for the tube thickness.

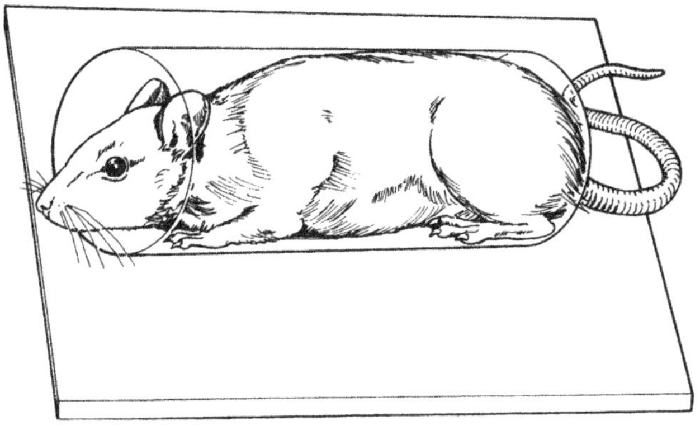

FIG. 13-9 Rodent positioning with Plexiglas radiolucent tube.

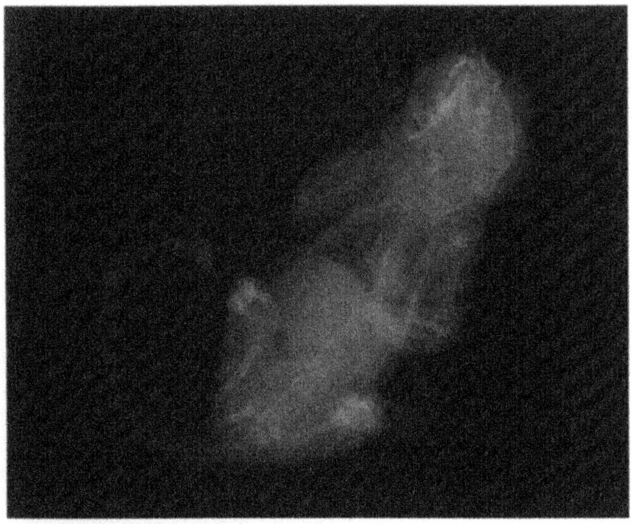

FIG. 13-10 Superimposition of limbs in dorsoventral radiograph of sugar glider.

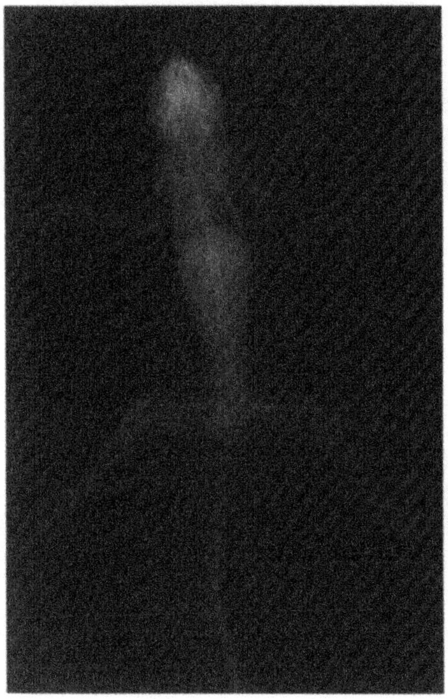

FIG. 13-11 Correct limb position in dorsoventral radiograph of sugar glider.

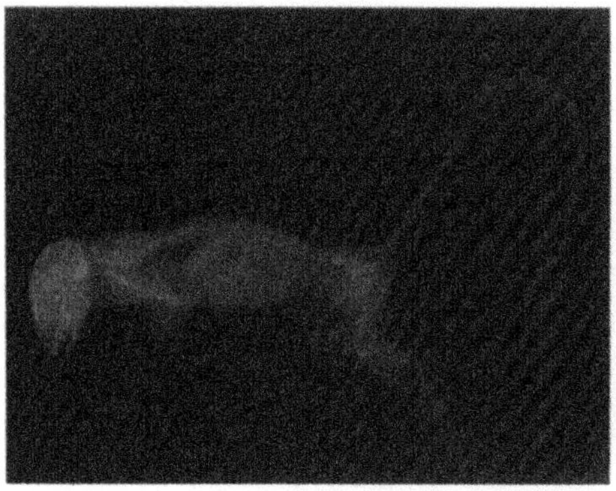

FIG. 13-12 Lateral radiograph of sugar glider.

Entire body lateral radiolucent tube view

For the lateral view the tube may be turned until the patient is in lateral recumbency and then taped into place directly onto the cassette. Center on the thoracolumbar area and collimate to include the entire animal.

Another option for the lateral radiolucent tube view is a *horizontal beam technique.* Place the patient inside the tube in a dorsoventral position. Elevate the tube on a foam pad. Place the cassette perpendicular to the x-ray table, directly against the right lateral side of the patient. Direct the beam horizontally toward the left side of the radiolucent tube. Measure from the cassette to the left outside edge of the tube. Center on the thoracolumbar area and collimate to include the entire animal.

Guinea Pig and Rabbit Radiography

Guinea pigs and rabbits present their own unique set of problems because of their relatively small thoracic cavities in relation to their much larger abdominal cavities. Great care must be taken during restraint to avoid injury to the thorax and vertebral column. A rabbit's powerful hindquarters can pull or kick hard enough during restraint to cause damage to the spinal cord.

With the exception of critically ill patients, chemical restraint is an absolute necessity. In the case of larger rabbits, a grid technique instead of tabletop technique may be warranted.

> A rabbit can be momentarily "hypnotized" by covering the eyes and stroking the ventral midline.

Dorsoventral-ventrodorsal view

Place sedated or anesthetized animal directly onto the cassette in sternal or dorsal recumbency. Tape the head to the cassette, placing adhesive tape across the base of the skull. Tape all four legs to the cassette with front legs extended out cranially and rear legs extended back caudally. Center over the heart for a thoracic view and over the liver for an abdominal view, and collimate accordingly. Measure over the highest point on the patient's body. For smaller guinea pigs and rabbits, whole body views are preferred, centering over the thoracolumbar area and collimating to include the entire animal (Figures 13-13, 13-14, and 13-15).

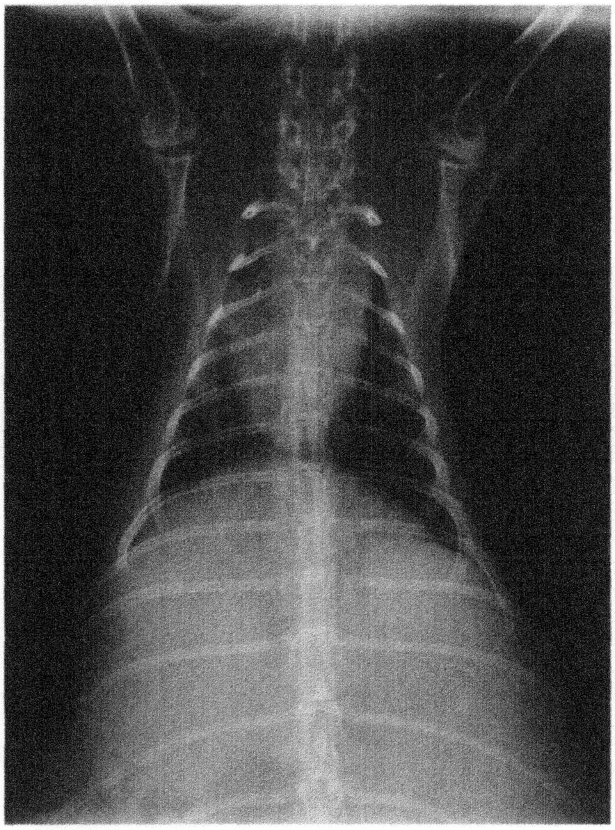

FIG. 13-13 Ventrodorsal radiograph of rabbit thorax.

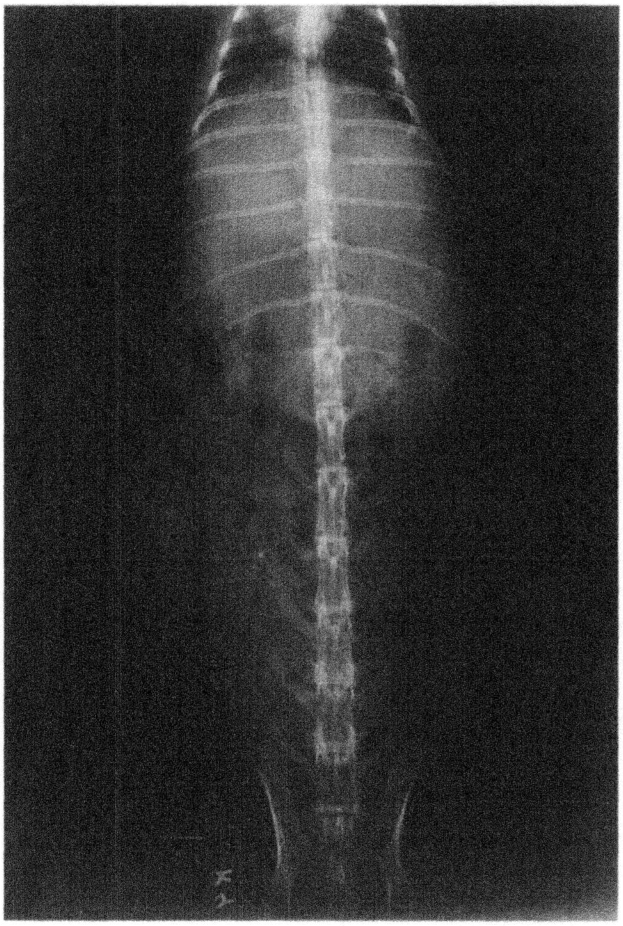

FIG. 13-14 Ventrodorsal radiograph of rabbit abdomen.

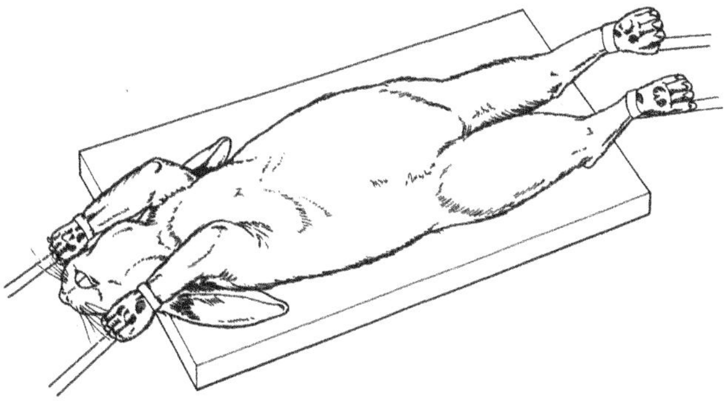

FIG. 13-15 Ventrodorsal positioning of rabbit.

Lateral view

Place anesthetized or sedated patient directly on the cassette in right lateral recumbency. Tape across the head and neck just behind the base of the skull. Tape all four legs to the cassette, extending front limbs cranially and rear limbs caudally. If necessary, use a small amount of padding to prevent obliquing. Padding can consist of roll cotton or foam wedges placed between the legs or under the dorsal or ventral aspect of the patient's thorax or abdomen as needed. Center over the heart for thoracic radiographs and the liver for abdominal radiographs, and collimate accordingly. Measure over the highest point of the animal's body. For smaller guinea pigs and rabbits, whole body radiographs can be taken (Figures 13-16, 13-17, and 13-18).

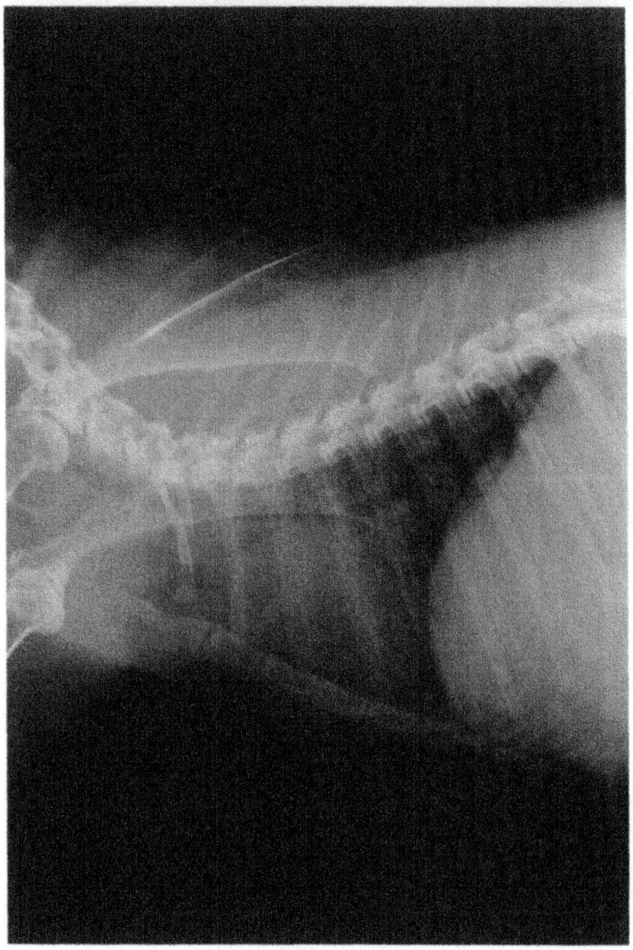

FIG. 13-16 Lateral radiograph of rabbit thorax.

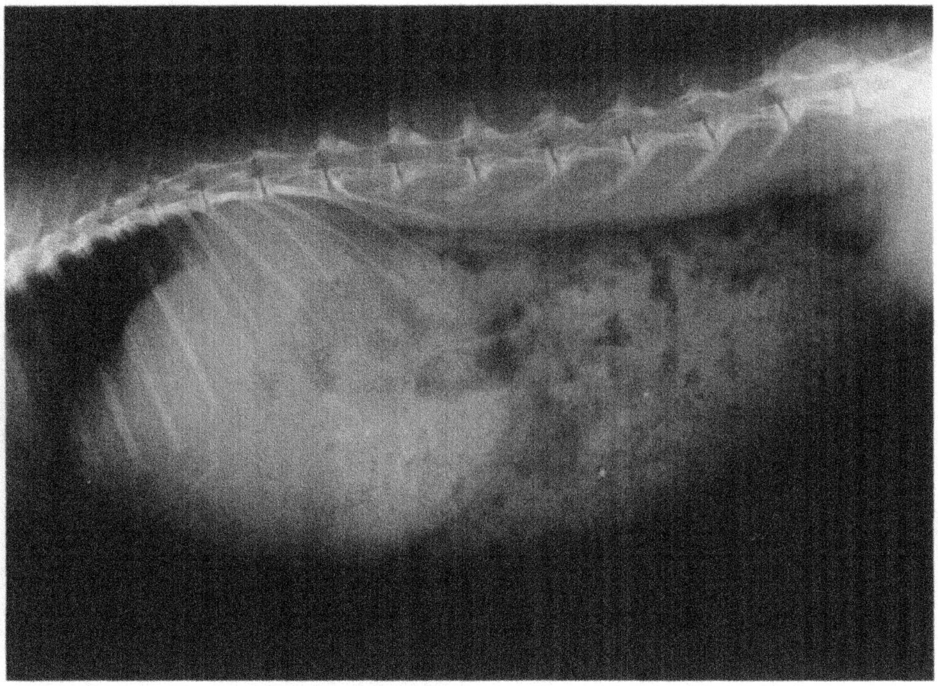

FIG. 13-17 Lateral radiograph of rabbit abdomen.

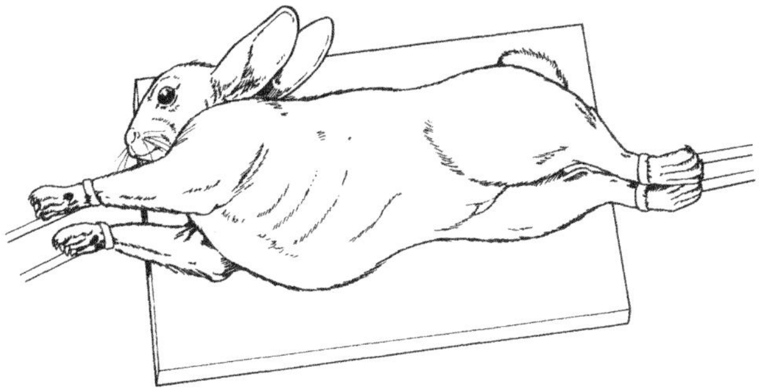

FIG. 13-18 Lateral positioning of rabbit.

Ferret Radiography

Because of a ferret's extreme agility and high activity level, radiographic positioning can be quite challenging. Radiolucent tube radiography is one option. A combination of manual restraint (gowned and gloved assistants) and physical restraint (tape stirrups on legs) is also sometimes successful. However, ferrets often twist and contort into less-than-desirable positions. For this reason, chemical restraint is strongly recommended. A ferret can be "hypnotized" for temporary restraint by "scruffing" the back of the neck until it yawns and relaxes (Figures 13-19 and 13-20).

Ferrets can be "hypnotized" by scruffing the skin on the back of the neck.

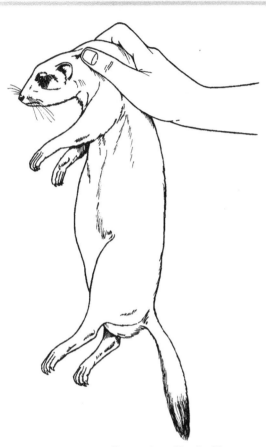

FIG. 13-19 Proper "scruffing" of ferret.

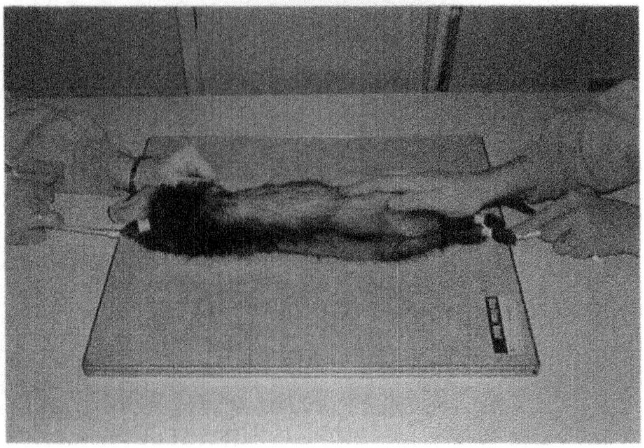

FIG. 13-20 "Scruffing" of ferret before taping into lateral position. Once the ferret is relaxed, only the tape will be used to restrain the animal.

Dorsoventral-ventrodorsal entire body view

Place properly restrained patient directly on the cassette in sternal or dorsal recumbency. Place tape across the head and neck at the base of the skull. Tape all four legs to the cassette, extending front limbs cranially and rear limbs caudally. Measure over the highest point on the patient. Center on the thoracolumbar area and collimate to include the entire animal. With larger ferrets individual thoracic and abdominal views may be necessary. Tabletop technique is recommended, but a grid technique can be used with larger patients (Figures 13-21 and 13-22).

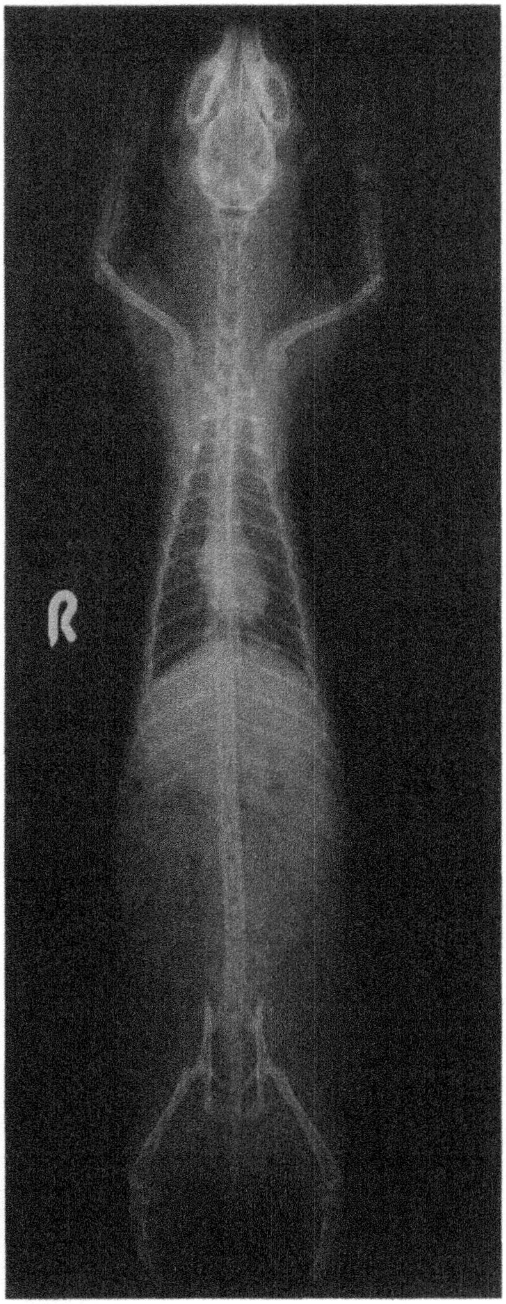

FIG. 13-21 Ventrodorsal radiograph of ferret.

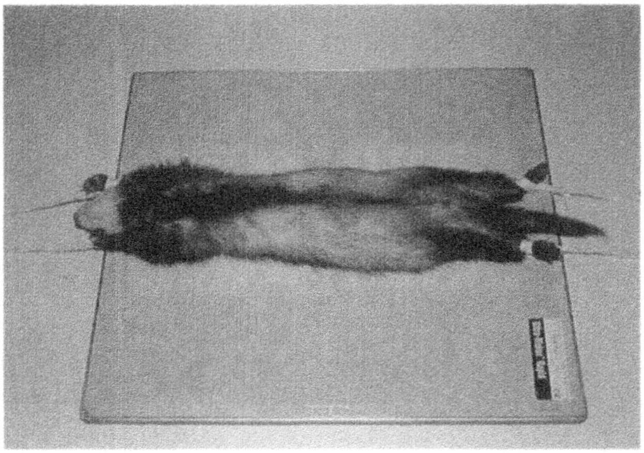

FIG. 13-22 Ventrodorsal positioning of ferret.

Lateral entire body view

Lay the anesthetized or sedated patient directly on the cassette in right lateral recumbency. Place tape across the head and neck at the base of the skull. Tape all four legs to the cassette, extending front limbs cranially and rear limbs caudally. If needed, use a small amount of padding between the legs or under the body to prevent obliquing. Using a tabletop technique, measure over the highest point on the patient. Center on the thoracolumbar area and collimate the beam to include the entire animal. When working with larger ferrets, individual thoracic and abdominal views may be necessary using a tabletop or grid technique (Figures 13-23 and 13-24).

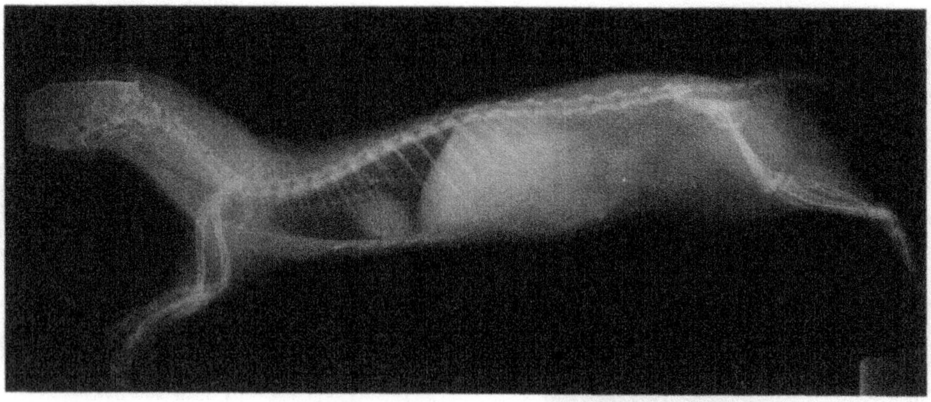

FIG. 13-23 Lateral radiograph of ferret.

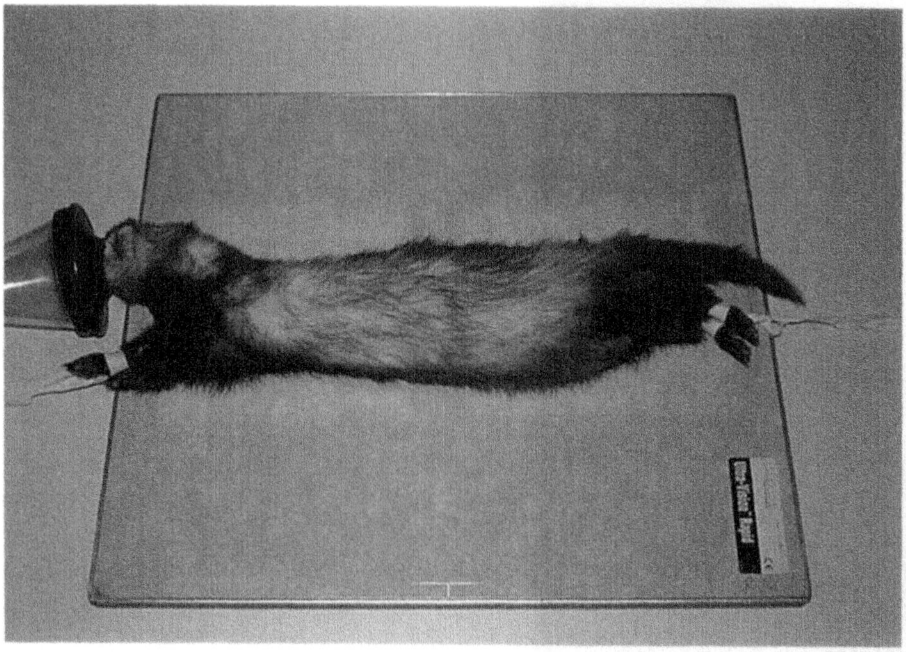

FIG. 13-24 Lateral positioning of ferret.

Reptile Radiography

This unique group of animals can present several radiographic challenges. A great deal of anatomic diversity exists among reptile species, and consequently, a variety of restraint methods, radiographic equipment, and exposure techniques can be used.

Of the three types of restraint methods (manual, physical, and chemical), physical restraint is most often used. Manual restraint (a gowned and gloved assistant holding the animal) usually is not practical with reptiles because most reptile radiographs are whole body views. However, one exception in which manual restraint may be useful is when taking sectional radiographs of large snakes.

Several types of physical restraint devices can be used to aid in reptile positioning. These include adhesive tape, rope, foam pads, Styrofoam, wood blocks, cloth bags, paper sacks, and cardboard boxes, as well as radiolucent Plexiglas tubes and containers (Figure 13-25).

Under most circumstances, chemical restraint is not necessary. It may be warranted, however, when working with large, uncooperative, or aggressive patients. Exposing a reptile to a cool environment such as the metal surface of an examination table can induce temporary lethargy and immobility. This "chilling" method, however, does not include refrigeration.

> Gently "chilling" a reptile can temporarily induce immobility.

Most exposures are made using a tabletop technique with the animal lying directly on the cassette. Nonscreen film, higher mA, and longer exposure time can be used to penetrate thick hides and bony shells because patient motion is not usually a factor.

Lizard Radiography

Many species of lizards, if calm and docile, can be radiographed using just adhesive tape as a restraint. Larger iguanas or monitors may require manual restraint as well. Chemical restraint may be necessary for aggressive animals, and in most cases it is wise to bind the mouths of these uncooperative patients to ensure the safety of all personnel involved. Some iguanas can be momentarily "hypnotized" by being placed in a ventrodorsal position and applying gentle, rhythmic strokes along the ventral midline.

Many types of lizards may also require tail restraint because of the tendency of these animals to whip their tails rapidly and powerfully in times of stress or fear. Sometimes it is possible to wedge the patient in a piece of precut foam or Styrofoam.

> Some iguanas can be "hypnotized" using gentle, rhythmic strokes along the ventral midline.

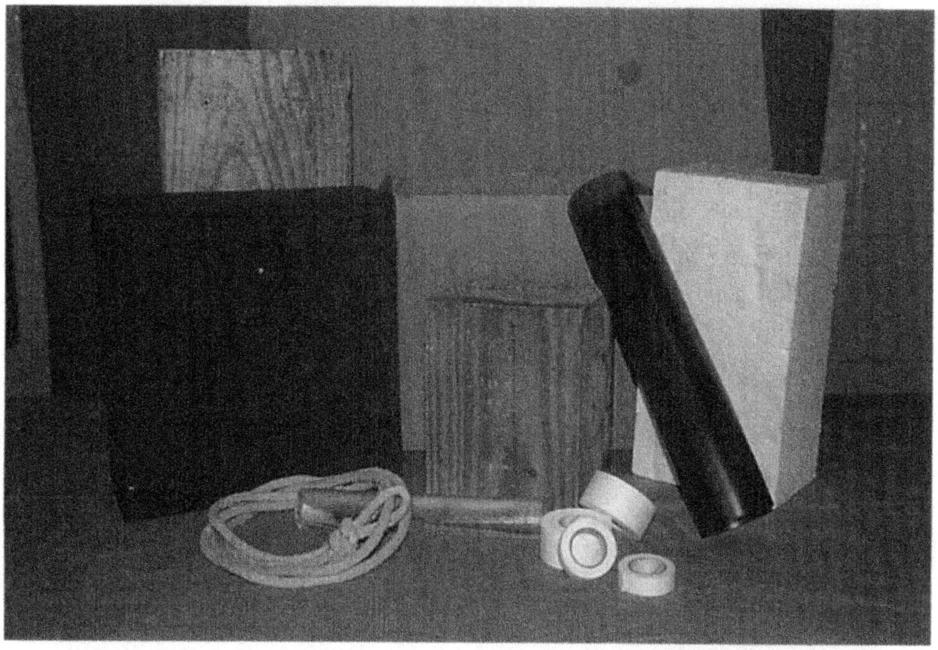

FIG. 13-25 Reptile positioning aids and restraint devices.

Entire body dorsoventral-ventrodorsal view

For dorsoventral view place adequately restrained patient directly on the cassette in sternal recumbency. Place adhesive tape across the top of the head and attach to the cassette. Gently stretch the body and extend the front limbs cranially and the rear limbs caudally. Tape limbs securely to cassette. Make certain that the dorsal spine is directly superimposed over the sternum. It may be necessary to place an additional piece of tape just cranial to the pelvic girdle. Finally, tape the tail to the cassette. Direct the center of the primary beam over the midabdomen and collimate to include the entire body. For ventrodorsal view place patient in dorsal recumbency with the sternum directly superimposed over the dorsal spine (Figures 13-26 and 13-27).

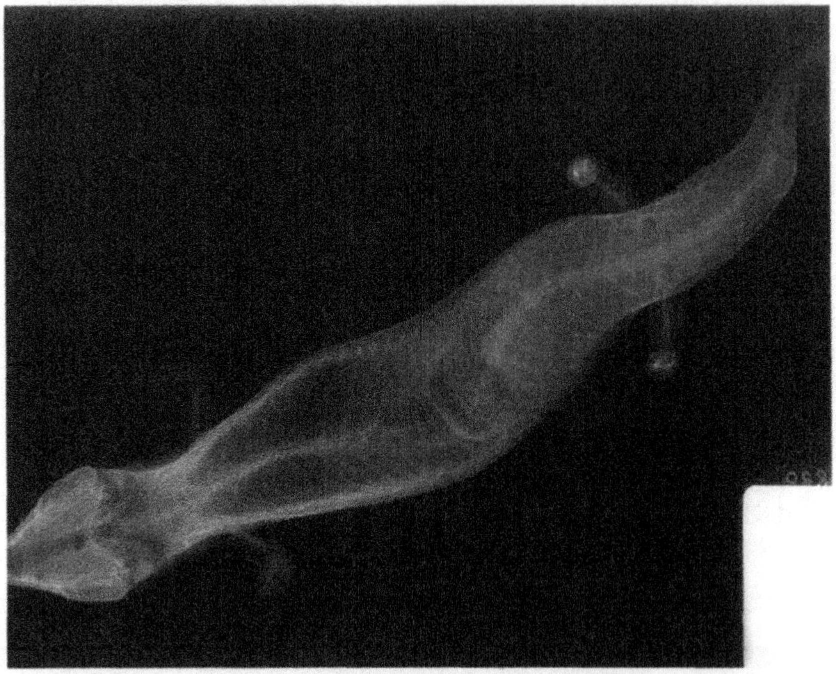

FIG. 13-26 Dorsoventral radiograph of skink.

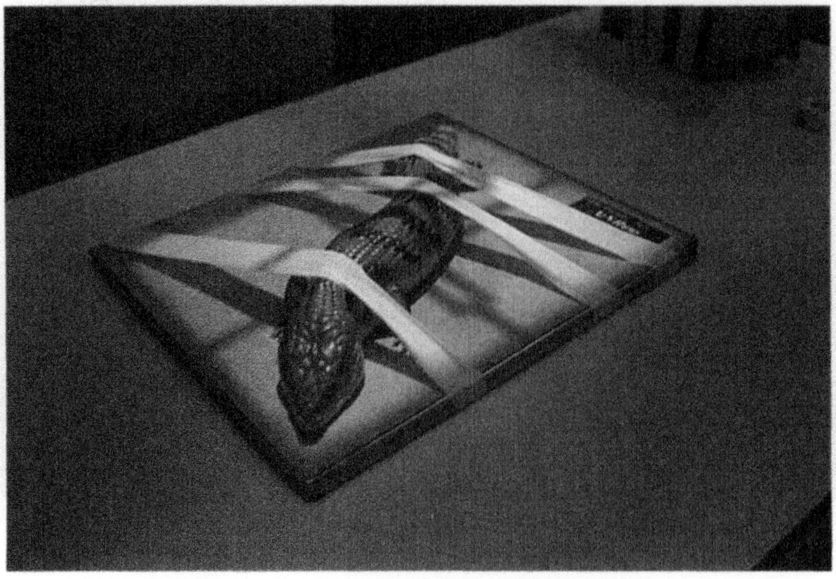

FIG. 13-27 Dorsoventral positioning of skink.

Entire body lateral view

Place the restrained patient directly on the cassette in right lateral recumbency. Place tape across the base of the skull, attaching the ends of the tape to the cassette. Tape all four legs to the cassette individually while gently extending front limbs cranially and rear limbs caudally. Place both right legs slightly forward and both left legs slightly back. Next, secure the tail to the cassette with adhesive tape. It may be necessary to place an additional piece of tape across the sternum, just caudal to the elbows, and possibly tape across the pelvic region. Direct the center of the primary beam over the midsection of the patient and collimate to include the entire body (Figures 13-28 and 13-29).

When positioning a lizard in right lateral recumbency, the left limbs are always caudal to the right limbs.

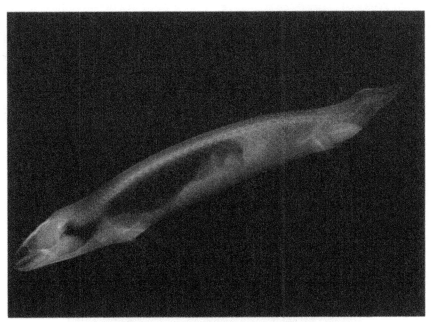

FIG. 13-28 Lateral radiograph of skink.

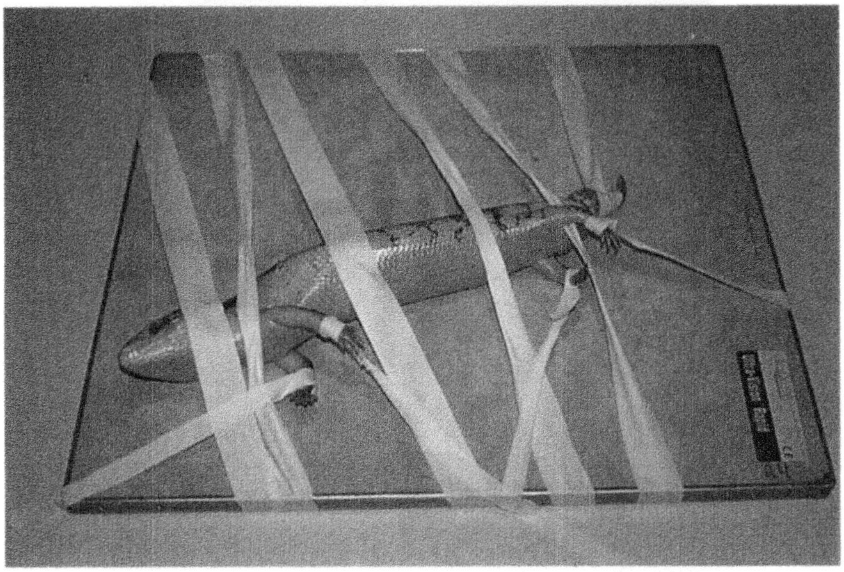

FIG. 13-29 Lateral positioning of skink.

Snake Radiography

Most snakes are relatively docile creatures, requiring only manual or physical restraint. Manual restraint is useful when it is necessary to radiograph only certain segments of a snake. Some effective methods of physical restraint include adhesive tape, rope, cardboard boxes, cloth bags, paper bags, foam pads, corks, radiolucent Plexiglas containers, and various diameters and lengths of radiolucent tubes. Snakes instinctively struggle and coil during any perceived threat, such as radiographic restraint. For this reason, chemical restraint may be necessary, especially with poisonous species or large, powerful boas or pythons.

Isolate snake patients from small mammal patients to prevent aggressive prey-seeking behaviors.

Tabletop technique is most always used, except with species whose girth exceeds 10 to 12 cm in diameter. At this point, a grid technique would be more effective.

Entire body dorsoventral-ventrodorsal view

Place the snake directly on the cassette in a naturally coiled position. If necessary, the patient can be physically restrained by laying it inside a cloth or paper bag, a cardboard box (metal staples removed), or a radiolucent container while in a dorsoventral coiled position, then placing it on the cassette (Figures 13-30 and 13-31). If the snake is still moving, it can be gently "chilled" into immobility by placing it in a cool environment for a short time, such as on the surface of a metal examination table. Do not use refrigeration as a chilling method.

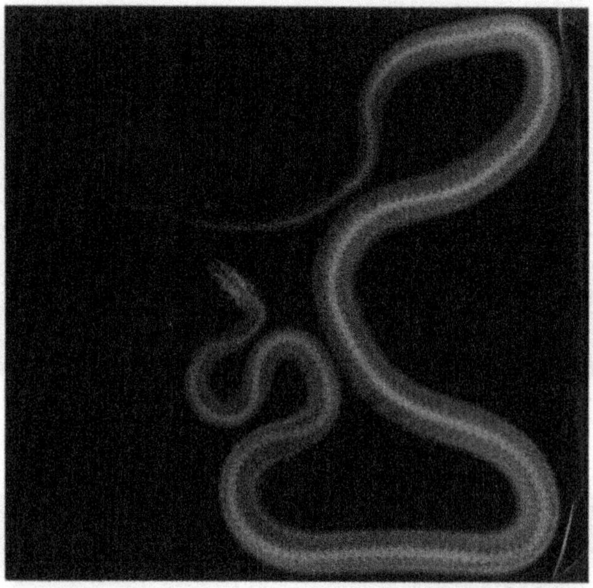

FIG. 13-30 Dorsoventral radiograph of coiled snake in box.

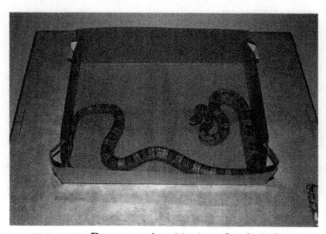

FIG. 13-31 Dorsoventral positioning of snake in box.

Using a tabletop technique, measure over the highest point of the snake's girth. Focus the beam on the center of the coil and collimate to include the entire body (Figure 13-32). A grid technique can be used on larger patients if necessary. If the patient is calm and exhibits no sign of movement, nonscreen film using a high mA and lower kVp produces a radiograph with increased detail.

A gowned and gloved individual can also restrain snakes in a dorsoventral position. For smaller snakes, grasp the patient at the base of the skull and the distal portion of the tail. Focus the primary beam on the patient's midsection and collimate to exclude the restrainer's gloved hands (Figure 13-33). Larger species of snakes can be radiographed in sections using this same technique.

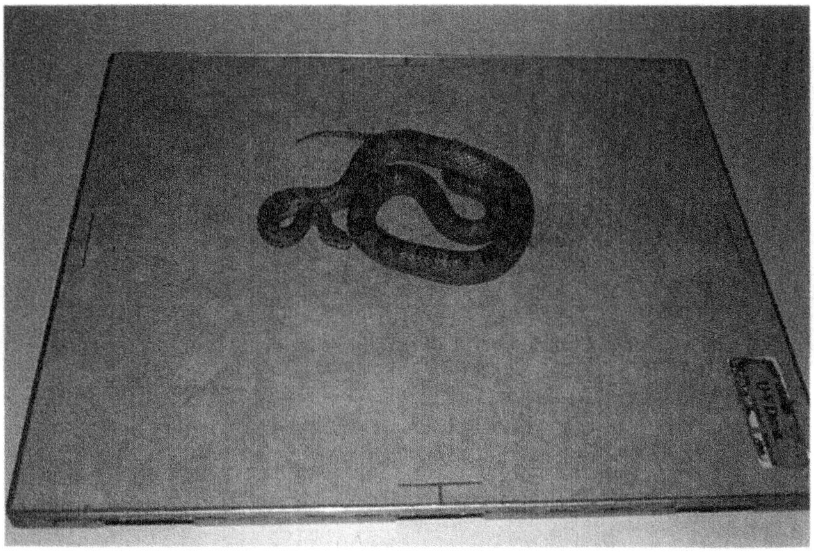

FIG. 13-32 Dorsoventral positioning of snake directly on cassette.

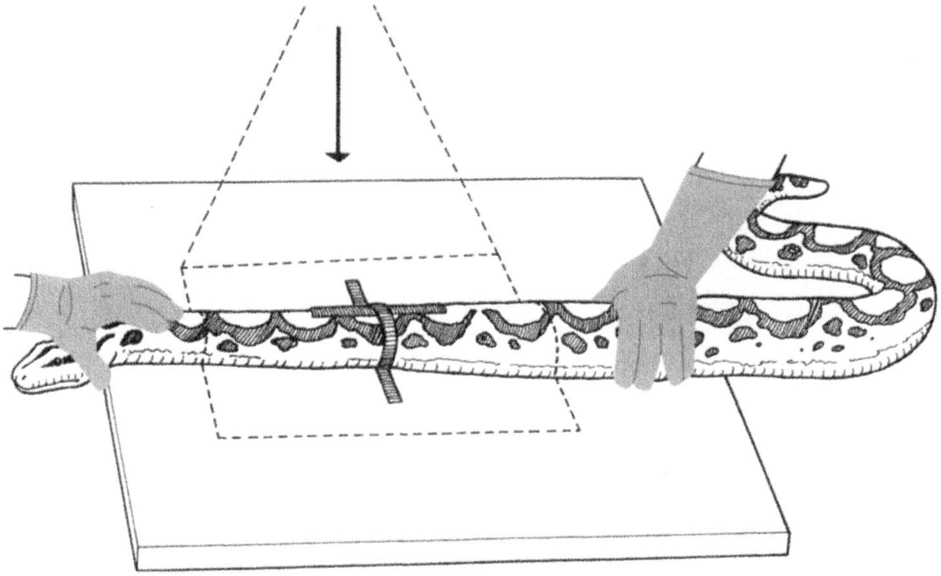

FIG. 13-33 Manual dorsoventral positioning of snake.

Another option for dorsoventral snake radiography is the use of a radiolucent tube. Gently guide the snake into the tube; most snakes crawl in on their own. The ends of the tube can then be plugged with porous corks to prevent escape. Place the tube directly on the cassette, and tape to prevent rolling. Center the primary beam on the midsection of the snake and collimate to include the entire body. Remember to add 2 to 4 kVp to the measurement to compensate for the tube thickness.

> For snakes, a piece of rolled film, (unexposed but developed) can be used in place of a Plexiglas tube.

If the snake is too long to fit completely inside the radiolucent tube, placing the snake partially inside the tube and radiographing it in sections can produce several different images (Figures 13-34 and 13-35).

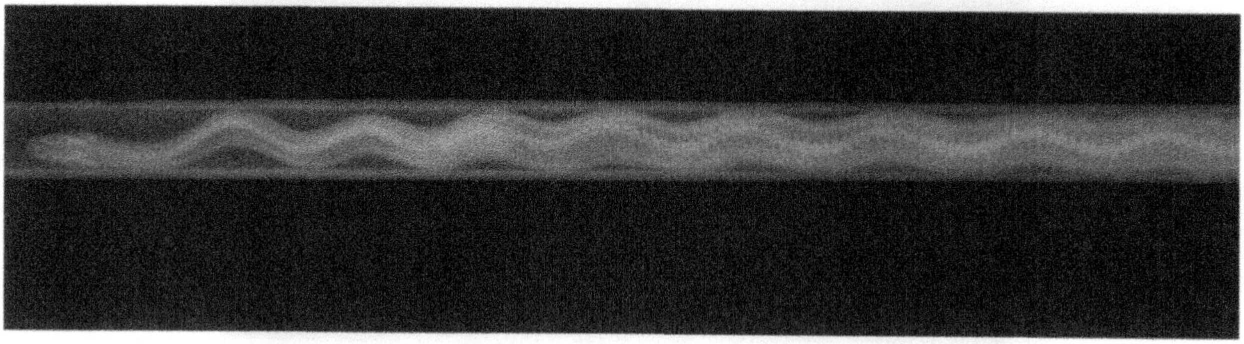

FIG. 13-34 Dorsoventral radiograph of snake in radiolucent Plexiglas tube.

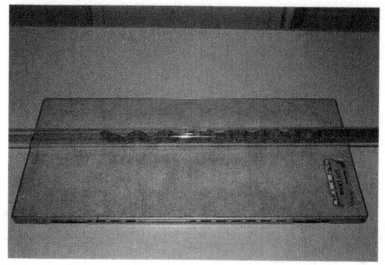

FIG. 13-35 Dorsoventral positioning of snake in radiolucent Plexiglas tube.

Unrestrained snakes do not coil or lie stretched in a "natural" ventrodorsal position. If this is the desired view, some form of manual, physical, or chemical restraint is essential. The snake can be held or placed inside a radiolucent tube in ventrodorsal position to be radiographed.

Entire body lateral view

While holding the base of the skull with one gloved hand and the distal portion of the tail with the other, gently stretch the snake across the cassette. Using a tabletop technique, measure over the highest point of the girth, center over the midsection of the snake, and collimate to include all but the head. Nonscreen film produces excellent detail, but it should be used on only quiet, sedate snakes because the absence of movement is essential.

> Use nonscreen film with only quiet, docile snakes, in which the likelihood of movement is minimal.

Many snakes are too long for even the largest cassettes; therefore, sectional views must be taken. A gowned and gloved assistant gently stretches the patient across the cassette. Starting at the proximal end, work distally until all portions of the snake are radiographed. Be sure to number and label each section in sequence for accurate identification of all views.

An additional option for lateral snake radiography is the use of a radiolucent Plexiglas tube. For small patients coax the snake into the tube (most crawl in on their own) and plug both ends with porous corks. Place the tube directly on the cassette, and turn the snake laterally. Using a tabletop method, center the primary beam on the snake's midsection and collimate to include the entire body.

For larger snakes cover only one end of the radiolucent tube when radiographing the head and upper body section. For the other sections slide the tube over the area of interest while a gowned and gloved assistant restrains the snake in a lateral position (Figure 13-36).

Turtle and Tortoise Radiography

Organ systems that are readily palpable in mammals are impossible to palpate in turtles and tortoises. The presence of a thick, bony shell can make even a radiographic examination challenging.

Turtles and tortoises are calm and docile creatures requiring minimal restraint. Manual restraint is not practical, because whole body radiographs are preferred and gloved hands would be exposed to the primary beam. Physical restraint is most often used to restrict movement. Some physical restraint devices include tape, cardboard boxes, radiolucent Plexiglas containers, foam pads, and wooden blocks. The use of chemical restraint is uncommon, except in the case of an uncooperative or aggressive snapping turtle.

Rapid screens using higher mAs and lower kVp work well, but nonscreen film or detail cassettes may be preferred because patient movement is unlikely. In addition, high detail is essential for imaging smaller turtles and tortoises.

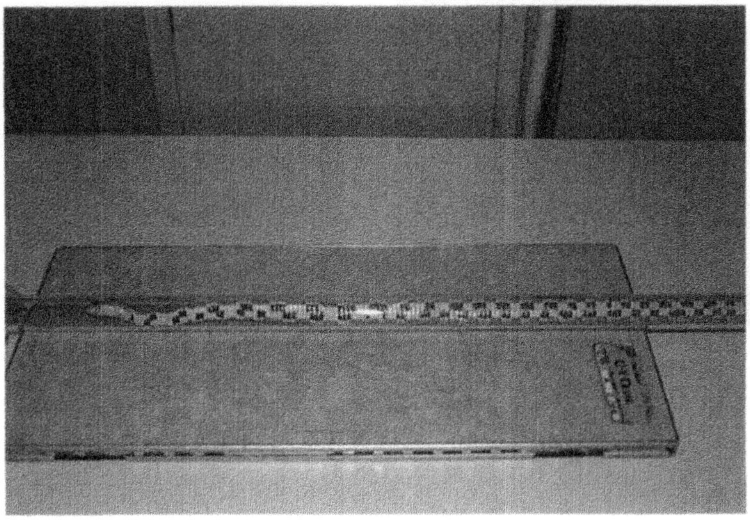

FIG. 13-36 Lateral positioning of snake in radiolucent Plexiglas tube.

Entire body dorsoventral-ventrodorsal view

Place the turtle or tortoise in dorsal recumbency for a moment to induce disorientation. Just before making the exposure, turn the patient back over into ventral recumbency and place the patient directly on the cassette. The turtle or tortoise momentarily extends its head, legs, and tail until it becomes reoriented. Make the exposure during this time to prevent superimposition of the extremities over the thorax and abdomen. Focus the primary beam over the center of the shell and collimate to include the entire body (Figures 13-37 and 13-38). For ventrodorsal views lay the patient in ventrodorsal position directly on the cassette, and tape to secure (Figure 13-39).

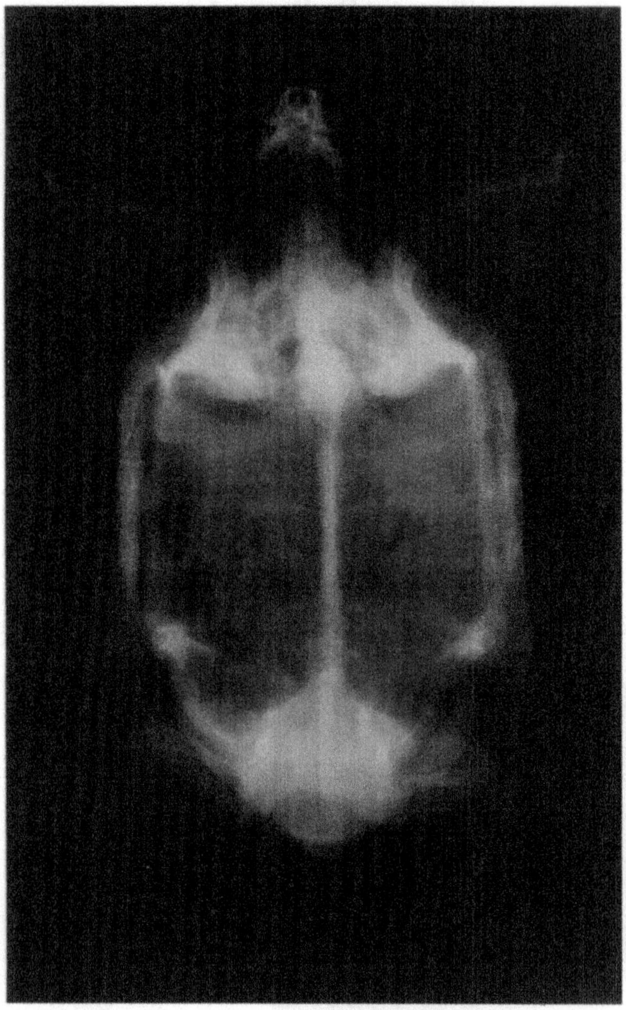

FIG. 13-37 Dorsoventral radiograph of turtle.

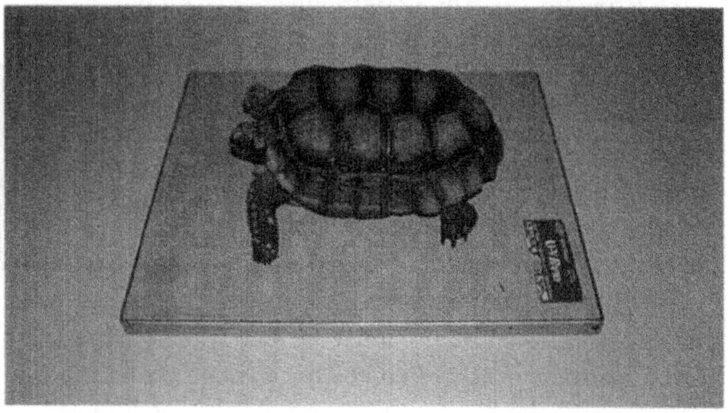

FIG. 13-38 Dorsoventral positioning of turtle.

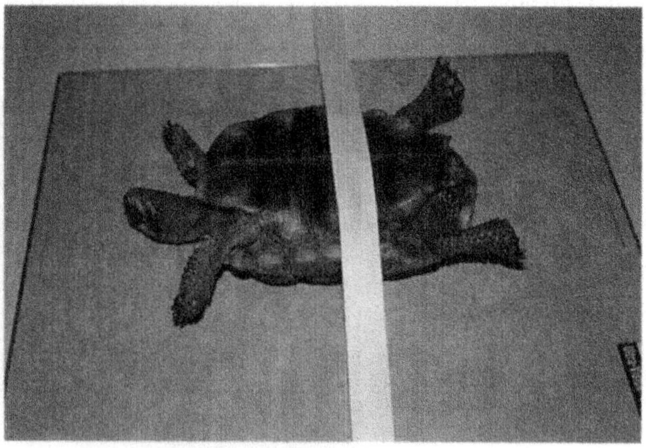

FIG. 13-39 Ventrodorsal positioning of turtle.

Entire body lateral view

Two positioning methods can be used when producing lateral radiographs of a turtle or tortoise. For the first view tape the turtle or tortoise to a thick wooden or foam block with the ventral side of the patient facing toward the block. Place the cassette on the table and the lateral side of the turtle and block perpendicular to the table, directly on the cassette. Direct the primary beam vertically so that it enters the patient's lateral side. Center over the turtle's midsection and collimate to include the entire body (Figures 13-40 and 13-41).

A second positioning option involves the use of an x-ray machine that can project the primary beam horizontally. Tape the turtle or tortoise to the top of a foam pad and place on the x-ray table. Position the cassette perpendicular to the table and secure directly against the turtle's lateral side. Angle the tube head parallel to the table surface and direct it toward the patient's lateral side. Center the primary beam on the midsection of the body and collimate to include the whole turtle (Figure 13-42).

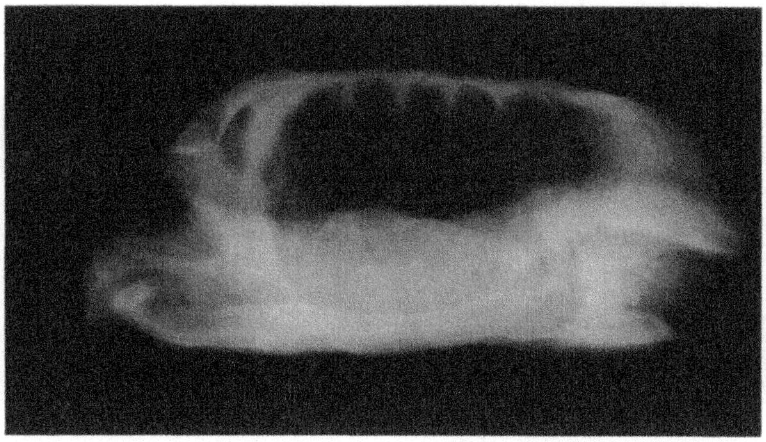

FIG. 13-40 Vertical beam lateral radiograph of turtle.

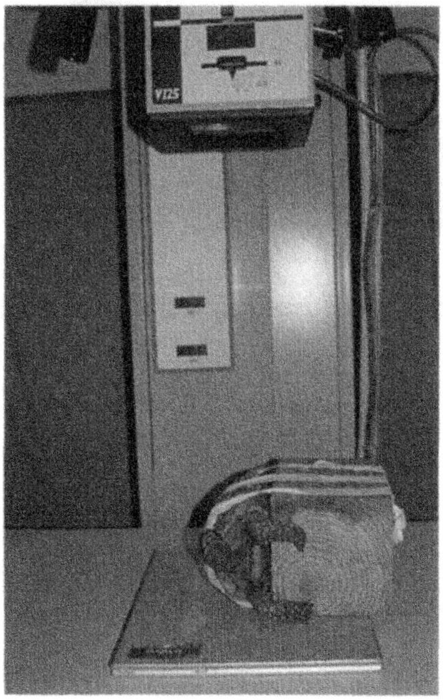

FIG. 13-41 Vertical beam lateral positioning of turtle.

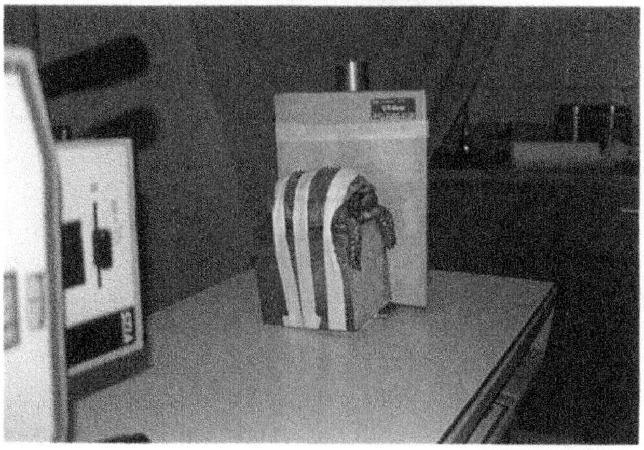

FIG. 13-42 Horizontal beam lateral positioning of turtle.

Entire body craniocaudal view

Two positioning options are available for the craniocaudal view. For the first option tape the turtle or tortoise to a thick foam pad or wooden block and turn vertically so that the patient is perpendicular to the table. Place the turtle and block on top of a cassette so that the most caudal portion of the shell rests on the cassette and the cranial aspect faces the tube head. Direct the primary beam vertically from the head through to the tail. Center the beam in the middle of the head and collimate to include the whole body (Figures 13-43 and 13-44). Occasionally, it is necessary to place a piece of tape gently across the turtle's nose to prevent the superimposition of the head across the lung field (Figure 13-45).

> Use adhesive tape across a turtle's nose if the head is in the path of the beam. Use only cloth or paper, not adhesive, tape on birds.

The second view involves the use of a horizontal beam method. Tape the ventral aspect of the tortoise to the top of a foam pad and place the tortoise and pad on the x-ray table. Position the cassette perpendicular to the table and directly behind the caudal aspect of the patient. Direct the primary beam horizontally toward the cranial aspect of the tortoise from the head through the tail. Center the beam in the middle of the head and collimate to include the entire body (Figure 13-46).

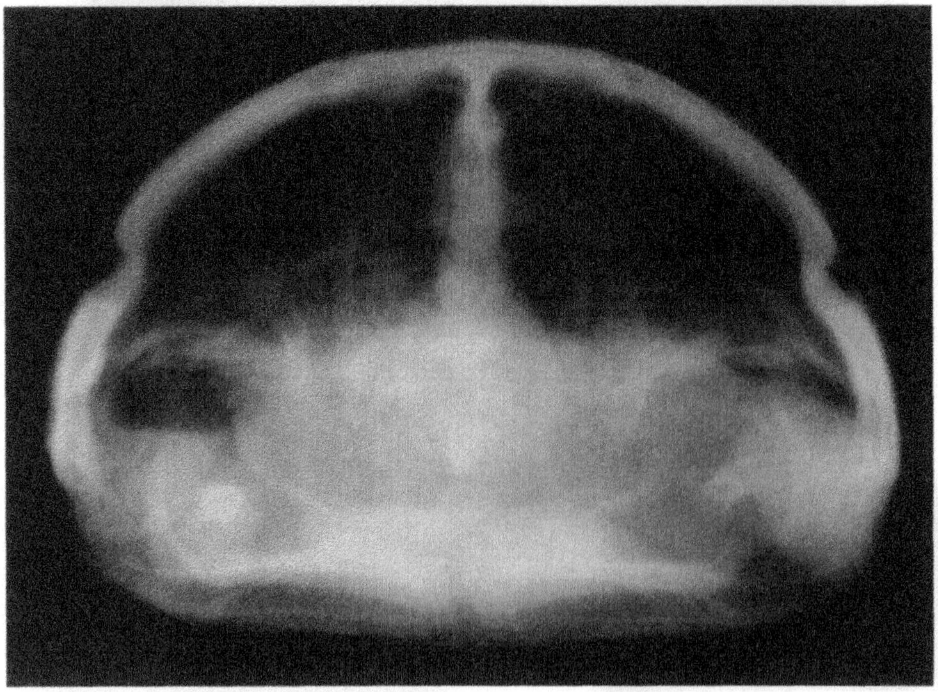

FIG. 13-43 Vertical beam craniocaudal radiograph of turtle.

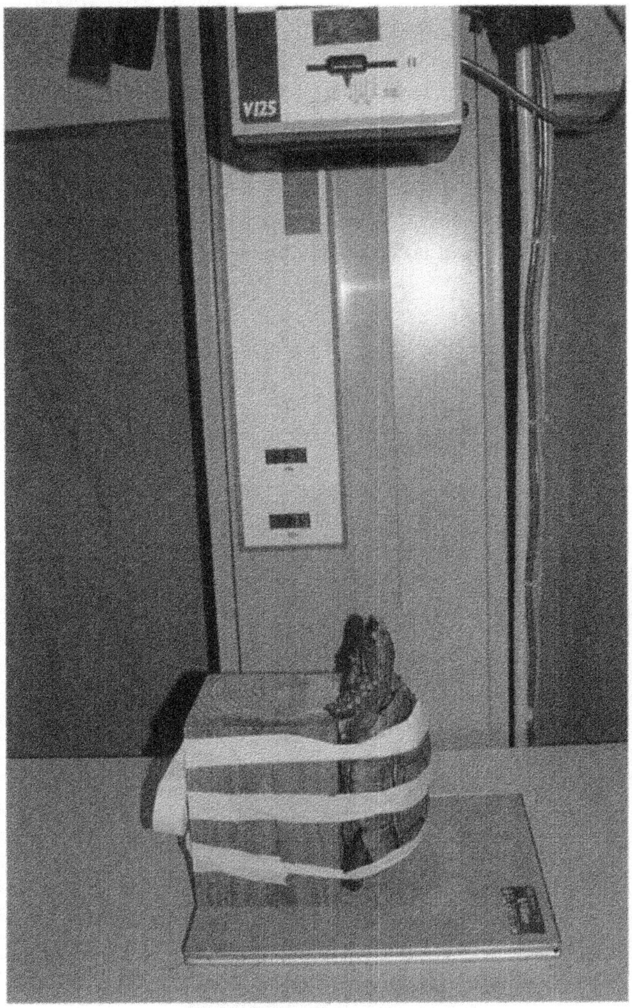

FIG. 13-44 Vertical beam craniocaudal positioning of turtle.

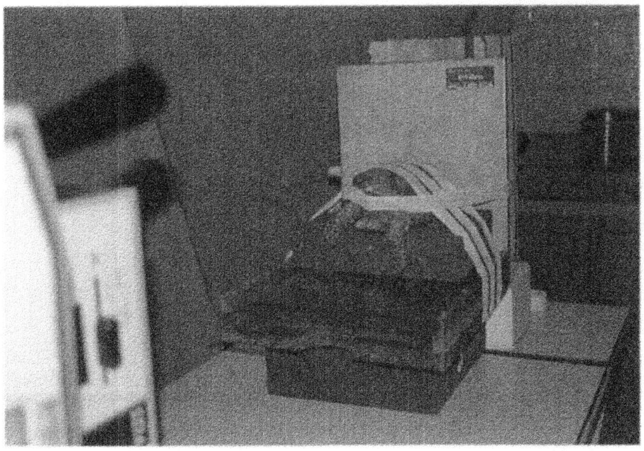

FIG. 13-45 Tape across nose of turtle to prevent superimposition of head.

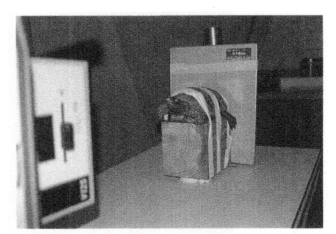

FIG. 13-46 Horizontal beam craniocaudal positioning of turtle.

Avian Radiography

Avian patients present some of the most interesting challenges in exotic radiography. Any conscious bird can struggle to the point of inducing self-trauma, so some form of chemical restraint is almost always essential. Manual restraint is not possible in most cases because whole body radiographs are preferred. Physical restraint devices that can be used include paper tape (e.g., 3M MicroPore), soft nylon or cotton ropes, Plexiglas plates, sheets of film cardboard, and intravenous (IV) tubing. Keep in mind that these devices can only be used in combination with chemical restraint (Figure 13-47).

Add 2 to 4 kVp to avian measurements when using film cardboard or a Plexiglas sheet over the cassette.

For a frightened, injured, or critically ill bird for which chemical restraint is not warranted, covering the head can sometimes be successful in calming the patient. When manually restraining a critical avian patient, the bird can be gently grasped by the mandibular articulation and tape stirrups attached to the feet. Do not grasp around the neck, which can cause tracheal collapse. The wings can then be secured with paper tape.

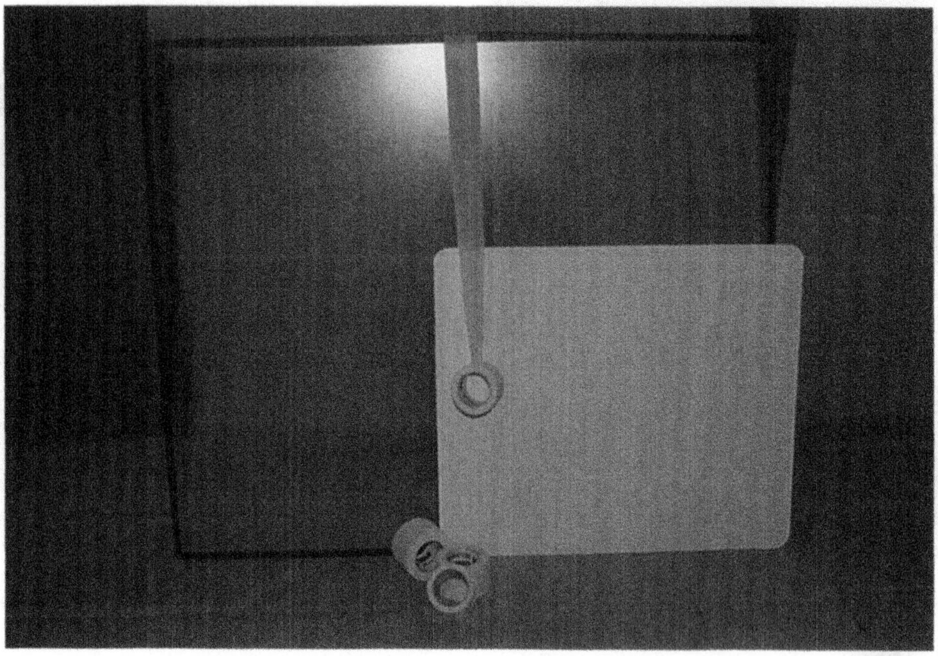

FIG. 13-47 Avian positioning aids and restraint devices.

Entire Body Ventrodorsal View

Lay the properly restrained patient in dorsal recumbency, directly on the surface of a radiolucent Plexiglas plate. A piece of film cardboard can also be used if working with small species such as finches, canaries, or cockatiels. Make sure the keel (sternum) is superimposed over the spine.

> For lateral avian views, the left wings and limbs are positioned caudally to the right wings and limbs.

Using specially designed paper tape, secure the bird to the radiolucent plate or cardboard sheet beginning with the head. Gently extend the head and neck cranially and place the tape across the mandibular articulation at the base of the skull. Do not tape too tightly, since this could collapse the trachea and compromise the patient's airway. Fully extend each wing by abducting laterally and taping to the Plexiglas or cardboard surface. Tape next to the body, across the humerus but not across the radius-ulna, to help prevent the possibility of wing fracture should the patient unexpectedly awake and begin struggling.

Caudally extend the limbs symmetrically and tape each leg individually, across the tarsometatarsal bones, securing them to the Plexiglas or cardboard. The tail can also be taped if necessary. Place the radiolucent or cardboard sheet on top of the cassette. Measure the bird across the keel, center the primary beam on the sternum, and collimate to include the entire body (Figures 13-48 and 13-49).

Another ventrodorsal option for securing an avian patient to a radiolucent Plexiglas plate is to devise what is commonly known as a "bird guillotine." A small dog or cat collar is attached to one end of the plate, and two small notches are cut out on the opposite edge. The bird's neck is placed in the collar and gently secured across the mandibular articulation. IV tubing is tied around the tarsometatarsal area, and the legs are extended caudally. The tubing is then pulled into the notches, and knots are tied in the tubes to prevent slipping. Lay the radiolucent plate on top of the cassette and measure across the keel. Center the primary beam on the sternum and collimate to include the whole body.

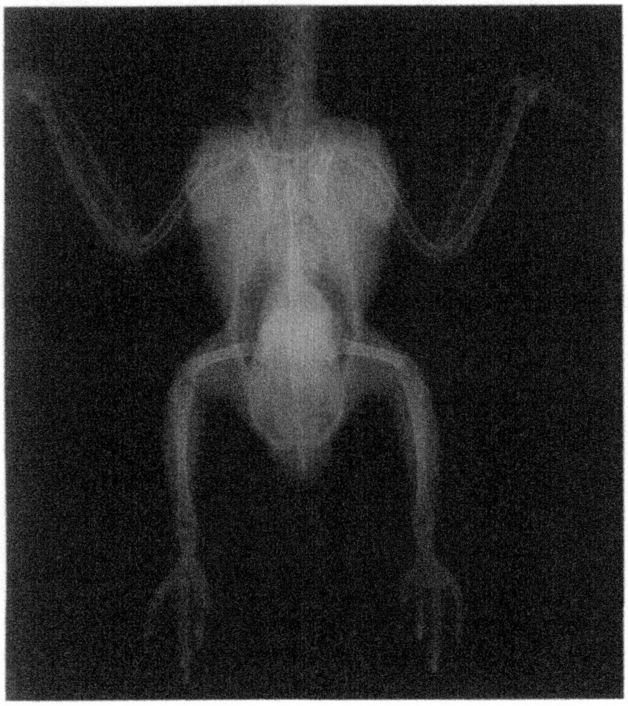

FIG. 13-48 Ventrodorsal radiograph of bird.

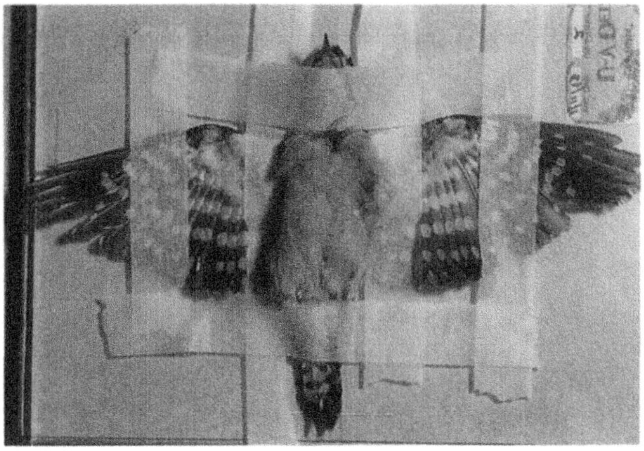

FIG. 13-49 Ventrodorsal positioning of bird.

Craniocaudal-Caudocranial Limb View

Craniocaudal and caudocranial appendicular skeletal radiographs may be desired for larger species of birds when fractures are suspected. Using a bird guillotine with IV tubing, secure the bird to a large, radiolucent Plexiglas plate and place it on a cassette, centering on only the area of interest. Focus the primary beam on this area and collimate accordingly. The limb can also be taped directly to the cassette, without the use of a Plexiglas plate. A detail cassette and tabletop bone technique can be used to produce good-quality skeletal radiographs, but nonscreen film also yields excellent bone detail.

When IV tubing and paper tape are not strong enough to secure particularly large bird species, such as trumpeter swans, peacocks, turkeys, and eagles, manual restraint by a gowned and gloved assistant can be used. If a distal limb fracture is suspected, the restrainer can place the limb directly on the cassette in a craniocaudal or caudocranial position. A gloved hand placed directly behind the hock can restrain the limb for the exposure. If a more proximal limb view is desired, adhesive tape or soft nylon or cotton rope can be gently secured to the distal limb, just proximal to the digits. The tape or rope can then be attached or tied to the x-ray table. If necessary, a gowned and gloved restrainer can carefully extend the limb to decrease "obliquing," which can produce the truest caudocranial-craniocaudal or craniocaudal-caudocranial image. Keep in mind that chemical restraint or general anesthesia is almost always required for birds when performing these types of radiographic procedures (Figure 13-50).

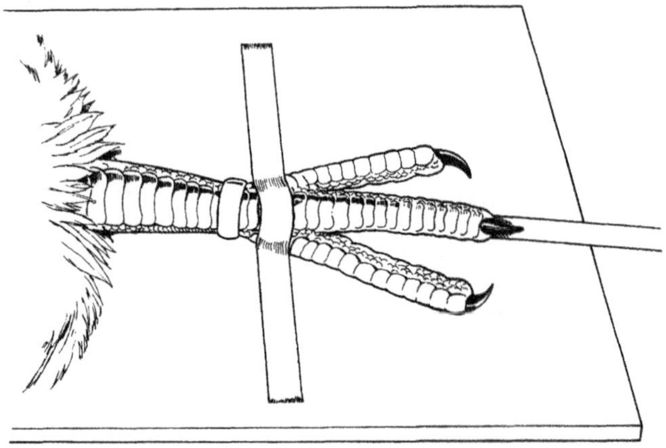

FIG. 13-50 Craniocaudal positioning of avian limb.

Entire Body Lateral View

Lay the restrained avian patient directly on a radiolucent or cardboard sheet in right lateral recumbency. Secure the bird's head to the sheet with paper tape by taping across the neck at the base of the skull. Do not tape too tightly because this could cause tracheal collapse. Abduct the wings dorsally, fully extending them above the dorsal spine, with the *down* (right) wing cranial to the *up* (left) wing. Tape the down wing first, followed by the up wing. Secure the wings across the humerus close to the body, not across the radius-ulna, to reduce the possibility of wing fracture in the event the patient awakens and struggles during the procedure. Extend the limbs ventral and caudal to the keel, and position the *dependent* (right) limb cranially to the *contralateral* (left) limb. Additional tape can be used to secure the body and tail if necessary.

Place the bird and the radiolucent plate directly on the cassette. Center the primary beam over the keel (sternum) and collimate to include the entire body (Figures 13-51 and 13-52).

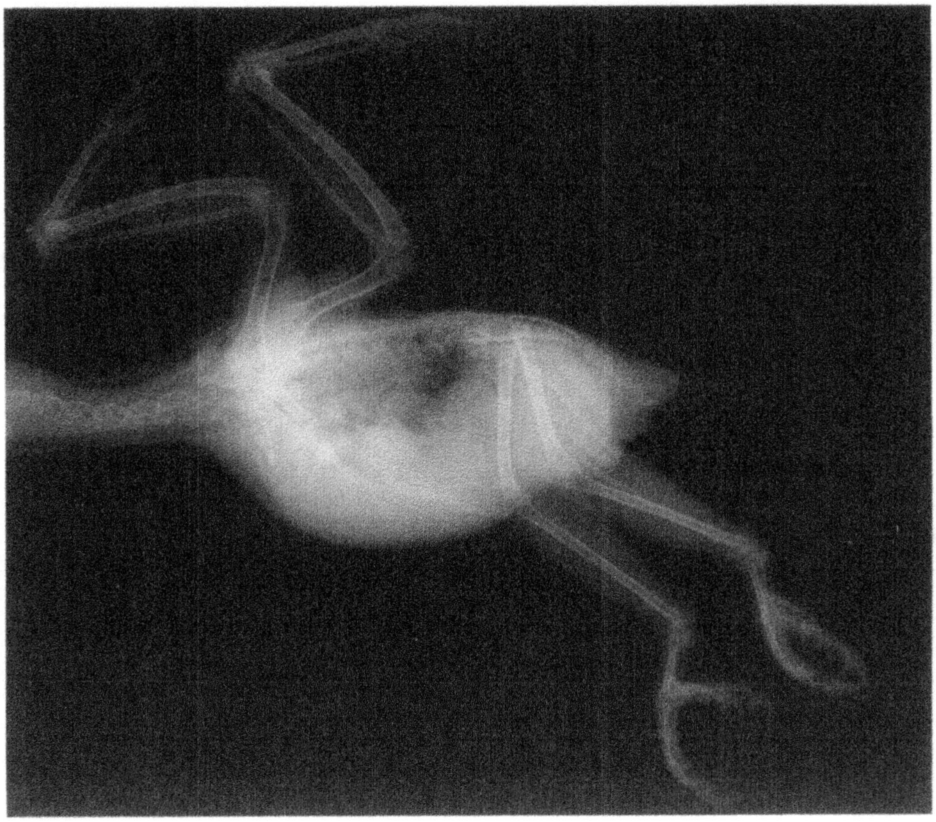

FIG. 13-51 Lateral radiograph of bird.

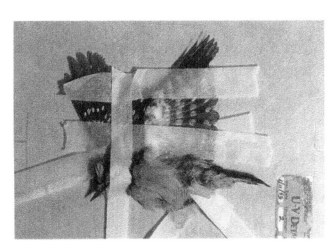

FIG. 13-52 Lateral positioning of bird.

Lateral Limb View

Lateral appendicular skeletal views may be required for larger avian species when a fracture is suspected. Using a detail cassette and tabletop bone technique, secure the area of interest to a radiolucent plate and position this area on top of the cassette. Focus the primary beam on the center of interest and collimate accordingly.

For the largest avian species, tape only the area of interest directly to the cassette. Focus the primary beam on that area, measuring over the highest point, and collimate. If paper tape will not adequately restrain the patient, manual restraint by a gowned and gloved assistant may be required. If a distal limb is to be imaged, the restrainer can place a gloved hand directly behind the patient's hock to hold the limb in a true lateral position. When a proximal limb fracture is suspected, adhesive tape or soft rope can be gently secured to the distal limb, just proximal to the digits. The tape or rope can then be attached or tied to the x-ray table. If needed, a gowned and gloved restrainer can carefully extend the limb to lessen obliquing and produce the truest lateral image. Chemical restraint or general anesthesia is a necessity when producing these types of views (Figure 13-53).

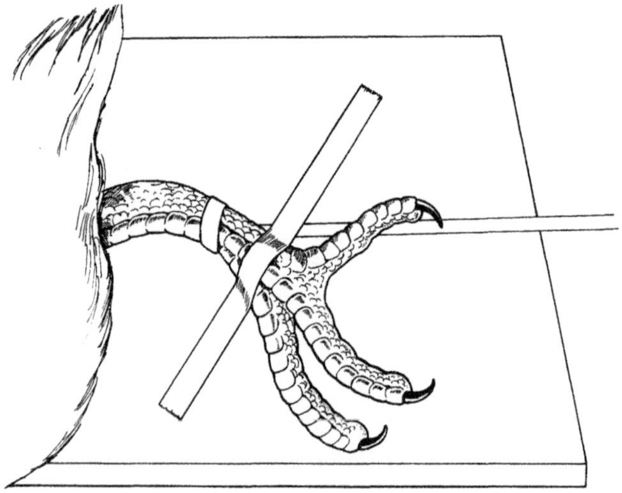

FIG. 13-53 Lateral positioning of avian limb.

Recommended Reading

Douglas SW et al: *Principles of veterinary radiography*, ed 4, London, 1987, Bailliere Tindall.

Lavin LM: *Radiography in veterinary technology*, Philadelphia, 1994, Saunders.

Rosenthal KL: *Practical exotic animal medicine*, Trenton, NJ, 1997, Veterinary Learning Systems.

Rubel GA et al: *Atlas of diagnostic radiology of exotic pets*, Philadelphia, 1991, Saunders.

14

Large Animal Radiography

CHERYL HURD

CHAPTER OBJECTIVES

- State the importance of proper hoof preparation before any view where the primary beam penetrates the hoof wall.
- Explain the purpose of packing the foot for any image where the primary beam is angled through the hoof wall.
- Define the terminology used for positioning in radiographic procedures.
- List the oblique projections and state how to label them.
- Read the written description, look at the line drawing, and produce a diagnostic radiograph for any area of interest.

The techniques described in this chapter are focused on positioning of horses. However, they are easily adapted to cattle, sheep, goats, and pigs. The descriptions are limited to the extremities because of the limited capability of portable or mobile x-ray machines. Views involving the skull, pelvis, and thorax require a machine with high-milliamperage (high-mA) capabilities and are beyond the scope of this text.

As with small animals, patient positioning is important for accomplishing diagnostic radiographs in large animals. The horse should be positioned squarely so that weight is evenly distributed on each limb. If the weight is not evenly distributed, the joint spaces may be inaccurately interpreted.

> To aid in obtaining a diagnostic radiograph, the horse must be standing squarely.

Radiographic Aids

Radiographic aids for large animal radiography can be custom made or made from items found around a farm.

Wooden Blocks

Wooden blocks are necessary to obtain certain positioning. The block should be constructed so that it is solid and large enough for the entire hoof to fit on comfortably. The foot must be elevated high enough so that when the distal phalanx is imaged, the cassette can be placed distal to the palmar or plantar surface of the hoof. When using the blocks to elevate the foot, the contralateral limb should also be elevated to the same height to ensure proper weight distribution.

Cassette Tunnel

The cassette tunnel is another aid that can be made (Figure 14-1). The cassette tunnel, a protective sleeve made of a radiolucent material such as Plexiglas, can withstand a horse's weight. Carbon sandpaper can be glued to the surface of the tunnel to prevent the hoof from slipping.

Navicular Box

A navicular box is useful when imaging the distal sesamoid bone (Figure 14-2). It is a box constructed to support the hoof in a position so that the dorsal aspect of the hoof is perpendicular to the floor and the palmar or plantar surface is parallel to the cassette. The part of the box supporting the hoof is made of Plexiglas, and the image is made through this surface.

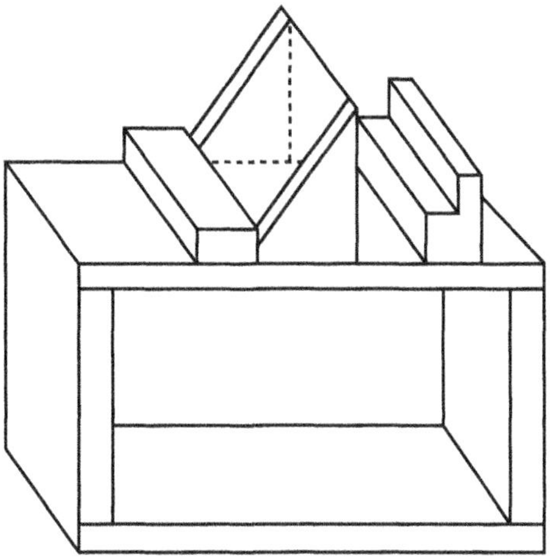

FIG. 14-2 Navicular box. (See also Figure 14-40.)

Cassette Holder

A cassette holder is an important tool for large animal radiography. By placing the cassette in this handle, the person holding the cassette can be positioned away from the animal and the primary beam. This greatly decreases the radiation exposure dose (Figure 14-3).

> The cassette should never be handheld during exposure.

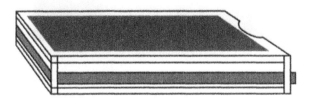

FIG. 14-1 Cassette tunnel.

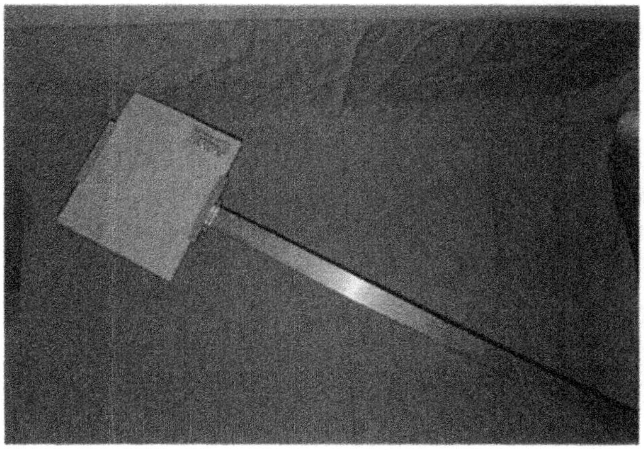

FIG. 14-3 Cassette holder.

Carpal Views

For standard radiographs of the carpus, position the horse squarely so that both feet are together and the leg being imaged is perpendicular to the ground (Figure 14-4).

Dorsopalmar View

Hold the cassette against the palmar aspect of the carpus. Position the primary beam parallel to the floor and centered on the middle of the carpal joint. The image should include the area from distal radius to proximal metacarpus. A true dorsopalmar view is achieved when the intercarpal space between the radial and the intermediate carpal bones has no other bone superimposed (Figures 14-4, *A*, and 14-5).

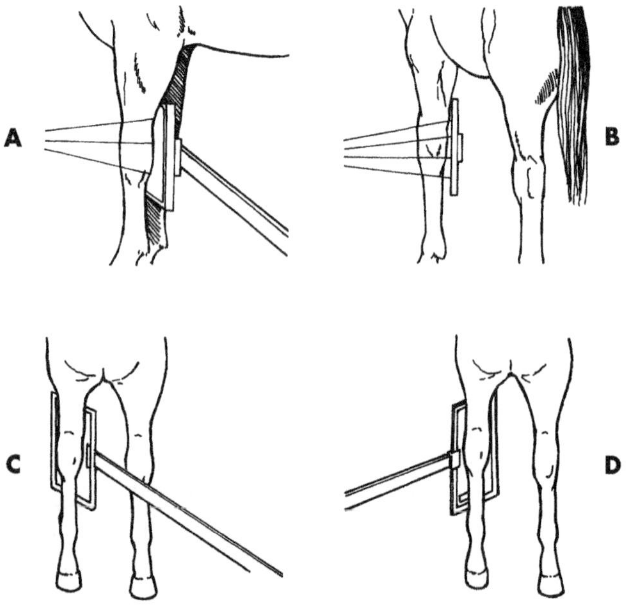

FIG. 14-4 Positioning for the standard projections of the carpus. **A,** Dorsopalmar; **B,** lateromedial; **C,** dorsolateral-palmaromedial; **D,** dorsomedial-palmarolateral.

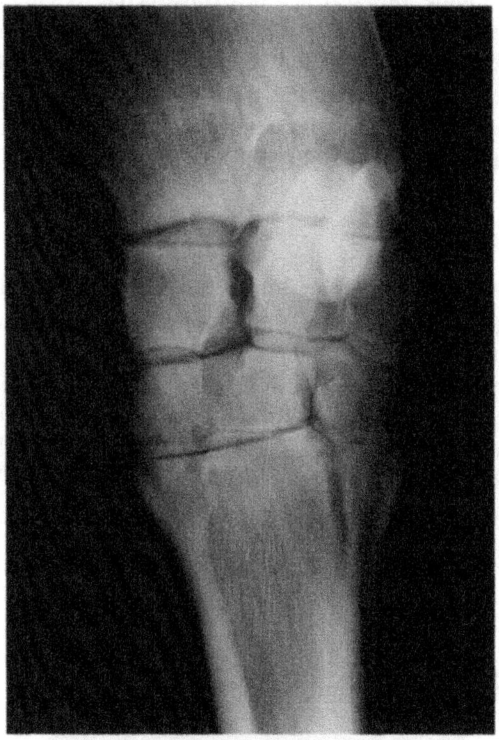

FIG. 14-5 Dorsopalmar projection of the carpus.

Lateromedial View

Hold the cassette against the medial aspect of the leg. Position the primary beam parallel to the floor and centered on the middle of the carpal joint. The image should include the area from distal radius to proximal metacarpus. A true lateromedial view is achieved when all the carpal bones are completely superimposed over one another. This allows the dorsal surface of the carpus to be viewed (Figures 14-4, *B*, and 14-6).

Dorsolateral-Palmaromedial Oblique View

Hold the cassette against the palmaromedial aspect of the leg. Position the primary beam parallel to the floor and centered on the middle of the carpal joint, 30 degrees off true lateromedial projection. The image should include the area from distal radius to proximal metacarpus. This oblique projection allows a clear view of the dorsomedial and palmarolateral surfaces of the carpal bones (Figures 14-4, *C*, and 14-7).

> Oblique views for the carpus are 30 degrees off true lateromedial or mediolateral position.

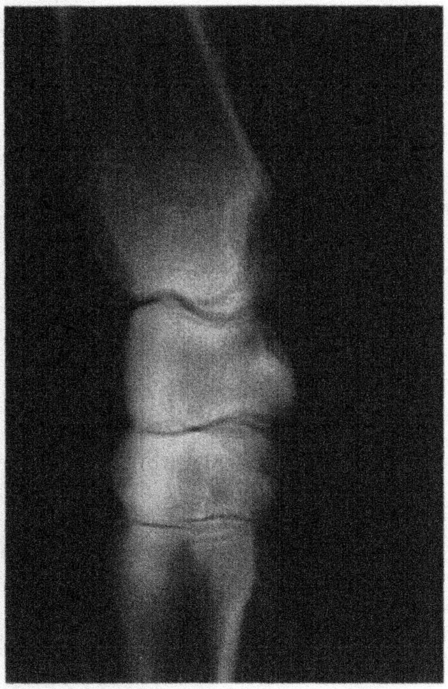

FIG. 14-6 Lateromedial projection of the carpus.

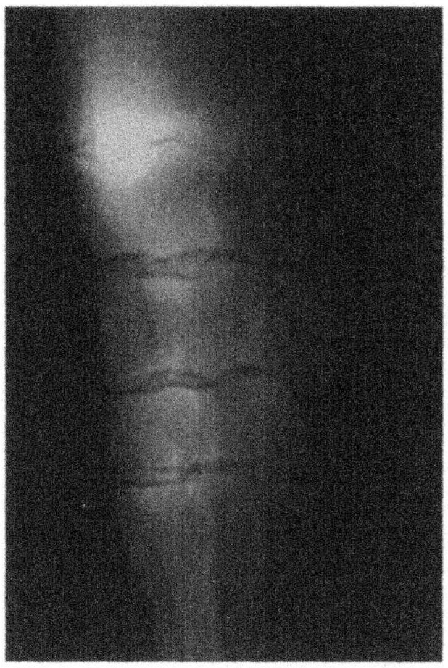

FIG. 14-7 Dorsolateral-palmaromedial projection of the carpus.

Dorsomedial-Palmarolateral Oblique View

Hold the cassette against the palmarolateral aspect of the leg. Position the primary beam parallel to the floor and centered on the middle of the carpal joint, 30 degrees off true mediolateral projection. The image should include the area from distal radius to the proximal metacarpus. This oblique projection allows a clear view of the dorsolateral and palmaromedial surfaces of the carpal bones (Figures 14-4, *D*, and 14-8).

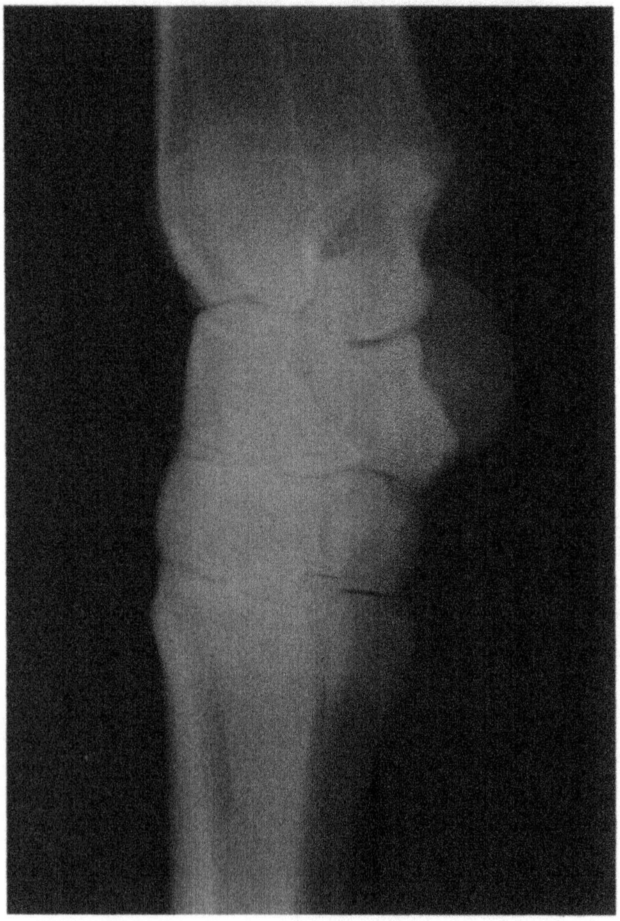

FIG. 14-8 Dorsomedial-palmarolateral projection of the carpus.

Flexed Lateromedial View

Flex the limb approximately 60 degrees, keeping the metacarpus parallel and the radius perpendicular to the ground. Hold the cassette against the medial surface of the carpal joint. It is important that the horse stands squarely on the remaining three limbs, allowing the flexed limb to be positioned perpendicular to the ground. Position the primary beam parallel to the floor, and center it on the space between the proximal and distal rows of carpal bones so that the interarticular spaces can be visualized (Figures 14-9, *C,* and 14-10).

When positioning for a flexed lateral carpus, keep the metacarpus parallel to the floor and the radius perpendicular to the floor

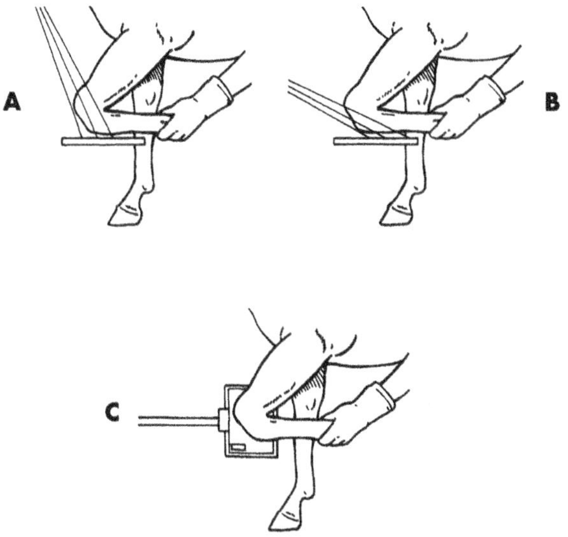

FIG. 14-9 Positioning for additional projections of the carpus. **A,** Dorsoproximal 60 degree-dorsodistal; **B,** dorsoproximal 20 degree-dorsodistal; **C,** flexed lateromedial.

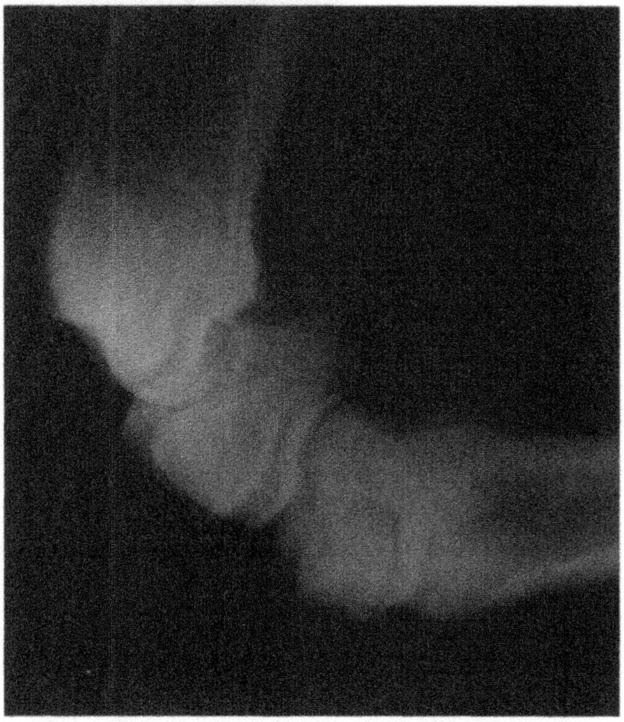

FIG. 14-10 Flexed lateromedial projection of the carpus.

Dorsoproximal 60 Degree-Dorsodistal Oblique View

Flex the limb, pushing the carpal joint cranially. Place the cassette on the dorsodistal aspect of the limb and parallel to the floor. Angle the primary beam 60 degrees in a proximal-to-distal direction, centering on the carpal joint. Because the cassette is not truly perpendicular to the primary beam, some elongation of the carpal joint occurs. This view is used to visualize the *proximal* row of carpal bones (Figures 14-9, *A*, and 14-11).

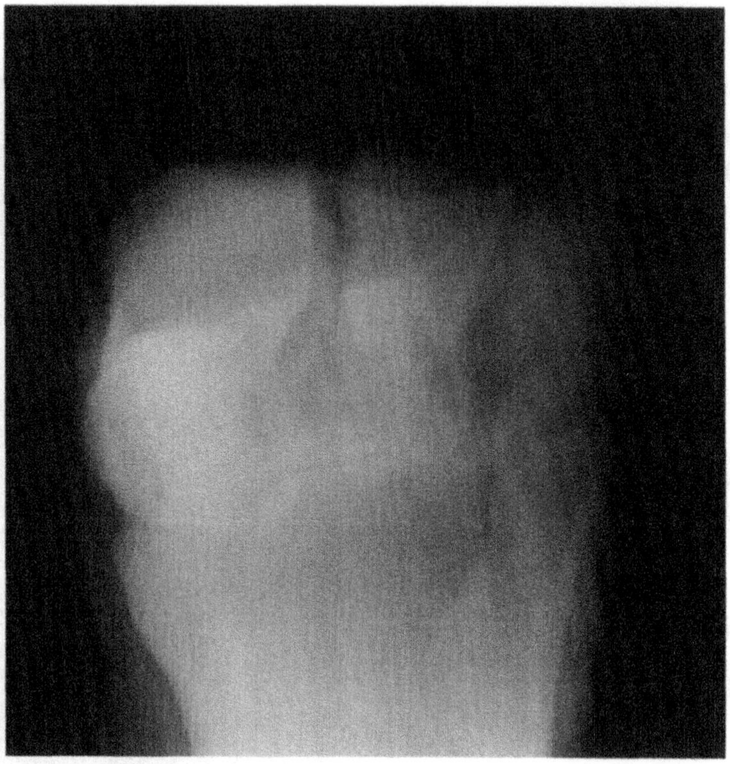

FIG. 14-11 Dorsoproximal 60 degree-dorsodistal projection of the proximal row of carpal bones.

Dorsoproximal 20 Degree-Dorsodistal Oblique View

Flex the limb, pushing slightly cranial and keeping the metacarpus parallel to the ground. Place the cassette on the dorsodistal aspect of the limb and parallel to the floor. Angle the primary beam 20 degrees in a proximal-to-distal direction, centering on the carpal joint. Because the cassette is not truly perpendicular to the primary beam, some elongation of the carpal joint occurs. This view is used to visualize the *distal* row of carpal bones (Figures 14-9, *B*, and 14-12).

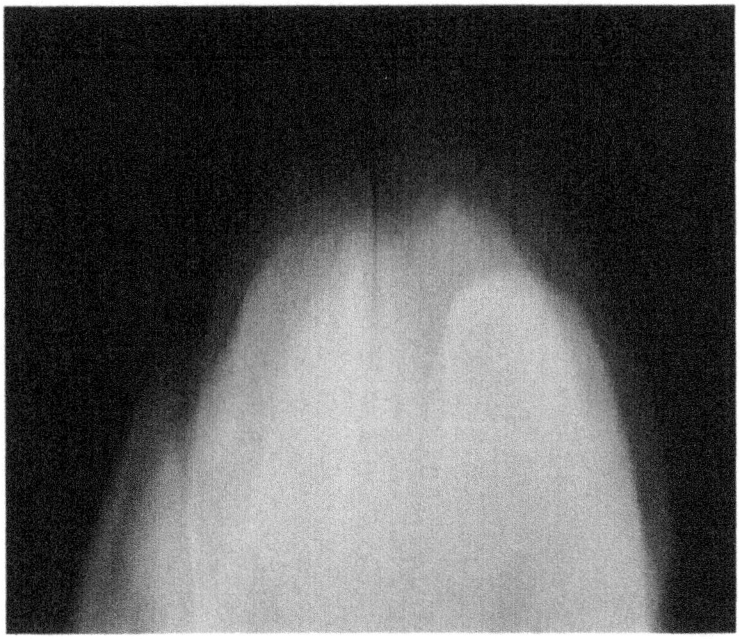

FIG. 14-12 Dorsoproximal 20 degree-dorsodistal projection of the distal row of carpal bones.

Tarsal Views

For standard radiographs of the tarsus, position the horse with its weight evenly distributed on all four legs. Position the limb so that the metatarsus is perpendicular to the ground (Figure 14-13).

Dorsoplantar View

Position the horse so that the limb of interest has a slight lateral rotation, allowing the primary beam to travel in a true dorsoplantar direction. If the horse is standing squarely, its body can obstruct the positioning of the x-ray tube. Hold the cassette on the plantar surface of the tarsal joint. Position the primary beam parallel to the floor and centered on the proximal intertarsal space. The image should include the area from distal tibia to proximal metatarsus (Figures 14-13, *A*, and 14-14).

When positioning the tarsus for a dorsoplantar view, position the limb of interest with a slight lateral rotation. This allows the x-ray tube to be positioned without interference from the horse's body.

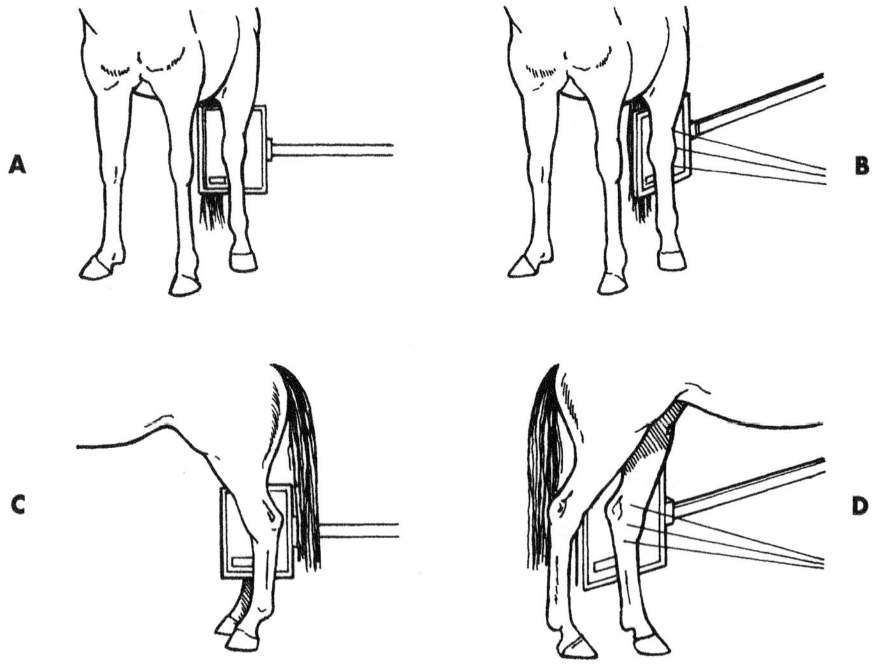

FIG. 14-13 Positioning for standard projections of the tarsus. **A,** Dorsoplantar; **B,** dorsolateral-plantaromedial; **C,** lateromedial; **D,** dorsomedial-plantarolateral.

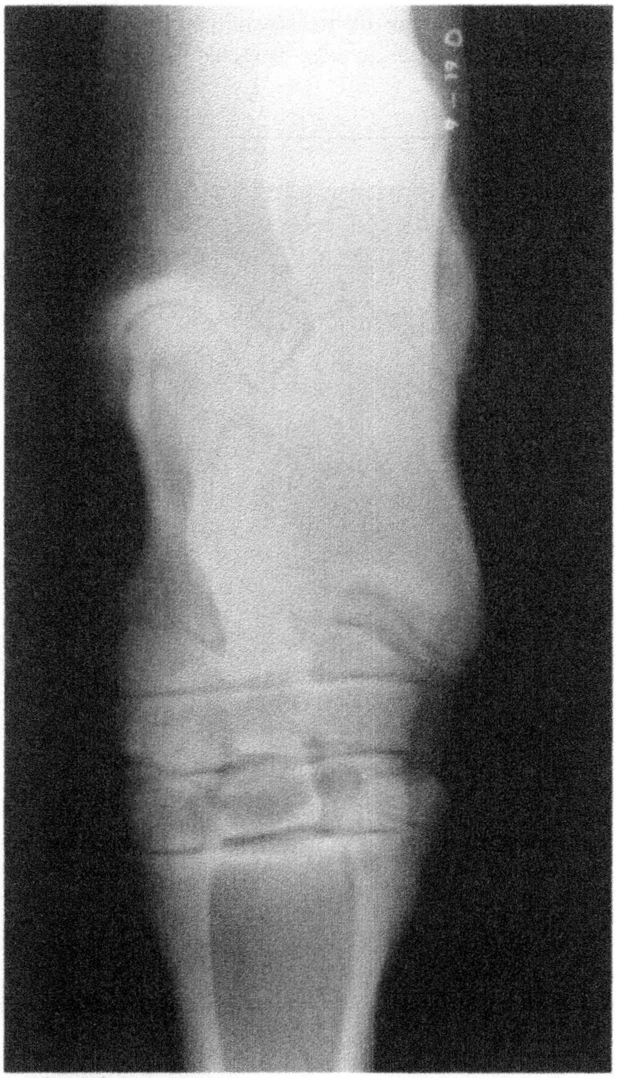

FIG. 14-14 Dorsoplantar projection of the tarsal joint.

Lateromedial View

Place the cassette on the medial surface of the tarsal joint. Position the primary beam parallel to the floor and centered on the proximal intertarsal joint. The image should include the area from distal tibia to proximal metatarsus. A true lateromedial view shows the trochlea of the talus superimposed so that only one trochlear ridge is visible (Figures 14-13, *C*, and 14-15).

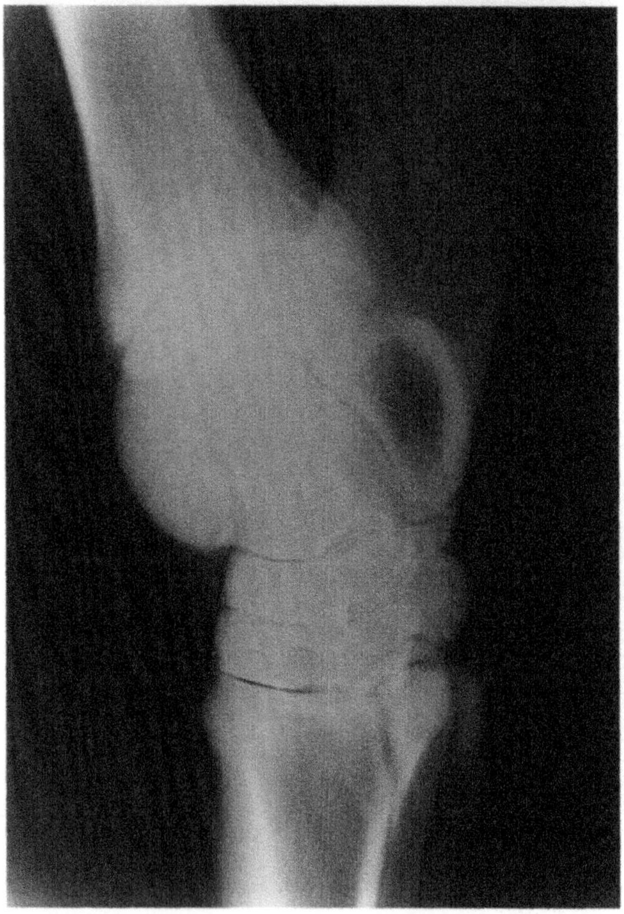

FIG. 14-15 Lateromedial projection of the tarsal joint.

Dorsolateral-Plantaromedial Oblique View

Place the cassette on the plantaromedial aspect of the tarsus. Position the primary beam parallel to the floor and centered on the proximal intertarsal joint, 45 degrees off true lateromedial projection. The image should include the area from distal tibia to proximal metatarsus. It is used to visualize the dorsomedial and plantarolateral surfaces of the tarsal bones (Figures 14-13, *B,* and 14-16).

Oblique views for the tarsus are 45 degrees off true lateromedial or mediolateral position.

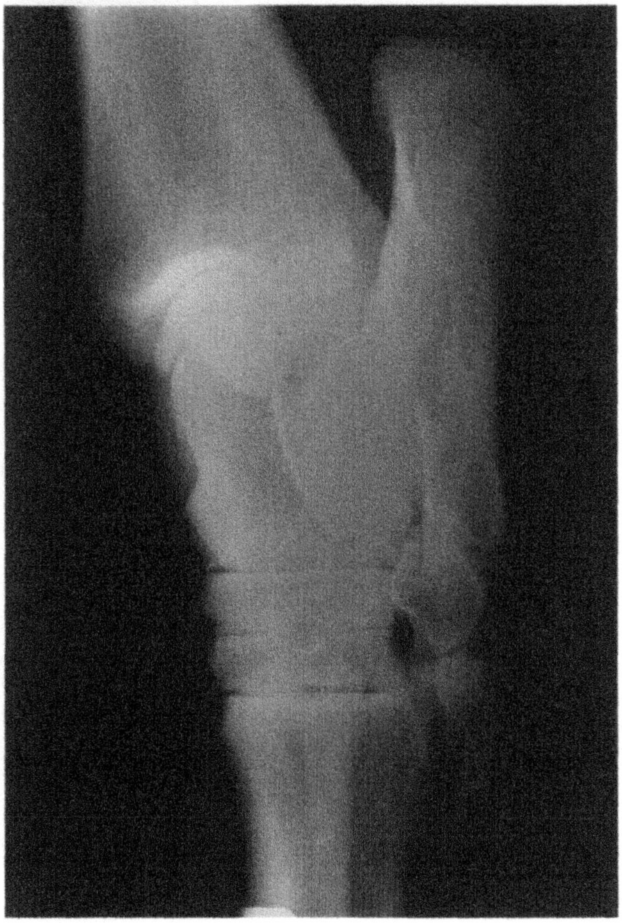

FIG. 14-16 Dorsolateral-plantaromedial projection of the tarsal joint.

Dorsomedial-Plantarolateral Oblique View

Place the cassette on the plantarolateral aspect of the tarsus. Position the primary beam parallel to the floor and centered on the proximal intertarsal joint, 45 degrees off true mediolateral. The image should include the area from distal tibia to proximal metatarsus. It is used to visualize the dorsolateral and plantaromedial surfaces of the tarsal bones (Figures 14-13, *D*, and 14-17).

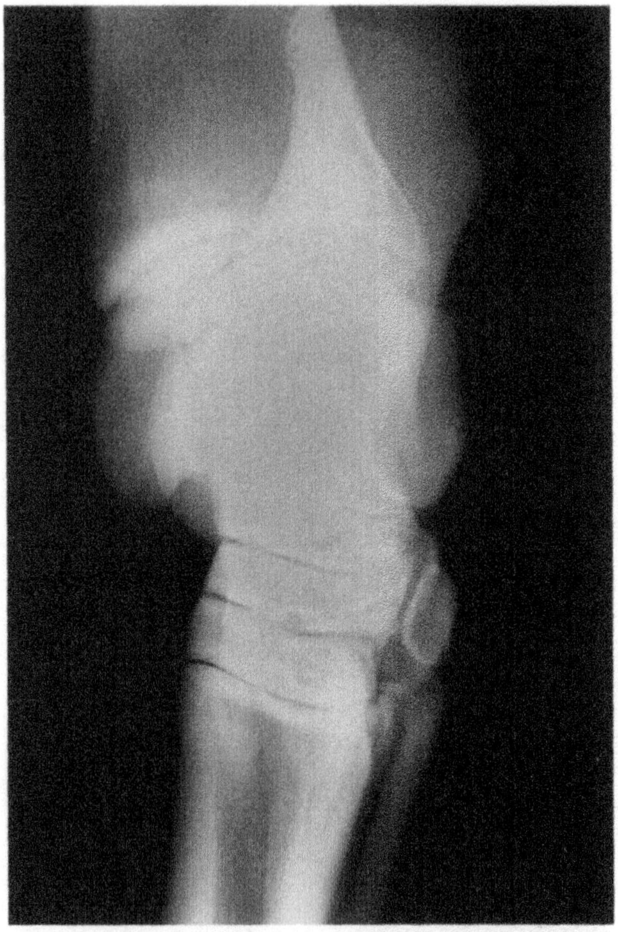

FIG. 14-17 Dorsomedial-plantarolateral projection of the tarsal joint.

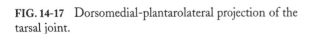

Flexed Dorsoplantar View

Flex the limb so that the metatarsus is parallel to the ground, pushing the whole limb caudally. Place the cassette on the distoplantar surface of the tarsus. Project the primary beam in a plantarodorsal direction at a 60-degree angle. This image isolates the calcaneus without superimposition of the tarsal bones (Figures 14-18 and 14-19).

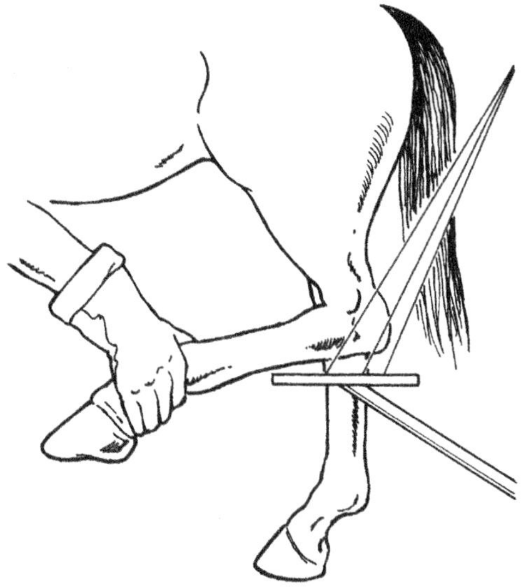

FIG. 14-18 Positioning for an additional projection of the talus. Plantaroproximal-plantarodistal flexed projection of tuber calcanei (tuberosity of calcaneus).

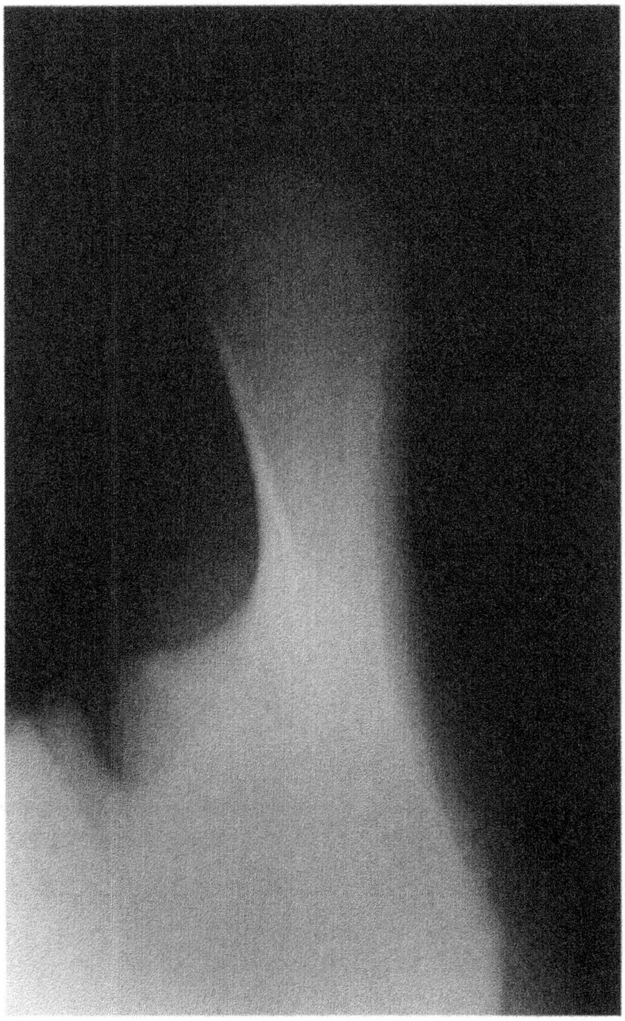

FIG. 14-19 Plantaroproximal-plantarodistal flexed projection of tuber calcanei.

Metacarpal Views

For standard radiographs of the metacarpus, position the horse squarely with its weight evenly distributed on all four limbs. The limb of interest should be perpendicular to the ground (Figure 14-20).

Dorsopalmar View

Place the cassette on the palmar surface of the metacarpus, keeping it parallel to the limb. Position the primary beam parallel to the floor and centered midway between the carpal and metacarpophalangeal joints. The image should include the carpal and metacarpophalangeal joints. The use of a 7 × 17–inch cassette is necessary to image the entire metacarpal region (Figures 14-20, *A,* and 14-21).

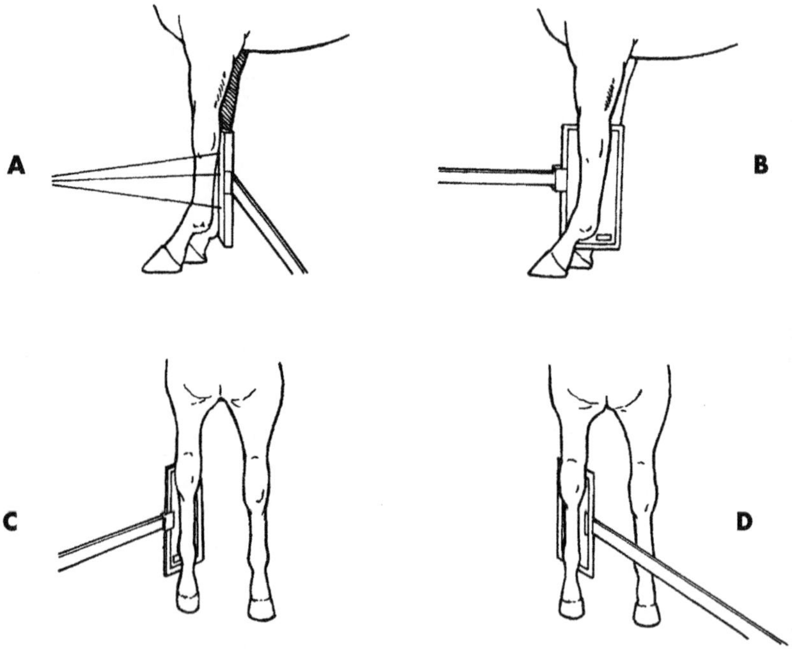

FIG. 14-20 Positioning for standard projections of the metacarpus. **A,** Dorsopalmar; **B,** lateromedial; **C,** dorsomedial-palmarolateral; **D,** dorsolateral-palmaromedial.

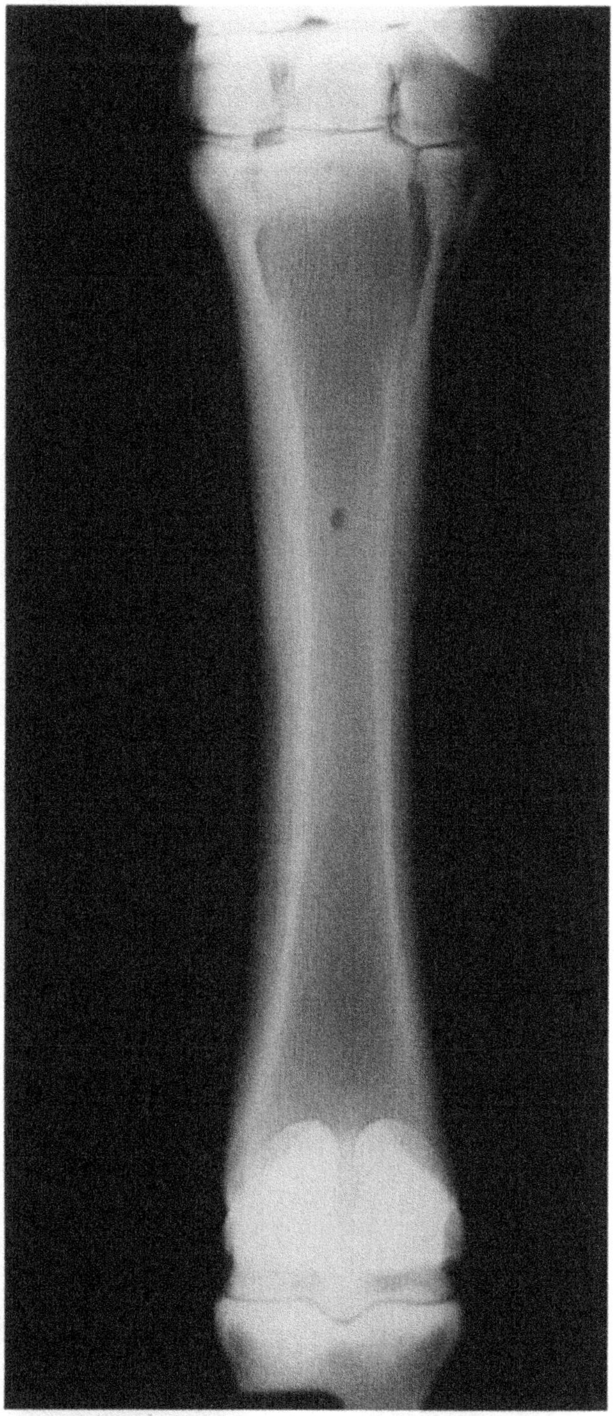

FIG. 14-21 Dorsopalmar projection of the metacarpus.

Lateromedial View

Place the cassette on the medial aspect of the metacarpus, keeping it parallel to the limb. Position the primary beam parallel to the floor and centered midway between the carpal and metacarpophalangeal joints. The image should include the carpal and metacarpophalangeal joints. A 7 × 17–inch cassette is necessary to image the entire metacarpal region. The true lateromedial image shows the second and fourth metacarpal bones superimposed over one another (Figures 14-20, *B*, and 14-22).

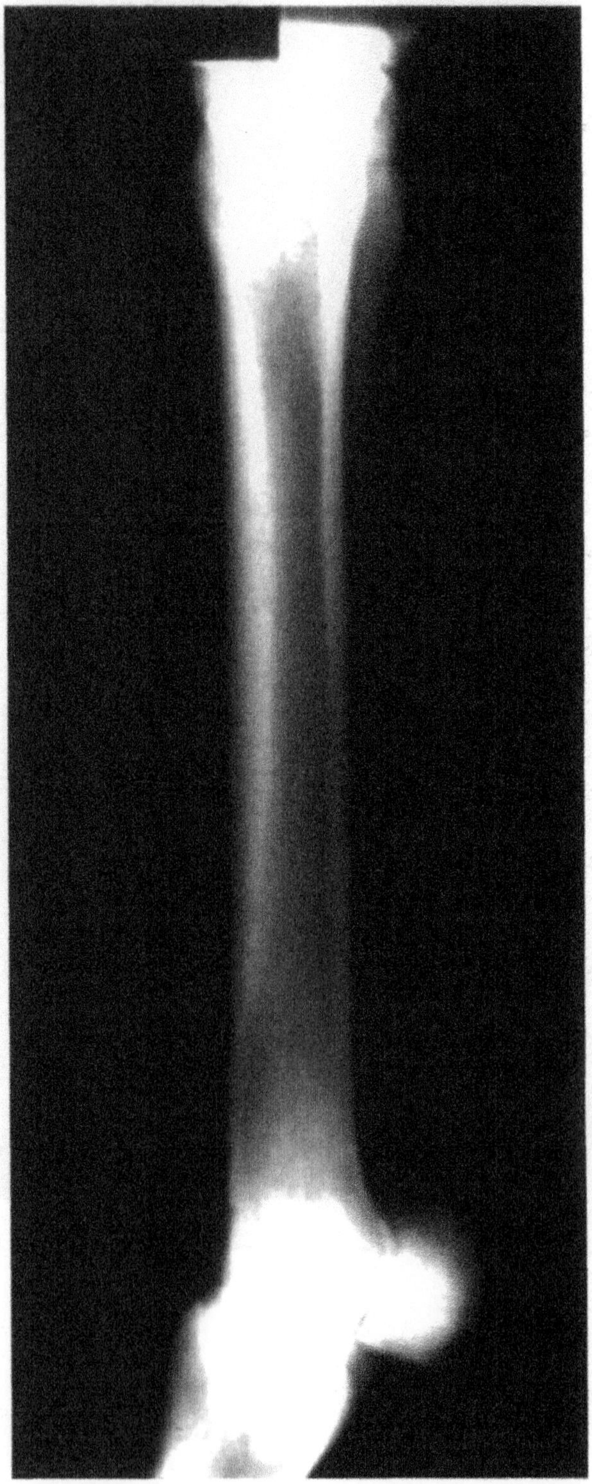

FIG. 14-22 Lateromedial projection of the metacarpus.

Dorsolateral-Palmaromedial Oblique View

Place the cassette on the palmaromedial aspect of the metacarpus, keeping it parallel to the limb. Position the primary beam parallel to the floor and centered midway between the carpal and metacarpophalangeal joints. Direct the primary beam dorsolaterally, 35 to 45 degrees off true dorsopalmar projection. The image should include the carpal and metacarpophalangeal joints. This image shows the fourth metacarpal bone without superimposition (Figures 14-20, *D*, and 14-23).

> Oblique views for the metacarpus are 35 to 45 degrees off true dorsopalmar position.

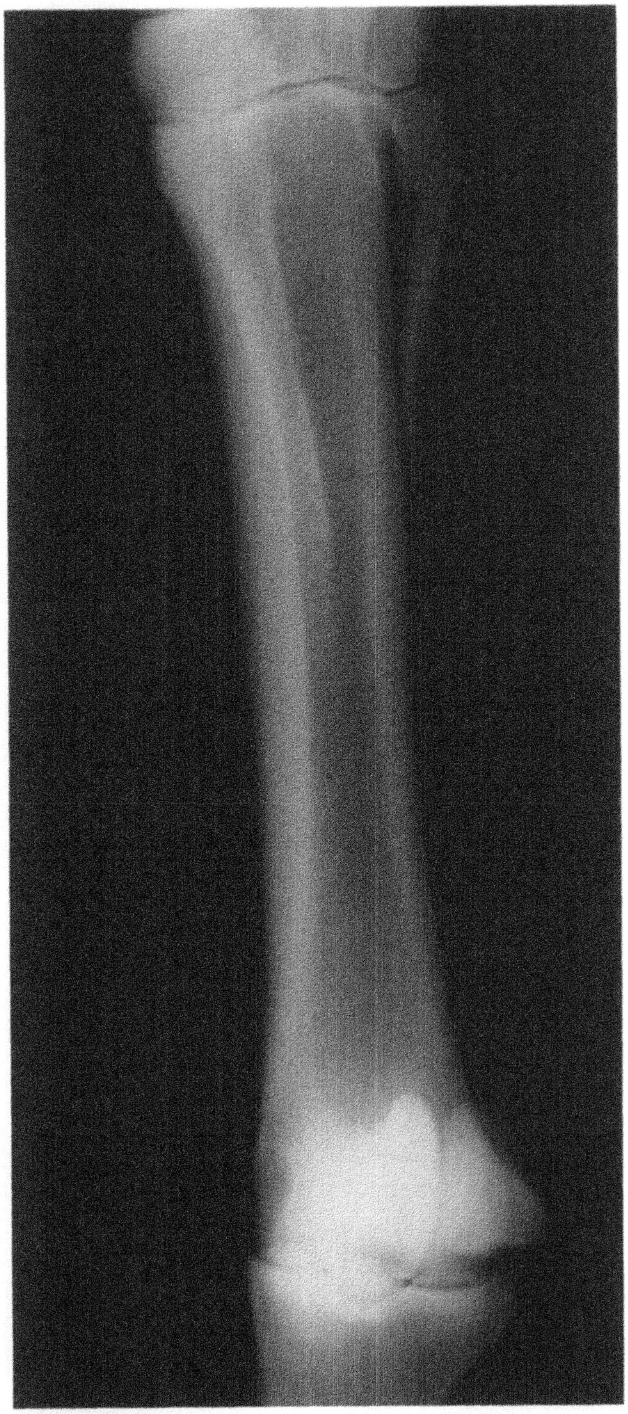

FIG. 14-23 Dorsolateral-palmaromedial projection of the metacarpus.

Dorsomedial-Palmarolateral Oblique View

Place the cassette on the palmarolateral aspect of the metacarpus, keeping it parallel to the limb. Position the primary beam parallel to the floor and center midway between the carpal and metacarpophalangeal joints. Direct the primary beam dorsomedially, 35 to 45 degrees off true dorsopalmar projection. The image should include the carpal and metacarpophalangeal joints. This image shows the second metacarpal bone without superimposition (Figures 14-20, *C*, and 14-24).

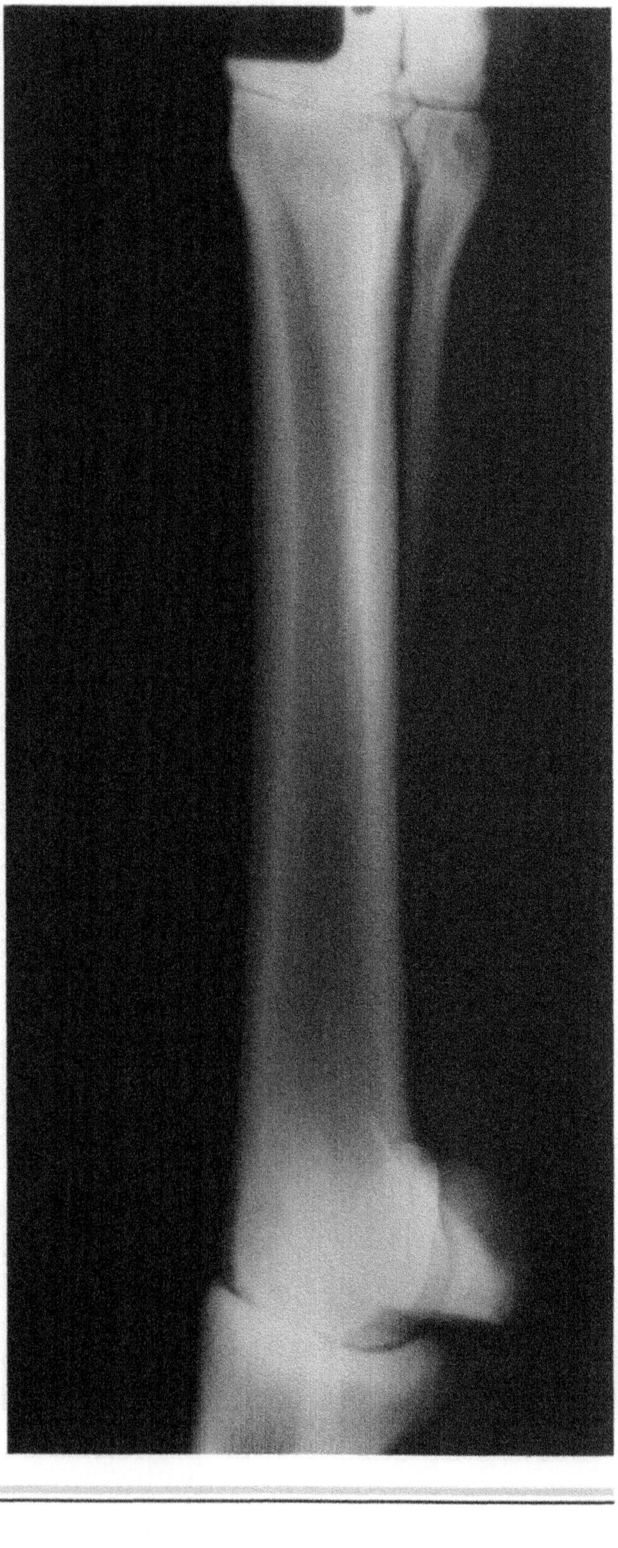

FIG. 14-24 Dorsomedial-palmarolateral projection of the metacarpus.

Metatarsal Views

Positioning for the metatarsus is identical to positioning for the metacarpus, with the exception that the term *palmar* is replaced with *plantar* when referring to the *rear limb*. It is also important that radiographs are labeled correctly as rear limb, left rear (LR), and right rear (RR).

Metacarpophalangeal Joint (Fetlock) Views

For standard radiographs of the metcarpophalangeal joint (fetlock joint), position the horse squarely with its weight distributed evenly on both legs. The leg must be perpendicular to the ground in a normal weight-bearing position (Figure 14-25). The horse may need to be placed on wood blocks if the x-ray machine cannot be moved close to the ground. In this case, both feet should be placed on blocks to ensure even weight bearing.

Dorsopalmar View

Angle the primary beam 20 degrees proximal to distal and centered on the midsagittal plane of the metacarpophalangeal joint. Place the cassette against the palmar surface of the limb, and position it so that it is perpendicular to the primary beam. The dorsopalmar view projects the sesamoids above the metacarpophalangeal joint space (Figures 14-25, *A*, and 14-26).

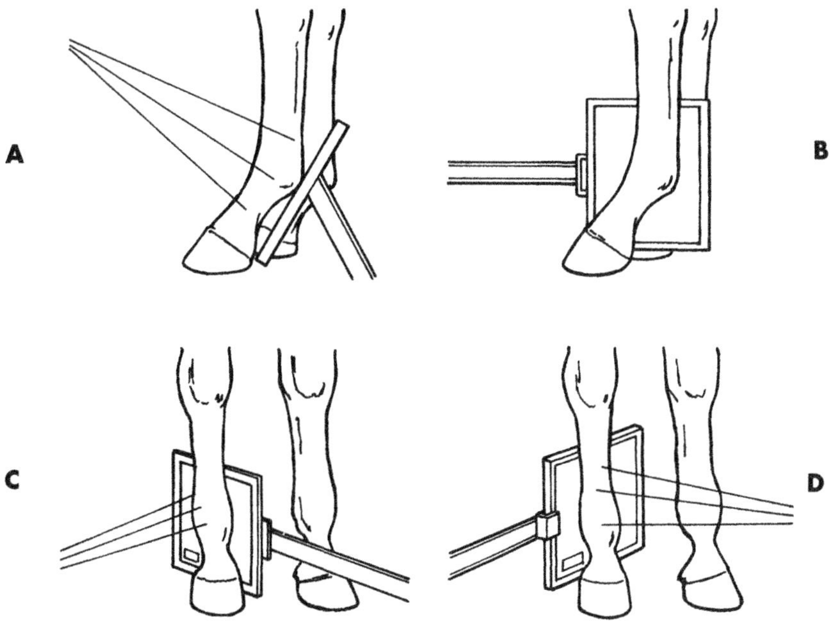

FIG. 14-25 Positioning for the standard projections of the metacarpophalangeal joint (fetlock). **A,** Dorsopalmar; **B,** lateromedial; **C,** dorsolateral-palmaromedial; **D,** dorsomedial-palmarolateral.

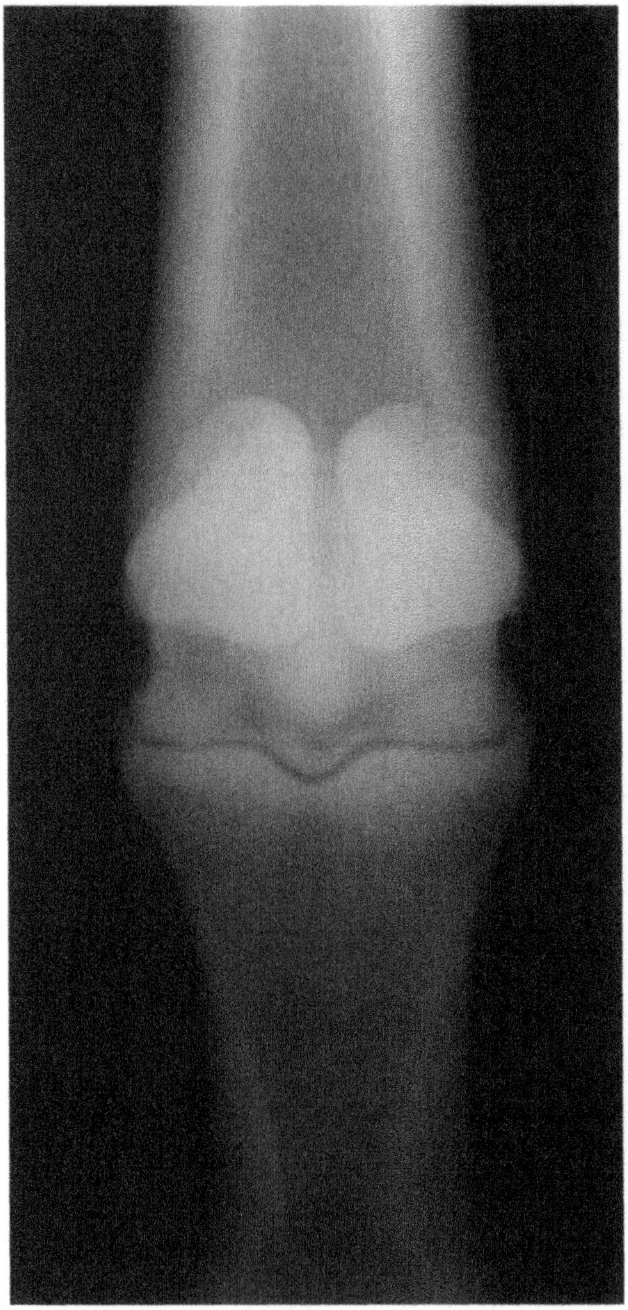

FIG. 14-26 Dorsopalmar projection of the metacarpophalangeal joint (fetlock).

Lateromedial View

Place the cassette on the medial aspect of the joint. Direct the primary beam parallel to the floor and center on the metacarpophalangeal joint. A true lateromedial view displays the metacarpal condyles and superimposed sesamoids, with a visible joint space (Figures 14-25, *B*, and 14-27).

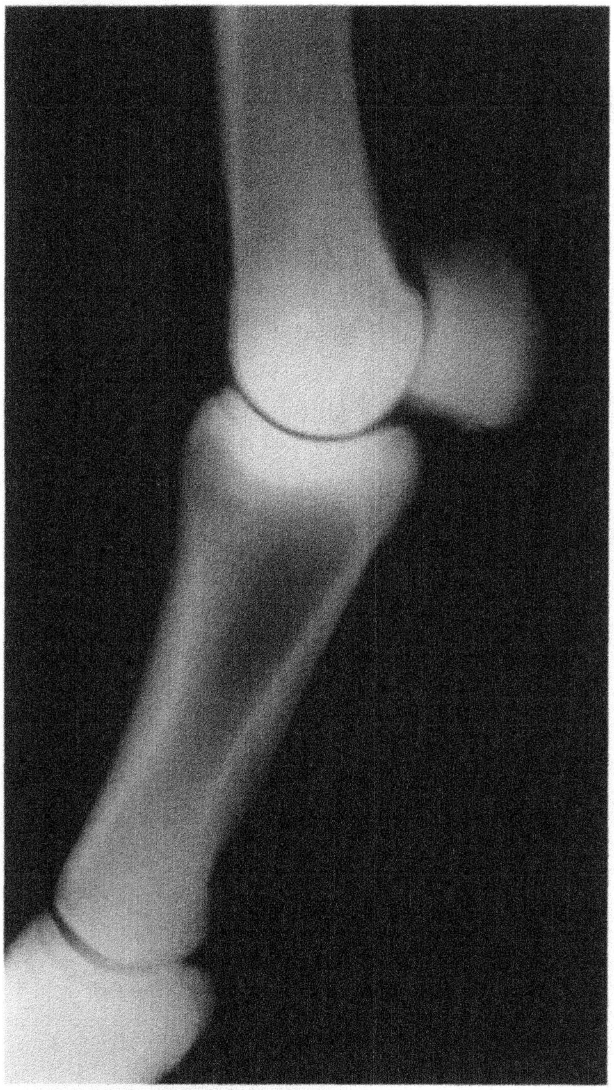

FIG. 14-27 Lateromedial projection of the metacarpophalangeal joint (fetlock).

Dorsolateral-Palmaromedial Oblique View

Place the cassette on the palmaromedial aspect of the joint. Position the primary beam parallel to the floor and centered on the metacarpophalangeal joint. Direct the primary beam dorsolaterally, 45 degrees off true dorsopalmar projection. This allows the lateral sesamoid to be visualized without the medial sesamoid bone superimposed (Figures 14-25, *C*, and 14-28).

Oblique views for the metacarpophalangeal joints are 45 degrees off true dorsopalmar position.

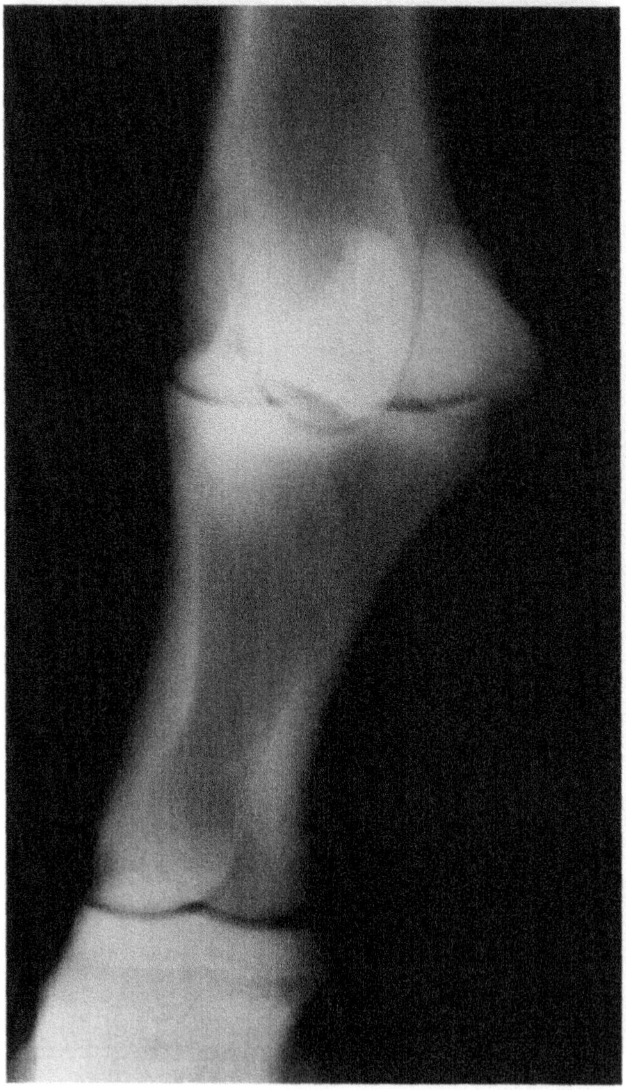

FIG. 14-28 Dorsolateral-palmaromedial projection of the metacarpophalangeal joint (fetlock).

Dorsomedial-Palmarolateral Oblique View

Place the cassette on the palmarolateral aspect of the joint. Position the primary beam parallel to the floor and centered on the metacarpophalangeal joint. Direct the primary beam dorsomedially, 45 degrees off true dorsopalmar projection. This allows the medial sesamoid to be visualized without the lateral sesamoid bone superimposed (Figures 14-25, *D,* and 14-29).

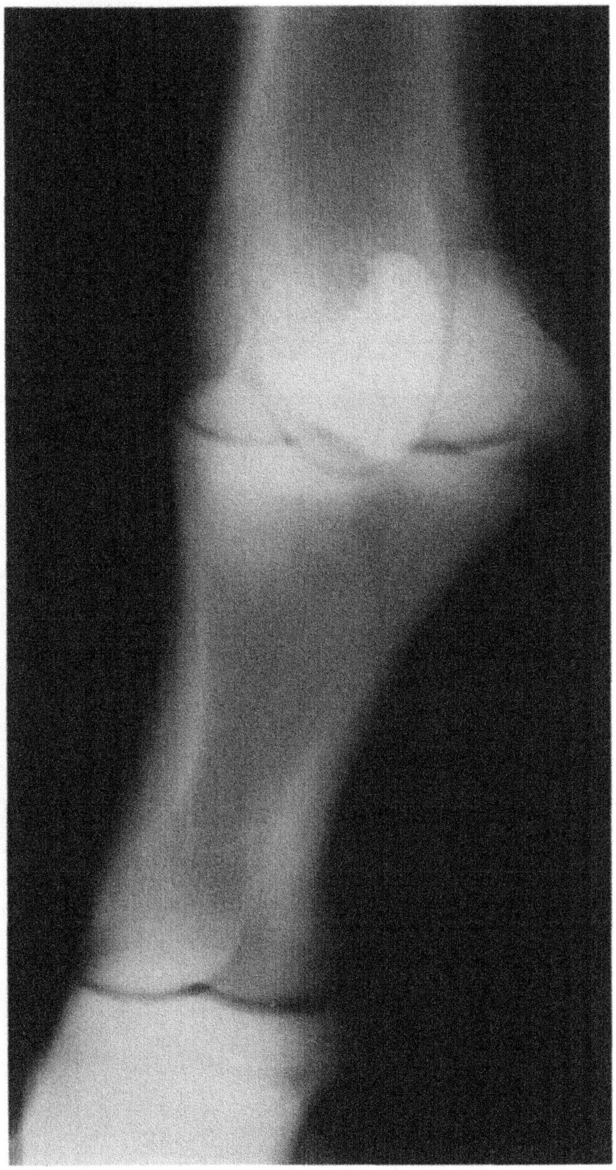

FIG. 14-29 Dorsomedial-palmarolateral projection of the metacarpophalangeal joint (fetlock).

Metatarsophalangeal Joint (Fetlock) Views

Positioning for the metatarsophalangeal joint is identical to that for the metacarpophalangeal joint, with the exception that the term *palmar* is replaced with *plantar* when referring to the rear limb. Because the anatomy is the same, it is important that the radiographs be labeled correctly as a rear limb, LR, and RR.

Proximal Interphalangeal Joint (Pastern) Views

For standard radiographs of the proximal interphalangeal joint (pastern joint) position the horse squarely with its weight distributed evenly on both legs. The leg must be perpendicular to the ground in a normal weight-bearing position (Figure 14-30). The feet may need to be placed on wood blocks if the x-ray machine cannot be moved close to the ground. In this case, both feet should be placed on blocks to ensure that they are evenly bearing weight.

Dorsopalmar View

Angle the primary beam 15 to 20 degrees proximal to distal and centered on the proximal interphalangeal joint. When positioning the horse, place the foot being imaged on the caudal aspect of the wood block. This allows the cassette to be placed on the ground perpendicular to the primary beam. Place the cassette on the palmar surface of the limb. The dorsopalmar image shows the proximal and middle phalanges (Figures 14-30, *A*, and 14-31).

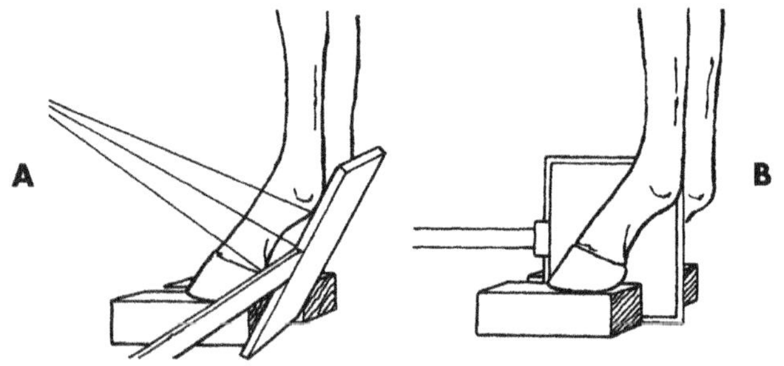

FIG. 14-30 Positioning for standard projections of the proximal interphalangeal joint (pastern). **A,** Dorsopalmar; **B,** lateromedial.

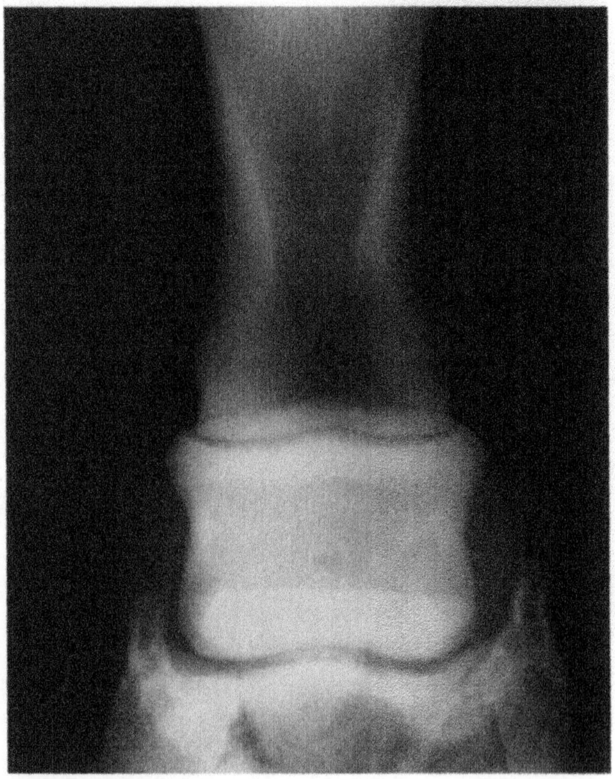

FIG. 14-31 Dorsopalmar projection of the proximal interphalangeal joint (pastern).

Lateromedial View

Place the cassette on the medial aspect of the joint. Position the primary beam parallel to the floor and centered on the proximal interphalangeal joint. The lateromedial image shows the proximal and middle phalanges (Figures 14-30, *B*, and 14-32).

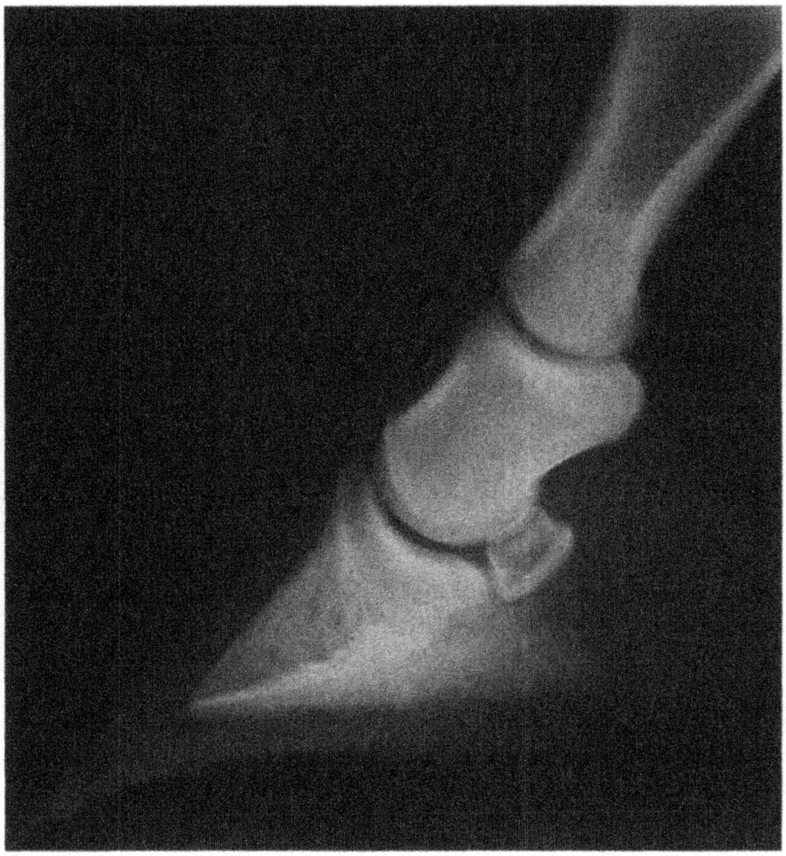

FIG. 14-32 Lateromedial projection of the proximal interphalangeal joint (pastern).

Distal Phalanx (Coffin Bone) Views

Preparation

If present, horseshoes should be pulled before radiographing the coffin bone. The hoof should then be cleaned and trimmed to new sole (Figures 14-33). This prevents ingrained debris from causing artifacts on the finished radiograph. Air trapped in the sulcus of the hoof may also cause an artifact. To prevent this, the sulcus should be packed with a radiolucent material, such as petroleum jelly or modeling clay (Figure 14-34). Place a paper towel or dry gauze over the bottom of the hoof to protect the packing (Figure 14-35).

Proper foot preparation is important when imaging through the hoof wall.

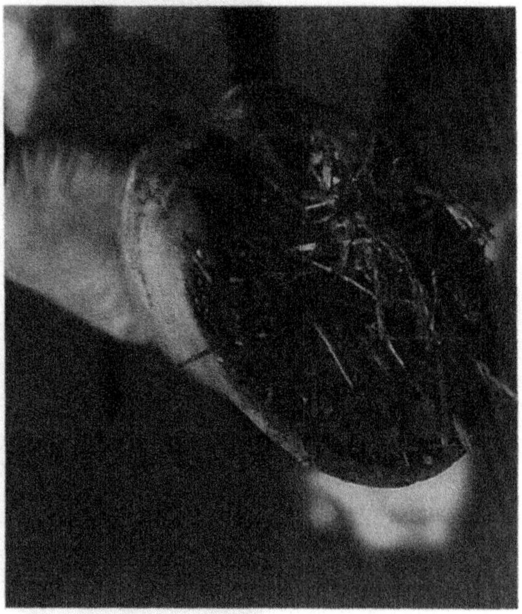

FIG. 14-33 The hoof must be prepared before imaging the distal phalanx and distal sesamoid. Pull the shoes, then clean and trim the hoof to new sole.

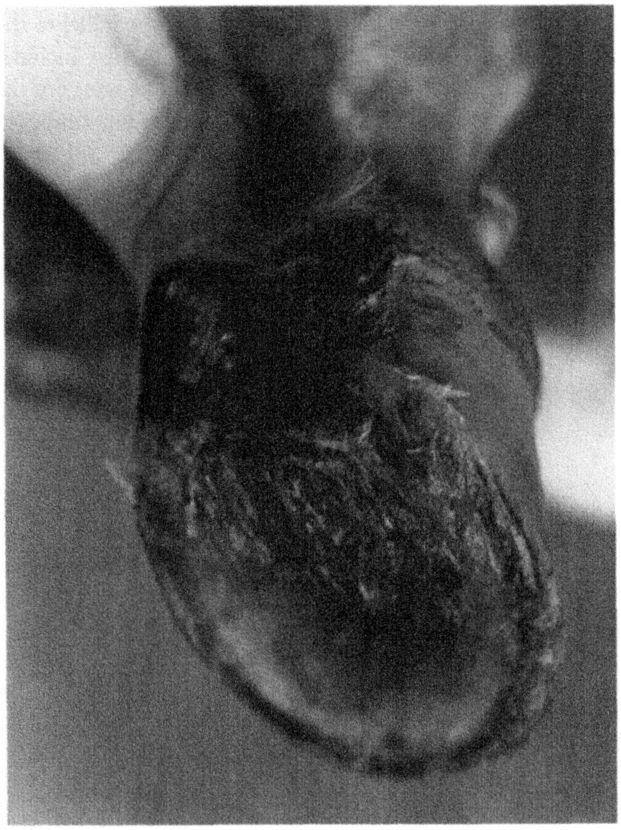

FIG. 14-34 Pack the hoof with a radiolucent material to remove air in the sulcus.

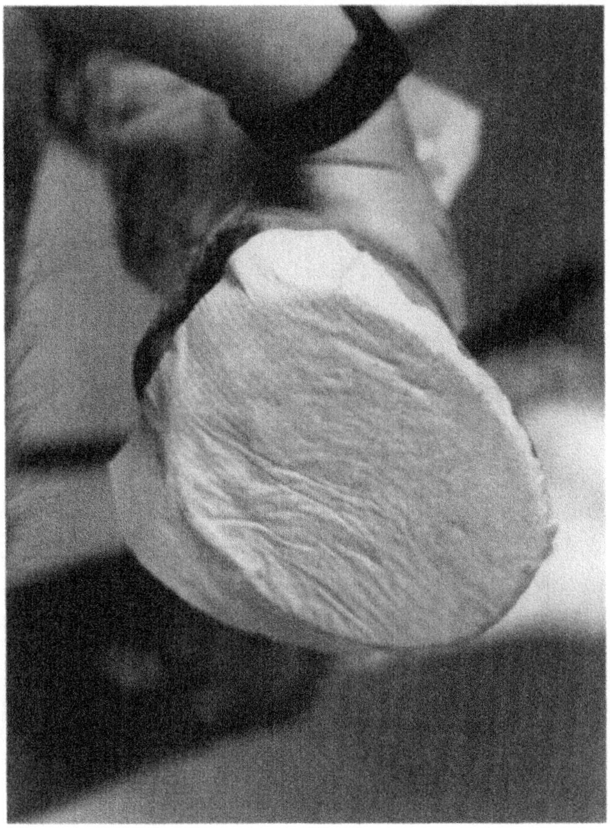

FIG. 14-35 Place a paper towel or dry gauze over the hoof packing for protection.

Lateromedial View

For lateromedial projections of the distal phalanx (coffin bone) place the horse with the foot of interest and the contralateral limb on wood blocks. This raises the distal limb off the floor so that the entire phalanx may be radiographed. Place the cassette on the medial aspect of the hoof, including the bulbs of the heel and the entire toe to evaluate rotation of the distal phalanx. Position the primary beam parallel to the floor and centered on the coronary band. This view includes the proximal, middle, and distal phalanges. The wings of the coffin bone and the navicular bone should be superimposed over one another (Figures 14-36, *A,* and 14-37).

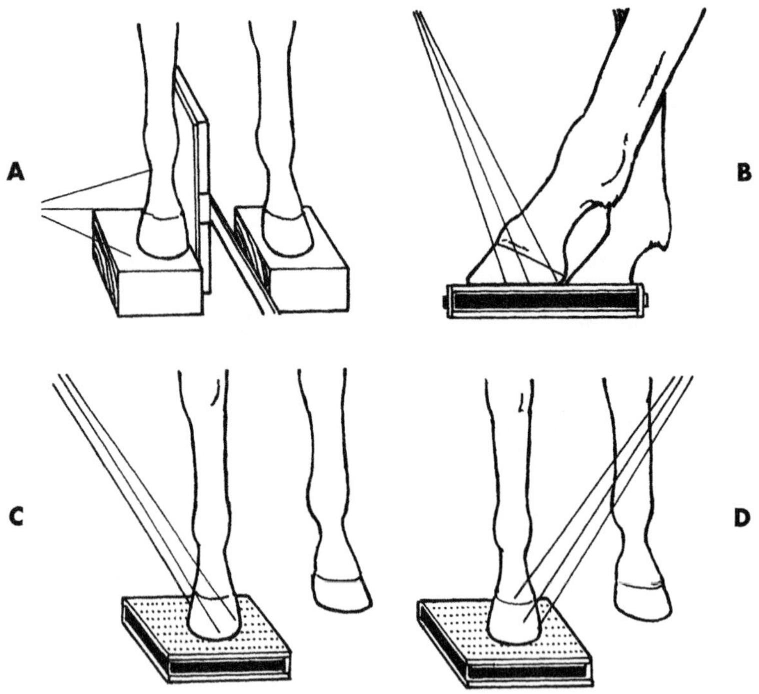

FIG. 14-36 Positioning for standard projections of the distal phalanx (coffin bone).
A, Lateromedial; **B,** dorsopalmar; **C,** dorsolateral-palmaromedial; **D,** dorsomedial-palmarolateral.

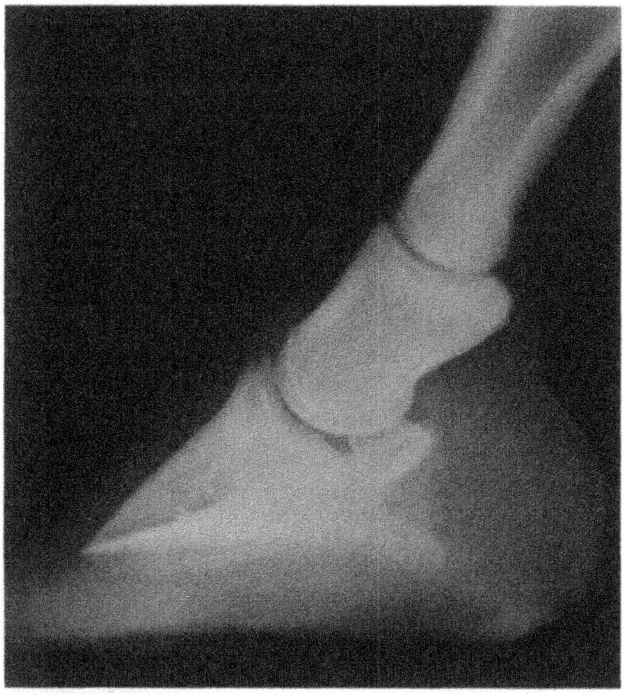

FIG. 14-37 Lateromedial projection of the distal phalanx (coffin bone).

Dorsopalmar View

Extend the limb cranially and place it on the cassette tunnel. Angle the primary beam proximodistally 60 degrees, and center it just distal to the coronary band. Because it is impossible to have the cassette perfectly perpendicular to the beam, there will be some distortion of the coffin bone on the radiograph. The resulting view should show equal proportions of each wing of the coffin bone (Figures 14-36, *B,* and 14-38).

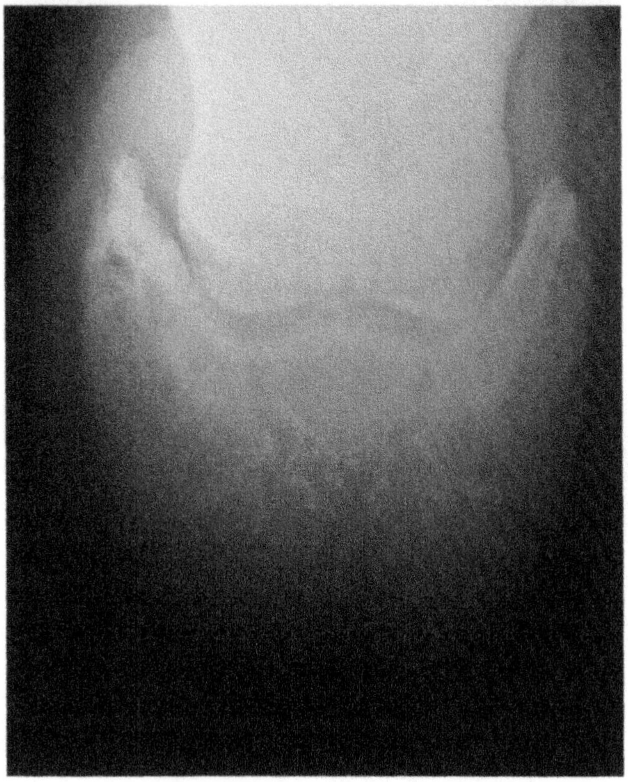

FIG. 14-38 Dorsopalmar projection of the distal phalanx (coffin bone).

Dorsolateral-Palmaromedial Oblique View

Place the cassette in the cassette tunnel. Extend the limb cranially and place it on the cassette tunnel. Angle the primary beam 60 degrees proximodistally so that it is perpendicular to the hoof wall. Direct the primary beam dorsolaterally, 45 degrees off true dorsopalmar projection, and center it just distal to the coronary band. This view is used to visualize the lateral wing of the coffin bone (Figures 14-36, *C* and 14-39).

Dorsomedial-Palmarolateral Oblique View

Place the cassette in the cassette tunnel. Extend the limb cranially and place it on the cassette tunnel. Angle the primary beam 60 degrees proximodistally so that it is perpendicular to the hoof wall. Direct the primary beam dorsomedially, 45 degrees off true dorsopalmar projection, and center it just distal to the coronary band. This view is used to visualize the medial wing of the coffin bone (Figure 14-36, *D*).

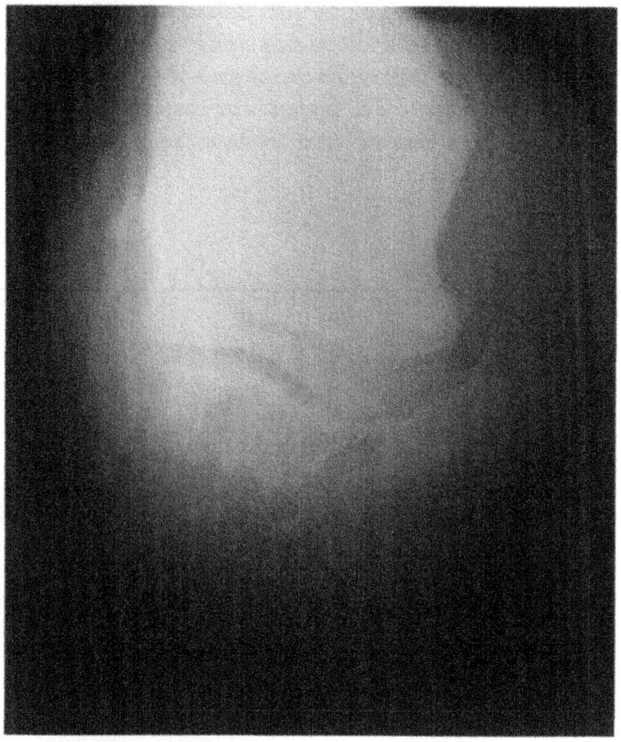

FIG. 14-39 Dorsolateral-palmaromedial projection of the distal phalanx (coffin bone).

Distal Sesamoid (Navicular Bone) Views

Preparation

If present, horseshoes should be pulled before radiographing the navicular bone. The hoof should then be cleaned and trimmed to new sole. This prevents ingrained debris from causing artifacts on the finished radiograph. Air trapped in the sulcus of the hoof may also cause an artifact. To prevent this, the sulcus should be packed with a radiolucent material such as liquid soap, petroleum jelly, or modeling clay. Place a paper towel or dry gauze over the bottom of the hoof to protect the packing (see Figures 14-33, 14-34, and 14-35).

Dorsoproximal-Palmarodistal Oblique View (Upright Pedal)

Have the horse bear weight on the opposite limb while the limb that is being radiographed is placed in a navicular box. This box has a groove to hold the hoof in an upright position so that the dorsal hoof wall is perpendicular to the floor. Position the primary beam parallel to the floor and centered on the coronary band. Place the cassette in the box behind the hoof so that it lies parallel to the dorsal hoof wall. The upright pedal position projects the navicular bone dorsal to the coffin joint for better evaluation (Figures 14-40, *A*, and 14-41).

Dorsopalmar-Dorsoplantar Oblique View

Place the cassette in the cassette tunnel. Have the horse stand on the cassette tunnel with the limb of interest positioned cranially while the horse is still bearing weight equally on all four limbs. Angle the x-ray machine 65 degrees toward the middle of the second phalanx. The dorsopalmar-dorsoplantar oblique projection will provide the same results as the dorsoproximal-palmarodistal oblique view.

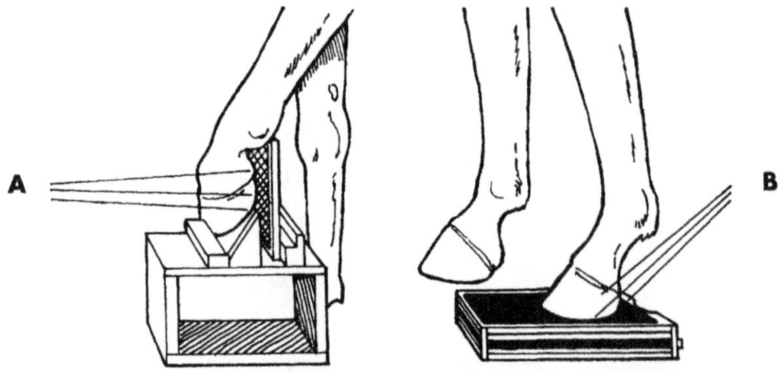

FIG. 14-40 Positioning for standard projections of the distal sesamoid (navicular bone).
A, Dorsoproximal-palmarodistal;
B, palmaroproximal-dorsodistal.

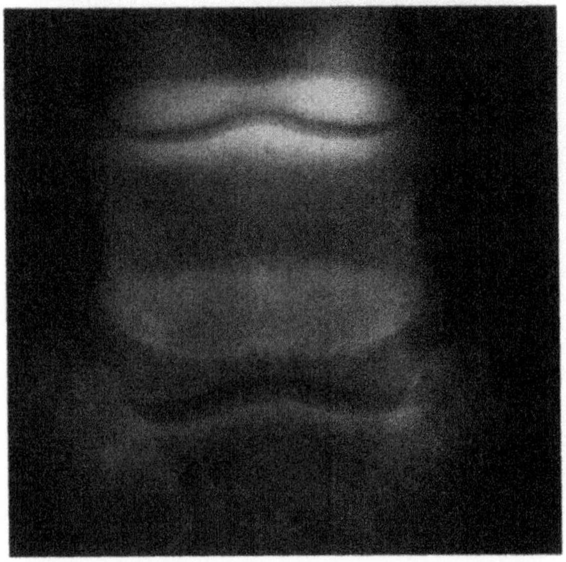

FIG. 14-41 Dorsoproximal-palmarodistal projection of the distal sesamoid (navicular bone).

Palmaroproximal-Dorsodistal Oblique View (Caudal Tangential)

Place the cassette in the cassette tunnel. Have the horse stand on the cassette tunnel with the limb of interest positioned caudally while the horse is still bearing weight equally on all four limbs. Angle the x-ray machine 45 degrees proximodistally, and position it underneath the horse's abdomen so that the beam may be directed in a palmar-to-dorsal direction. Center the primary beam between the bulbs of the heel. The caudal tangential image allows the palmar surface of the navicular bone to be visualized (Figures 14-40, *B,* and 14-42).

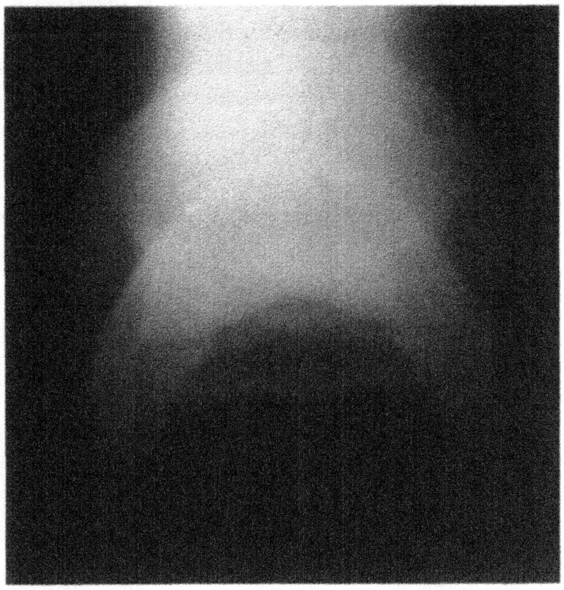

FIG. 14-42 Palmaroproximal-dorsodistal projection of the distal sesamoid (navicular bone).

Views of the Rear Feet

The views and positioning for the rear feet are identical to those for the front feet, except that the term *palmar* is replaced with *plantar* in all view descriptions. The radiographs must be labeled correctly as a rear limb, LR, and RR.

Femorotibial Joint (Stifle) Views

For standard radiographs of the femorotibial joint (stifle joint), have the horse stand squarely with its weight evenly distributed on all four legs (Figure 14-43). Caution should be used when radiographing this area; it is a sensitive region for the horse. The cassettes should be held in place with a cassette holder. Place the cassette firmly against the horse. A light touch is more irritating than a firm touch.

Caudocranial View

Place the cassette against the cranial aspect of the femorotibial joint. Because of the position of this joint, angle the primary beam slightly proximodistally. It is important to note that the femorotibial joint deviates laterally; this should be kept in mind when positioning the x-ray tube. Direct the primary beam toward the midsagittal plane of the limb, and center it on the joint. The caudocranial view visualizes the femoral condyles, proximal tibia, and patella (Figures 14-43, *A*, and 14-44).

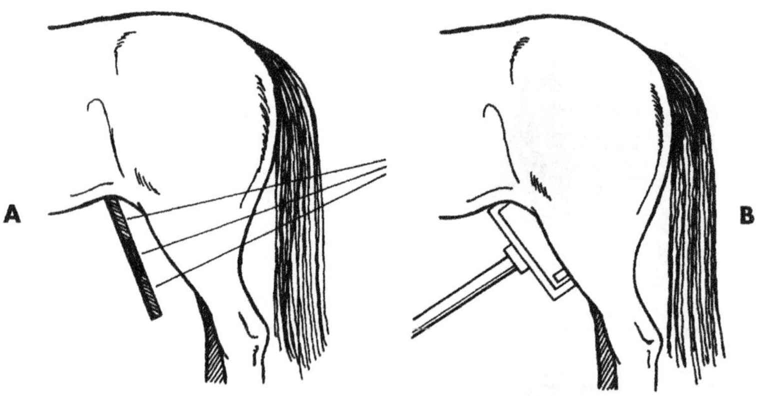

FIG. 14-43 Positioning for standard projections of the femorotibial joint (stifle). **A,** Caudocranial; **B,** lateromedial.

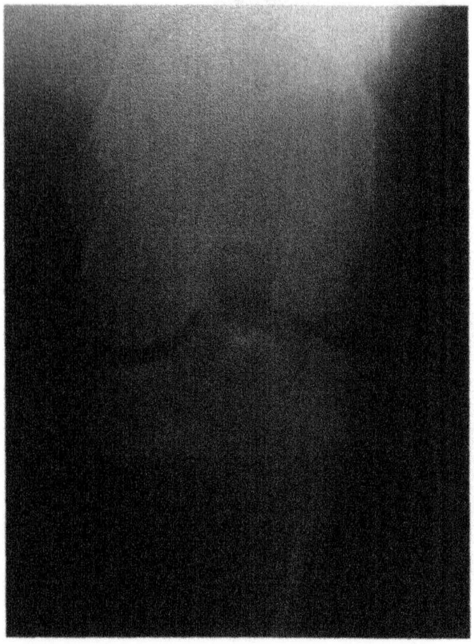

FIG. 14-44 Caudocranial projection of the femorotibial joint (stifle).

Lateromedial View

Place the cassette against the medial aspect of the joint as high (dorsal) in the flank as possible. Position the primary beam parallel to the floor and centered on the joint. The lateromedial image includes the femorotibial joint, proximal tibia, and patella. The femoral condyles should be superimposed so that only one condyle is visualized (Figures 14-43, *B,* and 14-45).

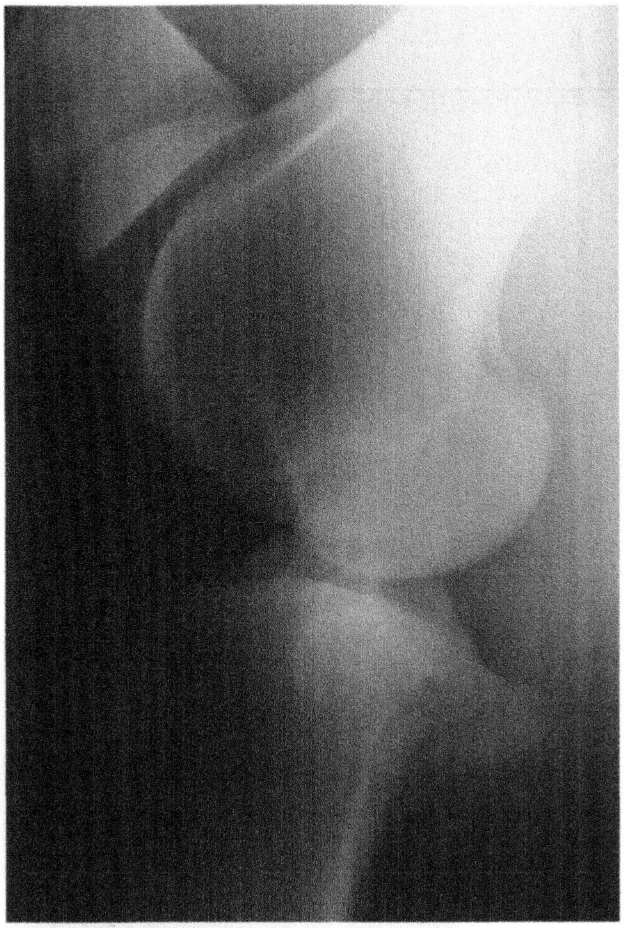

FIG. 14-45 Lateromedial projection of the femorotibial joint (stifle).

Brachioantebrachial Joint (Elbow) Views

Craniocaudal View

For craniocaudal radiographs of the brachioantebrachial joint (elbow joint), position the horse with the front limbs slightly abducted to separate the elbow from the thoracic musculature. Place the cassette diagonally on the caudal surface of the joint. Angling the cassette allows a larger portion of the medial surface to be captured on the radiograph. Position the primary beam parallel to the floor and centered on the joint. The resulting view should contain the distal humerus, brachioantebrachial joint, and proximal radius (Figures 14-46, *B*, and 14-47).

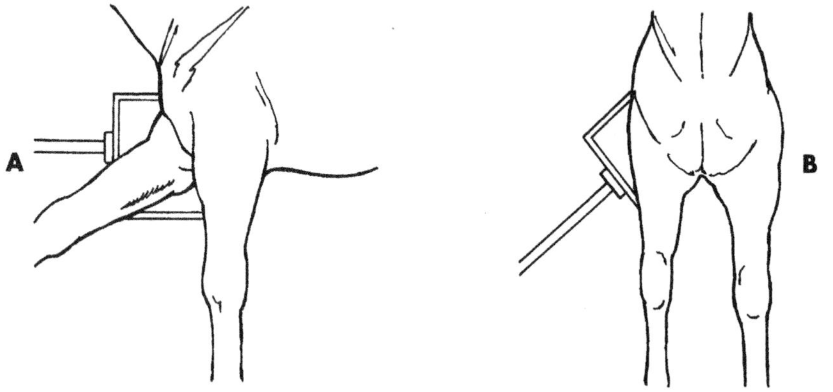

FIG. 14-46 Positioning for standard projections of the brachioantebrachial joint (elbow). **A,** Mediolateral; **B,** craniocaudal.

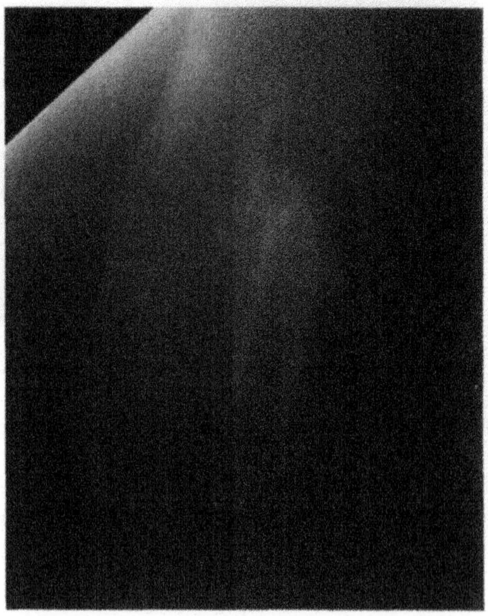

FIG. 14-47 Craniocaudal projection of the brachioantebrachial joint (elbow).

Mediolateral View

Extend the limb of interest cranially and have an assistant hold it. This minimizes the overlap of the pectoral muscles, improving the image. Place the cassette on the lateral aspect of the brachioantebrachial joint, parallel to the limb. Position the primary beam parallel to the floor and center on the joint. The mediolateral image visualizes from the distal humerus to the proximal radius (Figures 14-46, *A,* and 14-48).

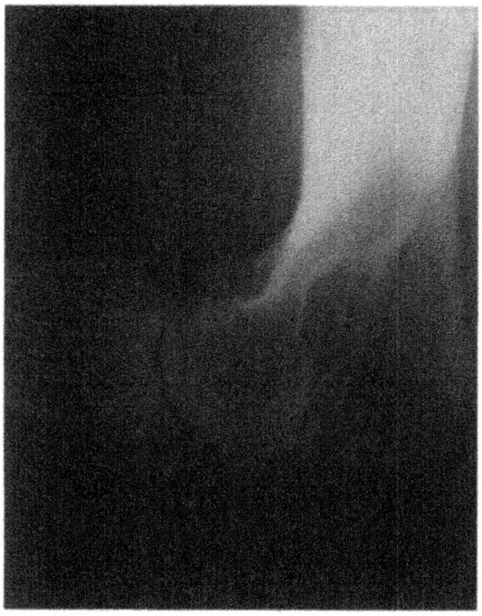

FIG. 14-48 Mediolateral projection of the brachioantebrachial joint (elbow).

Recommended Reading

Douglas SW et al: *Principles of veterinary radiography*, ed 4, London, 1987, Bailliere Tindall.

Feeney DA et al: A 200-centimeter focal spot-film distance (FFD) technique for equine radiography, *Vet Radiol* 23(1):13, 1982.

Mendenhall A, Cantwell HD: *Equine radiographic procedures*, Philadelphia, 1988, Lea & Febiger.

Morgan JP, Silverman S: *Techniques of veterinary radiography*, ed 5, Davis, Calif, 1982, Veterinary Radiology Associates.

Ticer JW: *Radiographic technique in veterinary practice*, ed 2, Philadelphia, 1984, Saunders.

15

Diagnostic Ultrasound

JEFFREY SIEMS

CHAPTER OBJECTIVES

- Explain how frequency and wavelength are related.
- Describe how acoustic impedance affects the production of the ultrasound image.
- List the terminology used to describe the ultrasound image.
- State how the patient must be prepared.
- Explain the importance of time gain compensation.
- Define the common artifacts that can be seen during a routine ultrasound scan.
- List the five transducer maneuvers and describe their implementation.
- Read a written description, look at the transducer position illustration, and produce an ultrasound image of the area of interest.

Use of diagnostic ultrasound in veterinary medicine is a noninvasive method of imaging soft tissues. A transducer sends low-intensity, high-frequency sound waves into the soft tissues, where the waves interact with the tissue interfaces. Some of the sound waves are reflected back to the transducer, and some are transmitted into deeper tissues. The sound waves that are reflected back to the transducer *(echoes)* are then analyzed by the computer to produce a gray-scale image. The use of ultrasound in conjunction with radiography gives the veterinarian an excellent diagnostic tool. Radiographs demonstrate the size, shape, and position of the organs. Ultrasound displays the findings on the radiographs, as well as the soft tissue textures and dynamics of some organs (e.g., motility of the bowel).

Basic Physics

Sound waves are classified by wavelength, frequency, and velocity. Ultrasound waveforms are similar to audible sound, except ultrasound has a shorter wavelength. As ultrasound travels through the tissues, it forms longitudinal waves consisting of compressions and rarefactions. The areas of *compression* force the molecules closer together, and the areas of *rarefaction* place them further apart (Figure 15-1). Sound waves can be compared with a transverse waveform (sine wave). With the pressure starting at zero, compression causes the pressure to rise to a peak, then fall back to zero. During rarefaction the pressure falls to a negative value before returning to zero. A *wavelength* is the distance from one band of compression or rarefaction to the next.

The *frequency* of a sound wave is the number of complete waveforms (cycles) per unit of time (Figure 15-2). Frequency

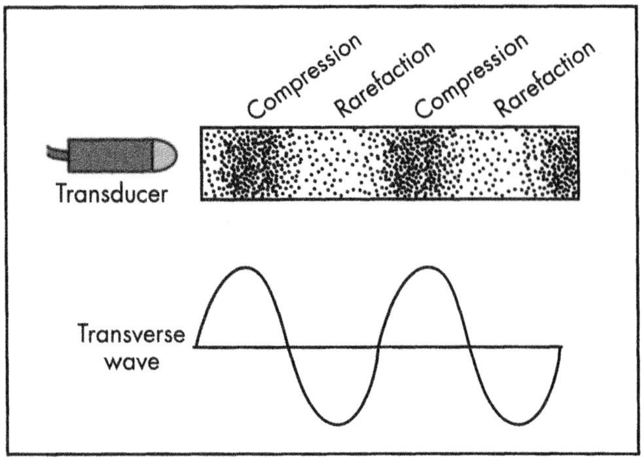

FIG. 15-1 Ultrasound waves traveling through the tissues form waves of compression and rarefaction of the tissue molecules. The areas of compression can be compared with the positive half of a sine wave. Rarefaction can be compared with the negative half of the sine wave.

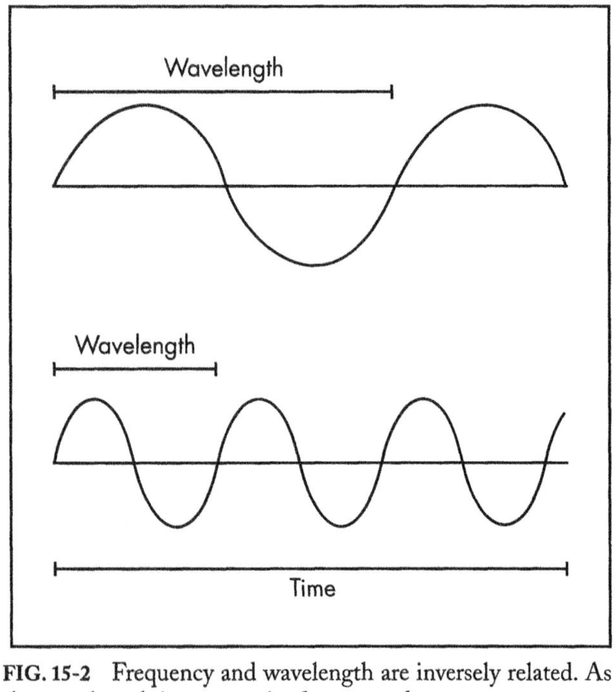

FIG. 15-2 Frequency and wavelength are inversely related. As the wavelength increases, the frequency decreases.

and wavelength are values that are inversely related. As the frequency increases, the wavelength decreases. Ultrasound uses high-frequency sound waves. The upper range of sound audible to humans has a frequency of around 20,000 hertz (Hz, cycles/second). The frequency of ultrasound waves varies from 2 to 10 million Hz, or 2 to 10 megahertz (MHz).

Velocity is the speed at which sound travels through a medium. The velocity of ultrasound is similar for all types of soft tissues. A velocity of 1540 meters per second (m/sec), the average speed in living tissue, is used by the computer software. The computer measures the time each sound wave takes to return to the transducer. It calculates the depth to where the sound was reflected and displays it accordingly on the monitor.

TABLE 15-1
ACOUSTIC IMPEDANCE OF DIFFERENT TISSUE TYPES

TISSUE TYPE	ACOUSTIC IMPEDANCE (RAYLS)
Fat	1.38×10^5
Water	1.48×10^5
Blood	1.61×10^5
Kidney	1.62×10^5
Soft tissue (average)	1.63×10^5
Liver	1.65×10^5
Muscle	1.70×10^5
Bone	1.80×10^5
Air	0.0004×10^5

Acoustic Impedance

Acoustic impedance is the ability of living tissue being imaged to resist or impede the transmission of sound. The interface between tissues with different acoustic impedance becomes a reflective surface for the sound waves. The acoustic impedance varies slightly among most tissues depending on the density and elasticity of the tissue (Table 15-1). Although the impedance of the various soft tissues varies only slightly, the difference allows one tissue to be distinguished from another while transmitting some sound to reflect off deeper tissues. It is when the acoustic impedance varies greatly that the reflector becomes nearly perfect. For example, interfaces between soft tissue and air and between soft tissue and bone vary greatly in acoustic impedance, thus reflecting almost all sound. This means that air-filled structures and bony structures are barriers to ultrasound waves.

Attenuation

As ultrasound travels through tissues, it loses intensity, or *attenuates.* The attenuation occurs through scatter and absorption. *Scattering* occurs when the sound reflects in many directions off the different tissue interfaces. Some of the sound is reflected in directions that never reach the transducer. *Absorption* occurs because of molecular friction from the sound passing through the tissues, producing heat. The molecular friction is caused by the compressions and rarefactions of the sound waves. The progressive loss of energy in the form of heat can eventually result in total absorption of the sound wave.

Sound that travels into and out of the tissues is subject to attenuation. This limits the depth of tissues that can be imaged. The amount of attenuation depends on the frequency of the transducer. Sound emitted from a high-frequency transducer attenuates faster than sound emitted from a lower-frequency transducer. Thus, lower-frequency transducers can image deeper tissues than can higher-frequency transducers.

Lower-frequency transducers allow for more depth but less resolution.

Higher-frequency transducers allow for more resolution but less depth.

Transducers

Ultrasound transducers emit a series of sound pulses and receive the returning echoes. A weak electrical current applied to the piezoelectric crystals incorporated in the transducer causes the crystals to vibrate and produce sound waves. After sending a series of pulses, the crystals are dampened to stop further vibrations. When struck by the returning echoes, the crystals vibrate again. This time the crystals convert the echoes into electrical energy.

Transducers are available in different configurations, which are mechanical or electronic. The scan plane can either be a sector scan (pie-shaped image) or a linear array scan (rectangular-shaped image). A mechanically driven *sector scan* can be produced by a belt and pulley used to wobble a single crystal or rotate multiple crystals across a scan plane. Another method of producing a sector scan is with the use of phased-array or annular array configurations. With a *phased array* the crystals are pulsed sequentially with a built-in delay to create a "pseudo-sector" scan plane. With an *annular array* the crystals are arranged in concentric rings. By using electronic phasing of the many crystals, annular array transducers produce a two-dimensional image by steering the entire array through a sector arc. Sector scanners are useful when imaging areas that are limited by ribs, gas-filled bowels, or lungs. The narrow near field and wide far field enable the transducer scan plane to be positioned between or around these structures.

The *linear array scanner* produces a scan plane by alternately firing groups of crystals in sequence. The pulsing of each group of crystals occurs so rapidly that individual pulses cannot be observed by the human eye. Linear array scanners are useful in areas with unrestricted window size. The rectangular-shaped scan plane is ideal for equine tendons or large or small animal transrectal imaging.

The frequency of the transducer determines the amount of detail or *resolution* of the image: the higher the frequency, the shorter the wavelength; the shorter the wavelength, the better the resolution of the image. The two types of resolution are axial and lateral. *Axial resolution* refers to the ability to differentiate between two reflecting interfaces that lie along the axis of the transmitted sound beam. If the wavelength of the sound is longer than the distance between the two interfaces, these are displayed as a single object. If the wavelength of the sound is shorter than the distance between the two interfaces, these are displayed as two separate objects. *Lateral resolution* refers to the ability to differentiate between two reflecting interfaces that lie in a plane perpendicular to the transmitted sound beam (Figure 15-3). Lateral resolution depends on the width of the sound beam. With a wide sound beam two separate reflective interfaces that lie within the width of that beam are displayed as only one reflection. A sound beam naturally diverges with a loss of lateral resolution in the far field. A method to compensate for this is to focus the sound beam in one area known as the *focal zone.* The sound beam can be focused either by use of an acoustic lens or by electronically transmitted means; both approaches improve the resolution in the focal zone.

Transducers are expensive and the most fragile part of the ultrasound equipment. Care must be taken when handling them. Hard impacts that can severely damage the sensitive crystals should be avoided. It is also advisable to prevent exposure to extreme temperature changes. Some transducers are sensitive to certain types of cleaning agents. Always refer to the manufacturer's instructions for appropriate cleaning products.

Display Modes

The three different display modes are A-mode (amplitude mode), B-mode (brightness mode), and M-mode (motion mode).

A-mode is the earliest form of ultrasound and requires the simplest form of computer software. With A-mode the returning echoes are displayed as a series of peaks on a graph: the higher the intensity of the returning sound, the higher the peak at that tissue depth. A-mode is not used to show

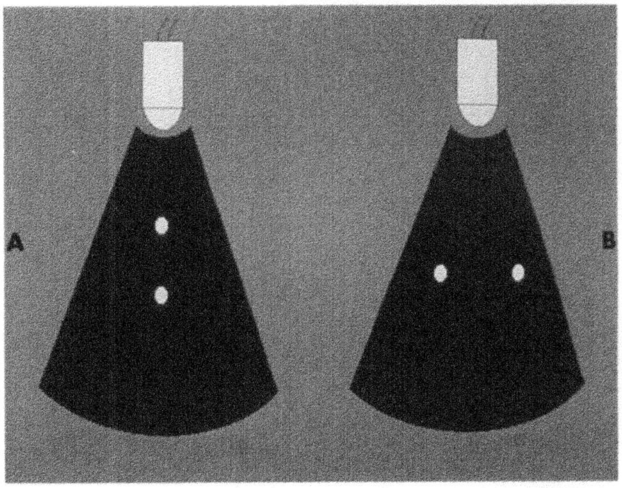

FIG. 15-3 **A,** Axial resolution is the machine's ability to differentiate between two closely spaced reflections parallel to the axis of the sound beam. **B,** Lateral resolution is the machine's ability to differentiate between two closely spaced reflections perpendicular to the axis of the sound beam.

tissue motion or anatomy. The first use in veterinary medicine was to measure the amount of subcutaneous fat in pigs.

B-mode uses bright pixels or dots on a screen, whereas A-mode uses peaks on a graph (Figure 15-4). With B-mode a dot is placed on a screen corresponding to the depth at which the echo was formed. The degree of brightness is proportional to the intensity of the returning echo: the higher the intensity, the brighter the dot. The image that is generated is a two-dimensional anatomic slice that is continually updated. B-mode is currently used for diagnostic applications.

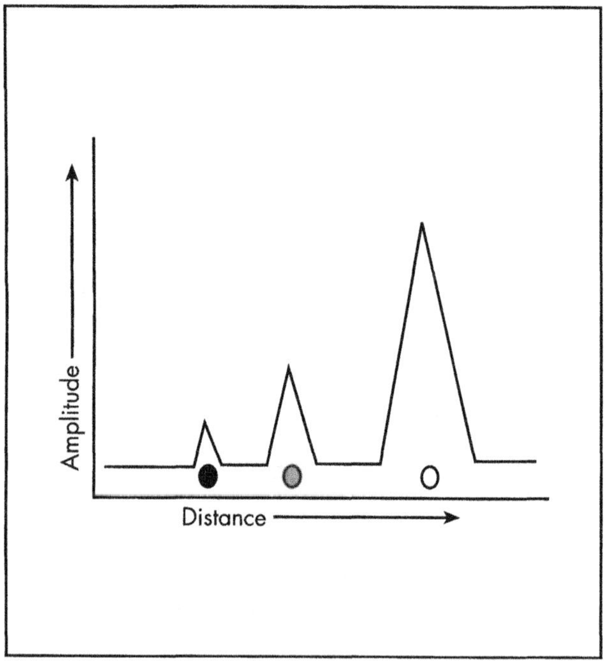

FIG. 15-4 Whereas A-mode uses peaks on a graph to depict the strength of the returning echoes, B-mode uses bright pixels on a monitor. The brighter the pixel, the stronger the returning echo.

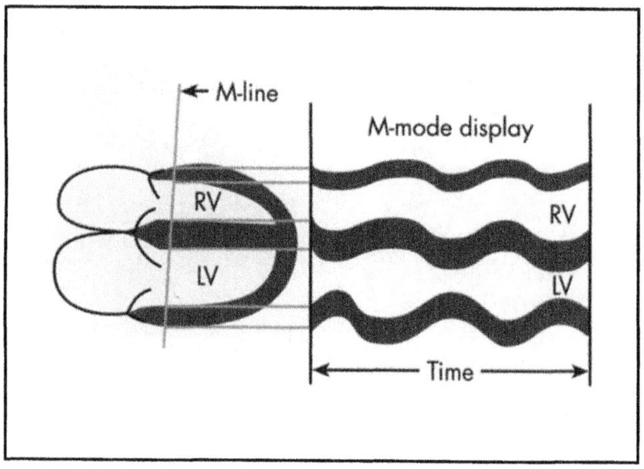

FIG. 15-5 M-mode displays the motion of a thin slice of an organ over time. *RV*, Right ventricle; *LV*, left ventricle.

M-mode is the continuous display of a thin slice of an organ over time. M-mode projects the echoes from a thin beam of sound over a time-oriented baseline (Figure 15-5). The main use is with echocardiography to assess the size of the heart chambers and the motion of the cardiac valves and walls.

Terminology Describing Echotexture

The terminology used to describe tissue texture within an ultrasound image is simple. *Echogenic* or *echoic* means that most of the sound is reflected back to the transducer. Echogenic areas appear white on the screen. *Sonolucent* means that most of the sound is transmitted to the deeper tissues, with only a few echoes reflected back to the transducer. Sonolucent areas appear dark on the screen. *Anechoic* describes the tissue that transmits all the sound to deeper tissues, reflecting none of the sound back to the transducer. Anechoic areas appear black on the screen and are generally fluid-filled structures (Figure 15-6).

The soft tissues are not only represented as black or white but also with many shades of gray in between. Additional terminology has been established to describe these areas. *Hyperechoic* describes tissues that reflect more sound back to the transducer than the surrounding tissues. Hyperechoic areas appear brighter than the surrounding tissues. *Hypoechoic* describes tissues that reflect less sound back to the transducer than the surrounding tissues. Hypoechoic areas appear darker than the surrounding tissues. *Isoechoic*

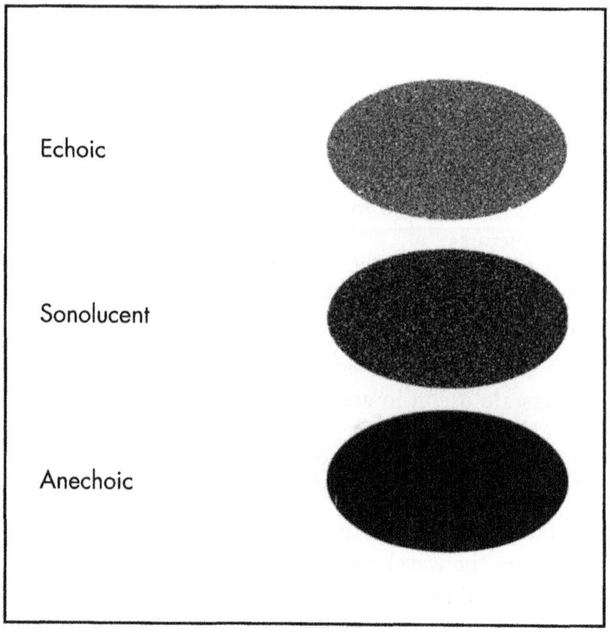

FIG. 15-6 *Echoic* tissue appears bright or white, *sonolucent* tissue appears dark, and *anechoic* tissue appears completely black on the monitor.

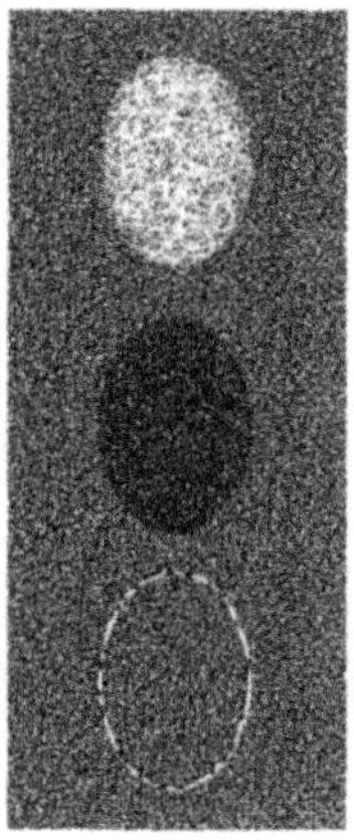

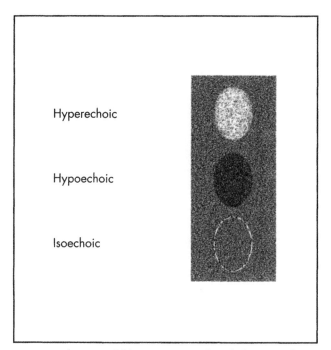

FIG. 15-7 An area within an organ or the whole organ that is brighter or whiter than the surrounding tissue is described as being *hyperechoic*. The areas that are darker than the surrounding tissue are described as hypoechoic. The areas that are the same as the surrounding tissues are described as *isoechoic*.

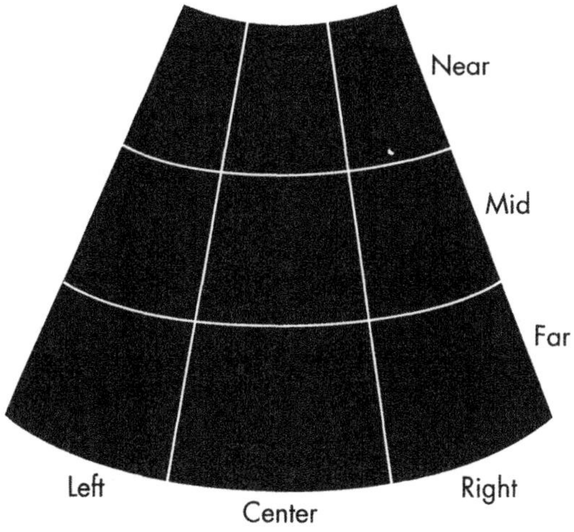

FIG. 15-8 The nine scan zones used to point out an area on the screen.

describes tissue that appears to have the same echotexture on the screen as the surrounding tissues (Figure 15-7).

At times it is impossible to point to areas on the screen, so terminology has been established to help with this problem. The screen is divided into nine zones, with each zone having its own label (Figure 15-8). Using this terminology, the sonographer can verbally point out the area of interest (e.g., midfield right or near field left).

Patient Preparation

To achieve an optimal acoustic window giving the best-quality image, close contact with the skin is necessary. Animals' hair must be clipped and in some cases shaved before the study. Occasionally, thin-coated animals can be imaged with minimal preparation. An acoustic coupling gel is used in all cases to eliminate the air interface and improve the acoustic window. Before applying the acoustic coupling gel, the area should be wiped with alcohol or generous amounts of soapy water to remove any loose hairs, dirt, and skin oils (Figure 15-9).

> Image quality increases as the acoustic coupling gel has time to work in.

Fasting of small animals before abdominal ultrasound is recommended. The ingesta and gas produced in the bowel decrease the amount of the abdomen that can be visualized.

Instrumentation

Ultrasound equipment has many controls for adjusting the quality of the image. Improper adjustment of any of these can greatly decrease the quality of the image.

Brightness and Contrast

The television monitor has controls that adjust the brightness and contrast for the image on the monitor. If the brightness has been adjusted too high or too low on the monitor, compensating with any other control cannot correct the brightness or darkness. Most machines have a gray bar, which displays the gray-scale capability. This capability varies from 16 to 128 shades of gray. The brightness and contrast should be adjusted so that black, white, and all the intermediate shades of gray can be seen.

Depth

The depth allows for adjustment of the amount of tissue being displayed on the monitor. The depth from the surface of the transducer is measured in centimeters (cm). The area of interest (e.g., kidney, heart) should cover at least two thirds of the screen. By decreasing the amount of depth being displayed, the area in the near field becomes larger (Figure 15-10).

> The organ of interest should fill three quarters of the monitor.

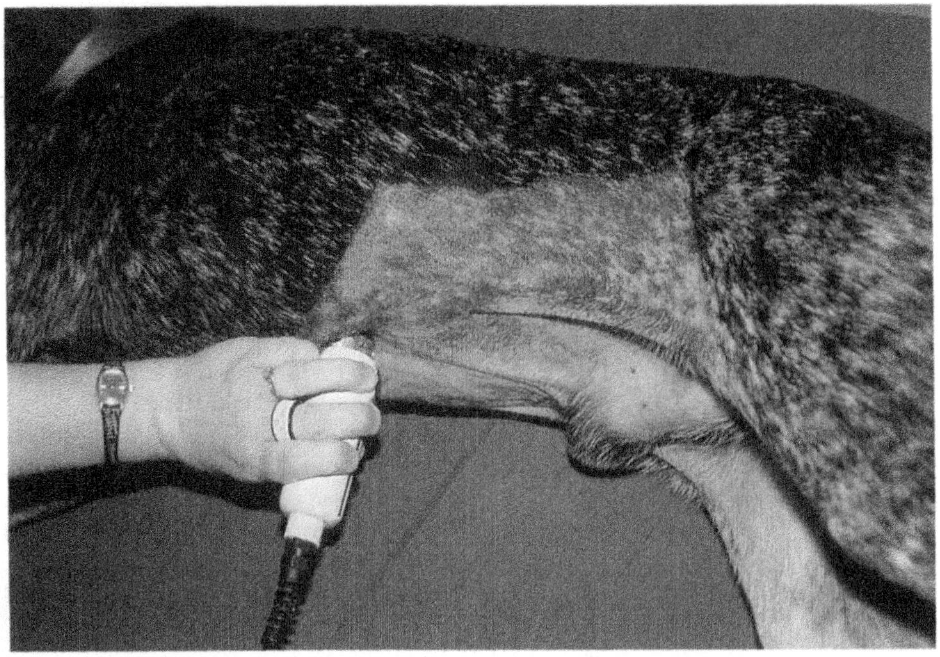

FIG. 15-9 Proper patient preparation is important before conducting an ultrasound examination. The hair should be clipped and the skin wiped with alcohol before the study begins.

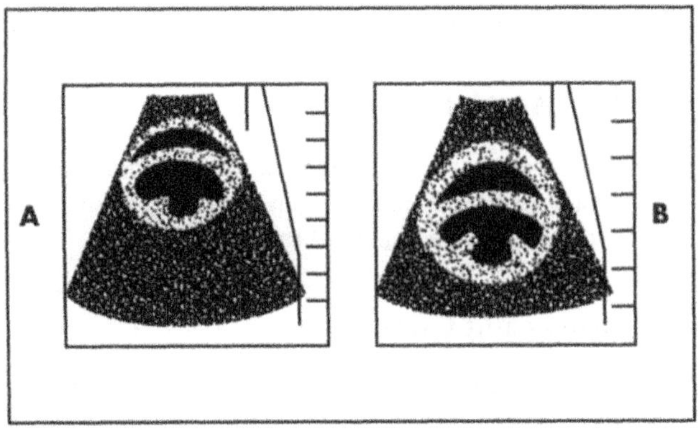

FIG. 15-10 The depth controls the amount of tissue displayed: **A,** 8 cm of depth; **B,** 6 cm of depth. The area of interest should cover at least two thirds of the screen.

Gain and Power

Gain (overall) and power (output) are two controls that can affect the overall brightness of the image (Figure 15-11). The gain and power are two ways to compensate for the attenuation of the sound beam as it travels through the tissues. Increasing the gain increases the *sensitivity* of the transducer to receiving the returning echoes. This can be compared with the volume on a hearing aid. Turning the volume up increases the hearing aid's ability to hear the incoming sounds. The power controls the *intensity* of the sound generated by the transducer. Increasing the power increases the intensity of the sound wave leaving the transducer. The sound wave is attenuated at the same rate; however, a higher-intensity sound wave transmitted into the tissues results in a higher-intensity sound wave returning to the transducer.

The image should display an even, overall brightness.

Time Gain Compensation

The controls that make up the time gain compensation (TGC) are the most important and also are the controls most often set improperly. The purpose of the TGC is to make like tissues look alike. The intensity of the sound decreases progressively as it returns from deeper tissues. When imaging the liver, for example, three similar reflectors located at 4 cm, 6 cm, and 8 cm of depth should have the same brightness on the monitor. Because of the attenuation of the echoes returning from the deeper tissues, however, the brightness gradually decreases (Figure 15-12, *A*). To compensate for the loss of energy, TGC adds increasing amounts of electronic gain to the returning echoes (Figure 15-12, *B*). The end product is three equal echoes that return from different depths, having the same brightness on the monitor (Figure 15-12, *C*).

TGC makes like tissues look similar to one another.

The typical controls that make up the TGC are near-field gain and far-field gain. The *near-field gain* controls the amount of electronic gain added to the sound returning from the near field (Figure 15-13). This should be set so that the echoes blend uniformly with those displayed in the midfield.

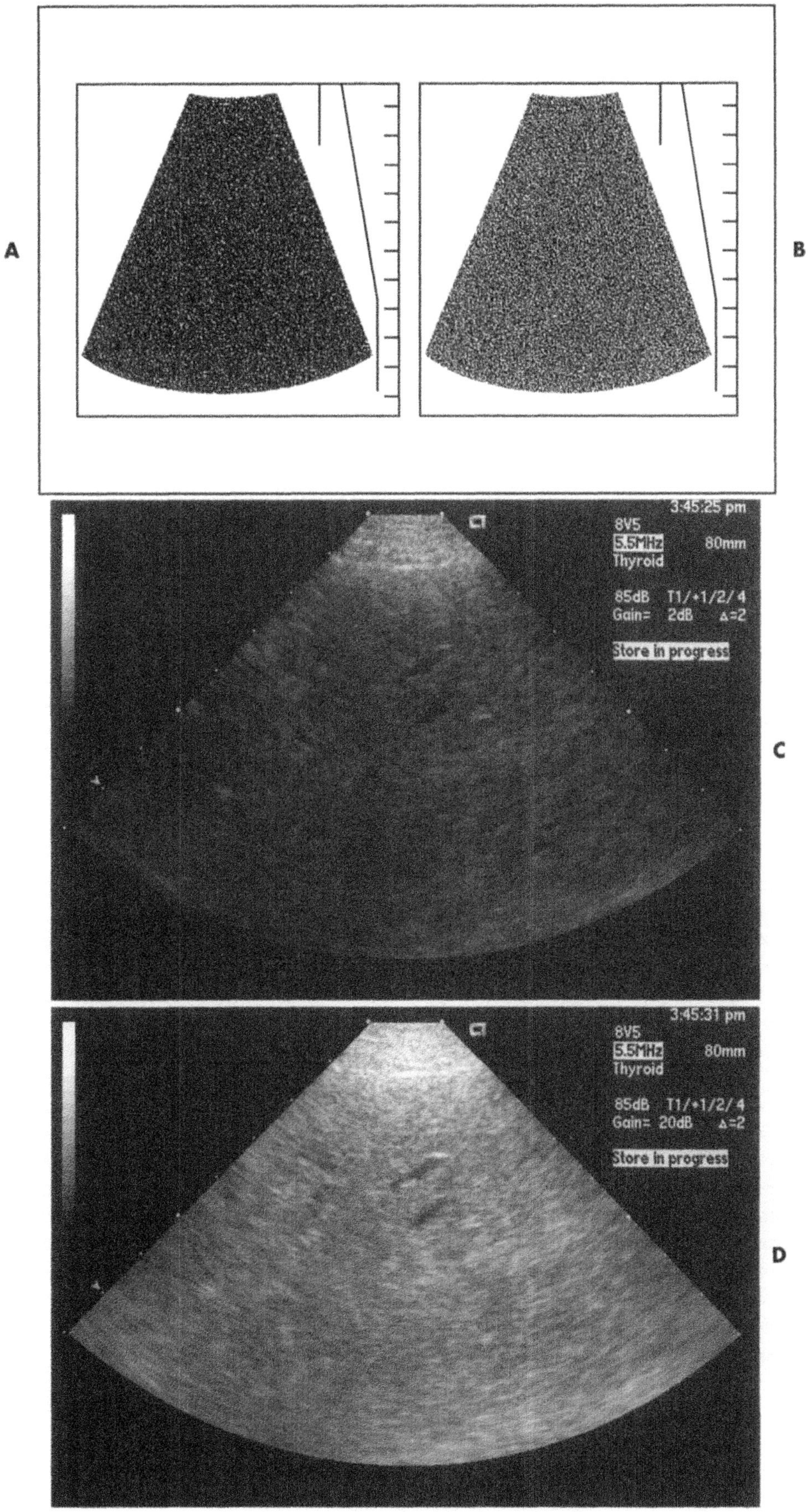

FIG. 15-11 Both overall gain and power controls affect the overall brightness of the screen. The higher the overall gain or the power, the brighter the image on the screen. **A** and **C** display adequate overall brightness, whereas **B** and **D** display increased brightness overall.

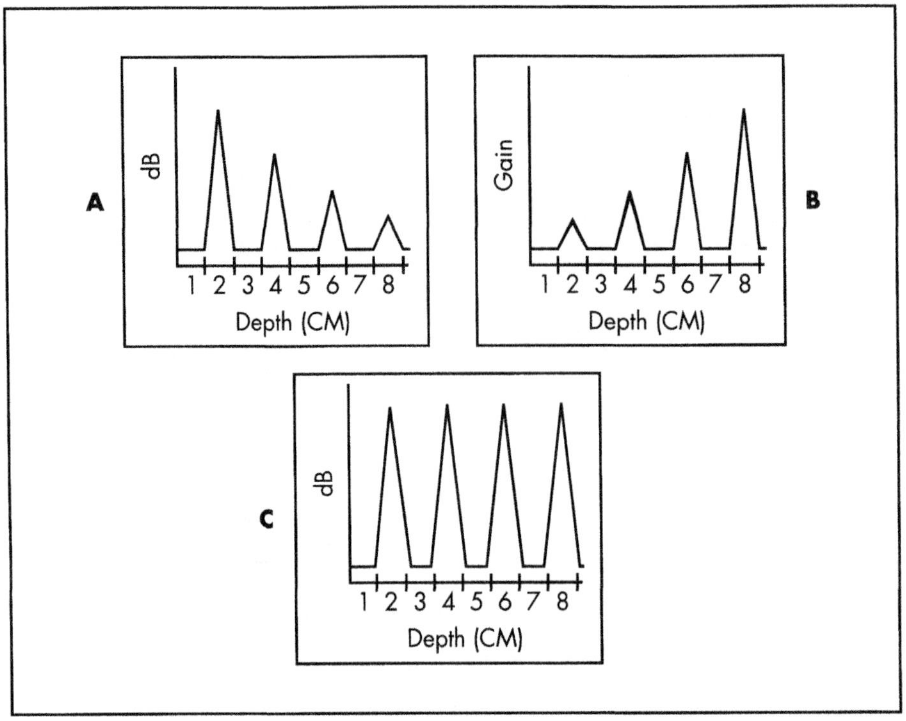

FIG. 15-12 Time gain compensation (TGC) makes like tissues look similar to one another. **A,** Decreasing intensity of returning echoes caused by attenuation of the sound beam from the deeper tissues. **B,** To compensate for loss in intensity, electronic gain or intensity is added in increasing amounts to the returning echoes. **C,** Results showing that echoes at all depths have the same intensity and appear to have equal brightness. *dB,* Decibels.

The *far-field gain* controls the amount of electronic gain added to the echoes returning from the far field (Figure 15-14). With some of the new ultrasound equipment the TGC is in the form of multiple slide pods. The pods at the top control the near-field gain, whereas the pods closer to the bottom control the midfield and far-field gain (Figure 15-15).

If proper brightness cannot be achieved, the following control factors should be verified. First, check the brightness and contrast of the monitor. If the brightness and contrast on the monitor are incorrectly set, changing the TGC cannot compensate for this error. Next, check the power setting to make sure it is not too low. If all the controls are set correctly, the next step is to attempt to improve the acoustic contact with the skin. This can be done by applying more coupling gel or shaving the clipped area with a razor. If none of these changes works, switching to a lower-frequency transducer may alleviate the problem. Some resolution will be lost, but it is a necessary trade-off when brightness cannot be achieved.

Artifacts

Artifacts can occur during any ultrasound study. Proper identification of these artifacts is important to prevent confusion or misinterpretation. The presence of some artifacts is beneficial when making a diagnosis. Two such artifacts include acoustic shadowing and distant enhancement. Others, if not readily identified, can be confused as part of the anatomy or a disease process.

Acoustic shadowing occurs when the sound is attenuated or reflected at an acoustic interface (Figure 15-16). This prevents the sound from being transmitted to the deeper tissues, resulting in lower-than-normal, or absence of, returning echoes from those areas. The structures that can cause acoustic shadowing include bone, calculus, mineralization, and occasionally fat. For acoustic shadowing to occur, the interface must be in the focal zone of the transducer. If not, the shadowed area may be filled in with echoes from the surrounding tissues as the sound beam diverges. This artifact is more pronounced with higher-frequency transducers.

Distant enhancement occurs when the sound beam traverses a cystic structure (Figure 15-17). The tissues deep toward the cystic structure appear brighter than the surrounding tissues. The enhancement occurs because the sound traveling through the fluid-filled areas is less attenuated than in the surrounding tissues. This artifact is useful in establishing that an anechoic or hypoechoic structure is in fact fluid-filled.

> Distant enhancement can be used to confirm the presence of fluid.

Many artifacts have no diagnostic usefulness, although if not identified as artifacts, they can lead to confusion. The *slice thickness* artifact, for example, occurs when imaging an

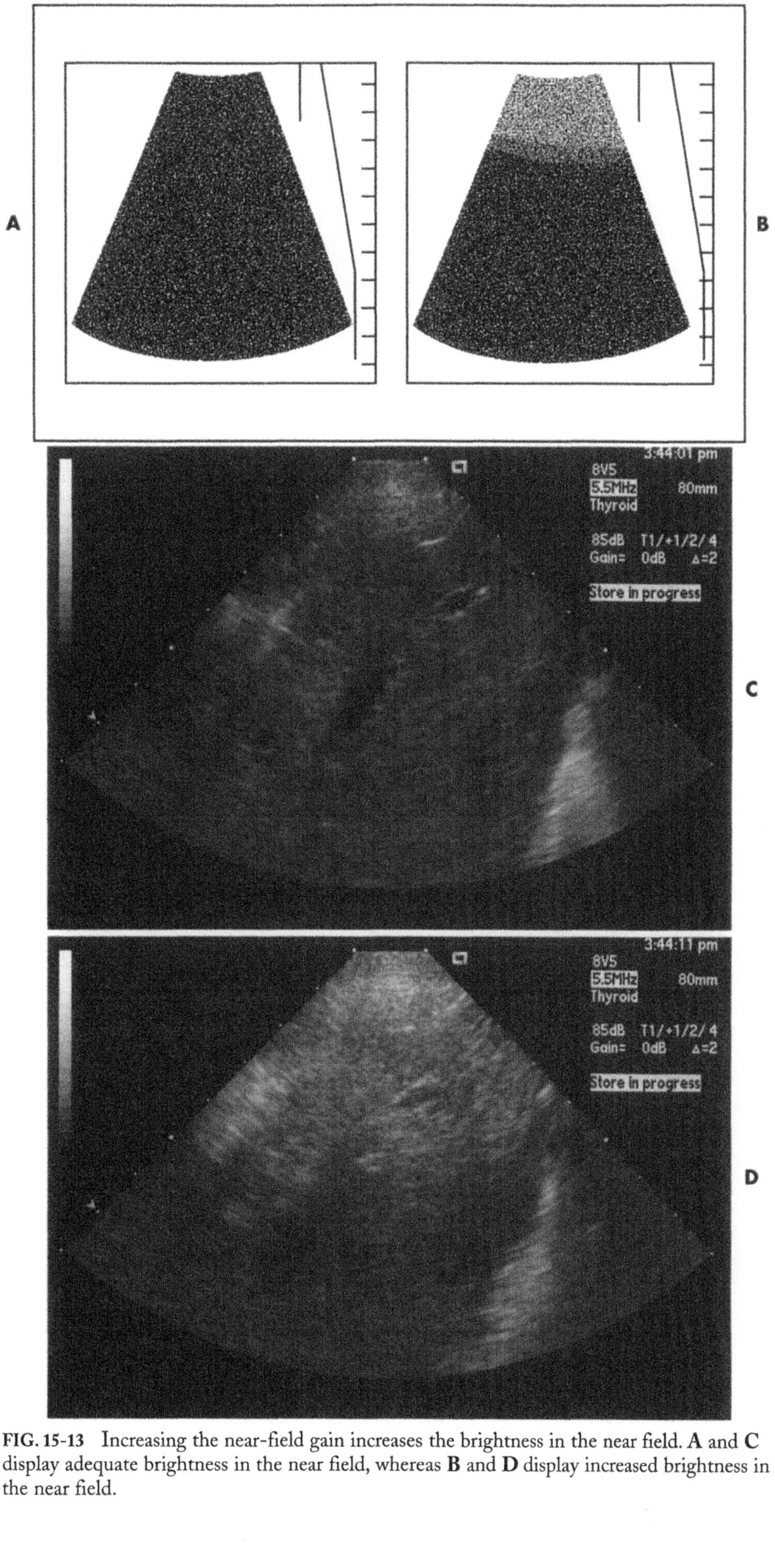

FIG. 15-13 Increasing the near-field gain increases the brightness in the near field. **A** and **C** display adequate brightness in the near field, whereas **B** and **D** display increased brightness in the near field.

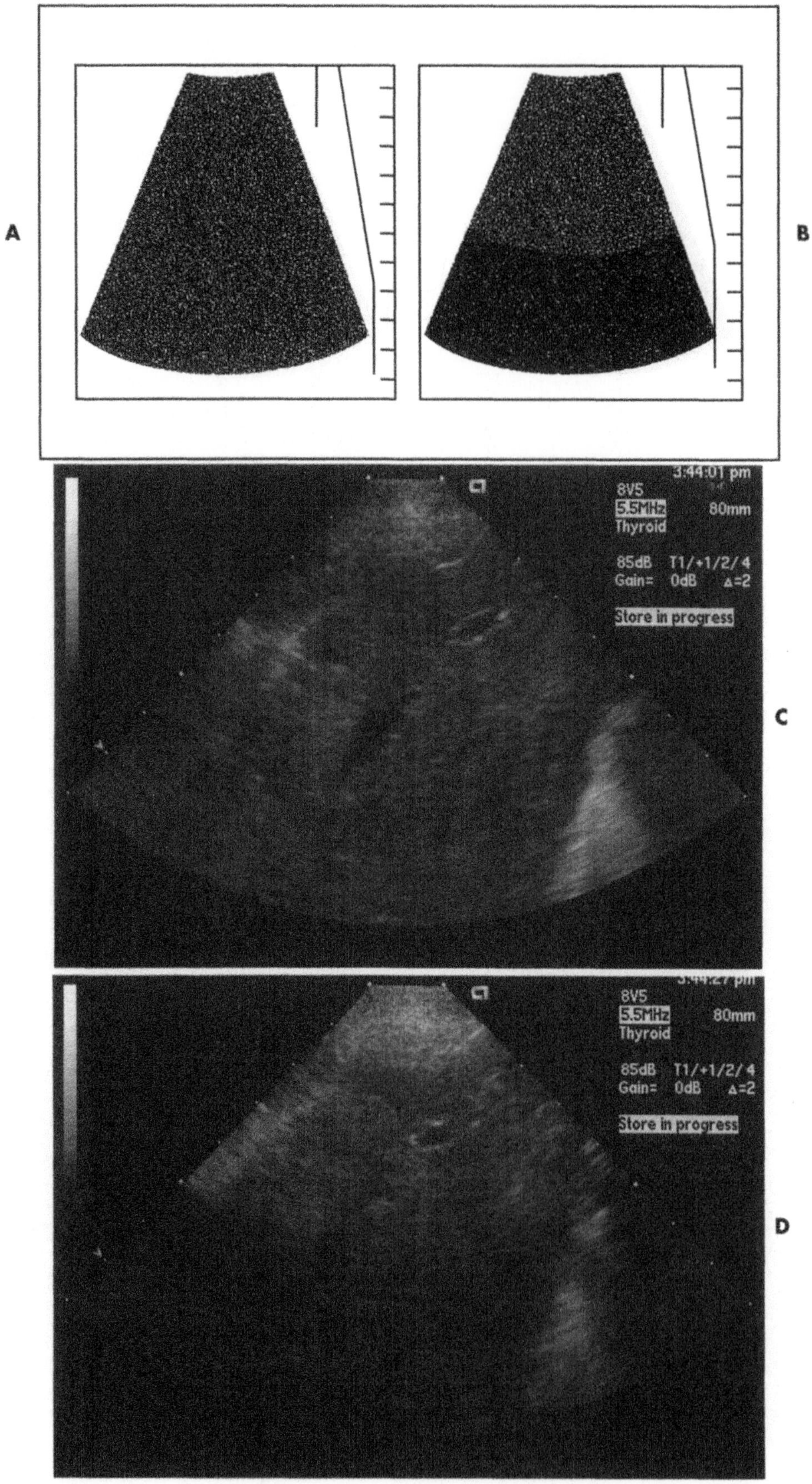

FIG. 15-14 Increasing the far-field gain increases the brightness in the far field. **A** and **C** display adequate brightness in the far field, whereas **B** and **D** display decreased brightness in the far field.

anechoic or hypoechoic structure. Echoes are added when the transducer receives echoes with different amplitudes from the same area at the same depth. The computer then averages these amplitudes and incorporates them in the two-dimensional image (Figure 15-18). The slice thickness artifact can be minimized by decreasing the overall gain; however; this does not totally eliminate it.

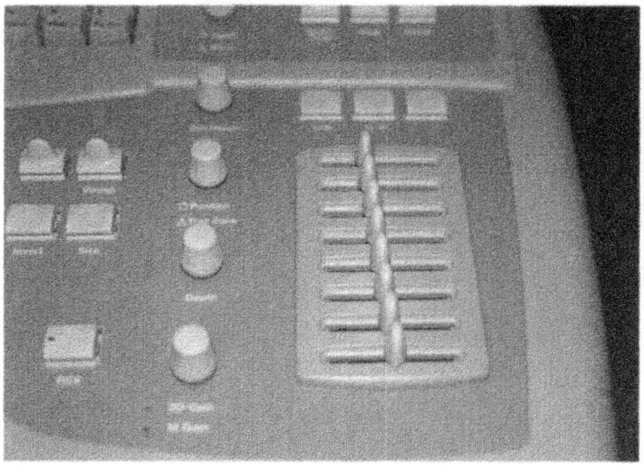

FIG. 15-15 Slide pods control the brightness in different parts of the field. The top pods control the near-field gain, whereas the pods closer to the bottom control the midfield and far-field gains.

Reverberation artifact occurs when the sound is reflected off a highly reflective interface (e.g., soft tissues to air or soft tissues to bone or metal) and then reflected back into the tissues by the surface of the transducer (Figure 15-19). This bouncing back and forth can continue until the sound energy has completely attenuated. Each time the sound returns to the transducer it produces an image at a location on the screen that is proportional to the time of travel between the transducer and the reflective interface. This creates a series of lines of equal distance on the screen.

The *mirror-image* artifact creates the illusion of liver on the thoracic side of the diaphragm or the appearance of a second heart beyond the lung interface (Figure 15-20). This artifact can be produced in areas with strongly reflective interfaces. The sound transmitted into the liver is reflected off the diaphragm. Some of those echoes are not reflected directly toward the transducer but back into the liver. In the liver some of the misdirected echoes are reflected back to the diaphragm and then to the transducer. The computer sees the misdirected echoes as being reflected from the other side of the diaphragm. One way that the mirror-image artifact can be minimized is by decreasing the depth to include only the area of interest.

To eliminate the mirror-image artifact, decrease the depth of the image.

Refraction artifact is produced when the transmitted sound is refracted at an interface between two tissues of different acoustic impedance. When a sound wave strikes an

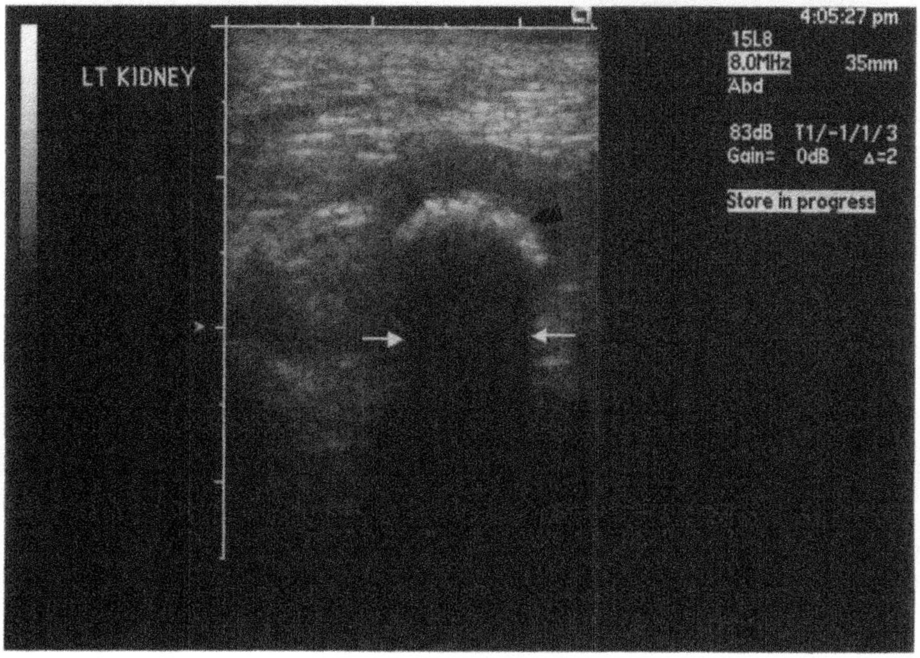

FIG. 15-16 Acoustic shadowing from a renal calculus. Black arrow indicates the highly reflective surface of the calculus. White arrows indicate the shadowing caused by the calculus.

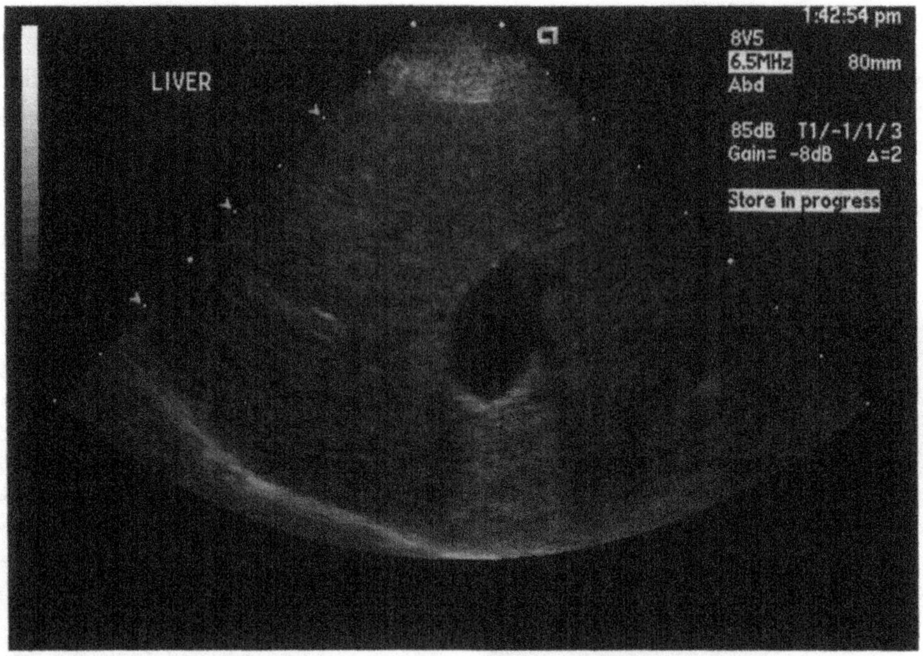

FIG. 15-17 Distance enhancement in the liver resulting from the sound waves passing through the fluid-filled gallbladder.

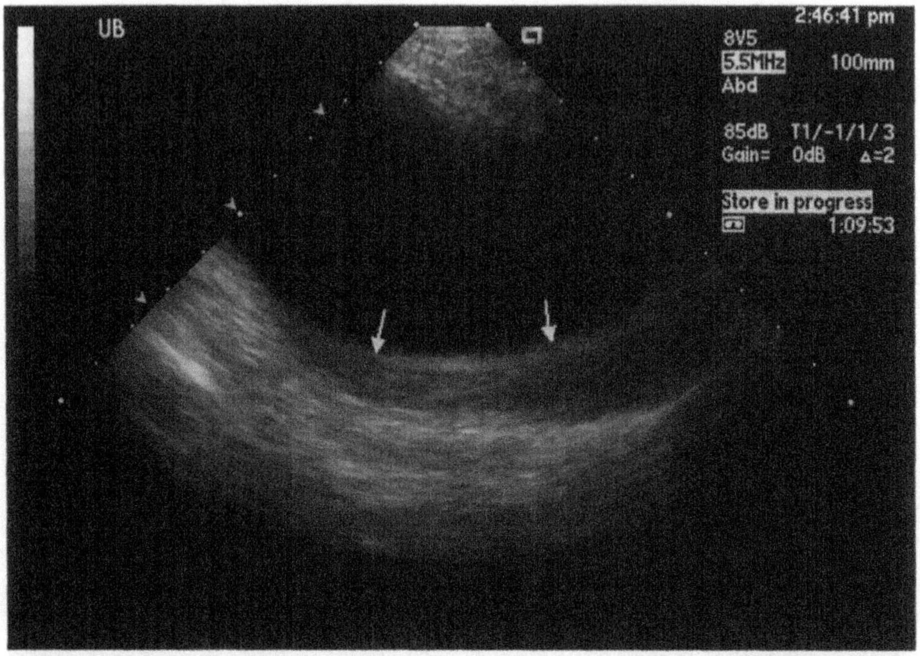

FIG. 15-18 Urinary bladder with a slice thickness artifact on the far wall of the bladder *(arrows)*.

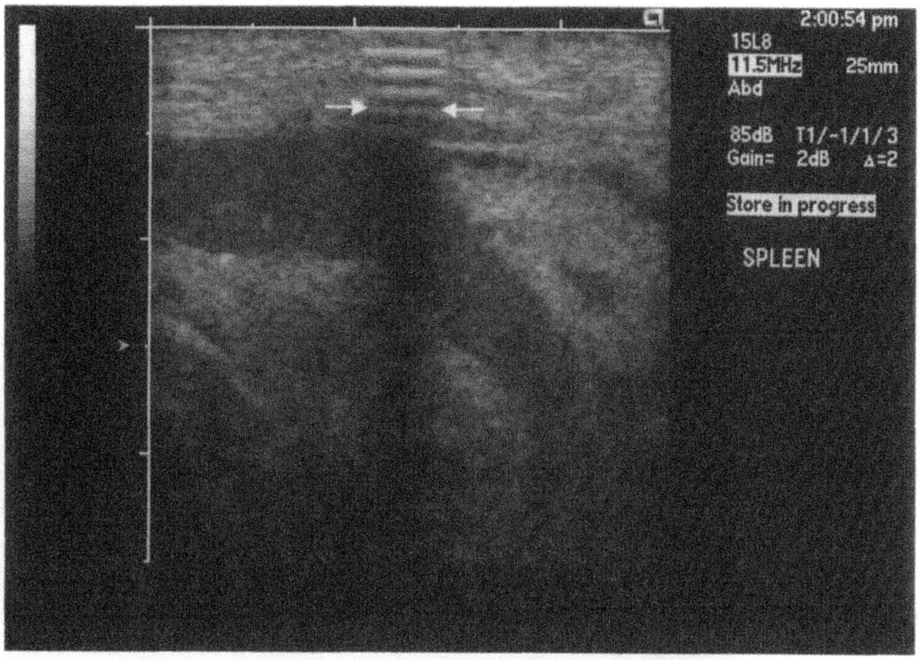

FIG. 15-19 Reverberation artifact resulting from poor contact with the skin. Notice the equally spaced echoic lines trailing from the white interface *(arrows).*

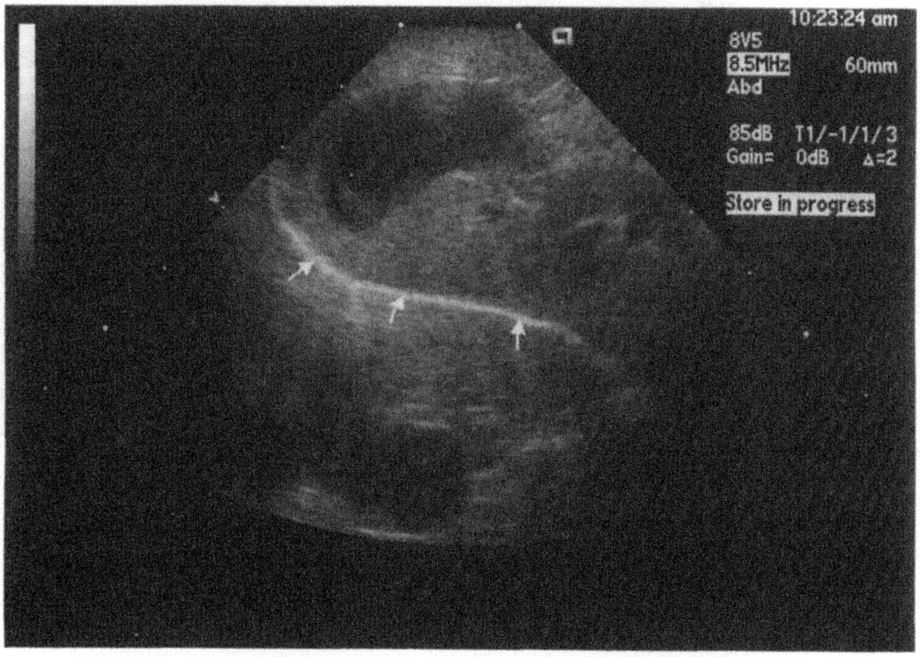

FIG. 15-20 Mirror-image artifact. The arrows indicate the liver/diaphragm-to-lung interface. The actual liver is in the near field to this line. The far field represents the mirror image of the liver.

interface that is perpendicular, part is reflected back to the transducer, and part is transmitted in a straight path into the deeper tissues. If the sound wave strikes an interface at an angle other than perpendicular, the transmitted sound is refracted. Refraction may cause an object to appear slightly shifted from its real position or may create a shadow adjacent to a curved structure (Figure 15-21).

Range ambiguity artifact is a group of echoic lines within a fluid-filled structure. When the sound is transmitted into a large fluid-filled area, it is reflected off the far wall of the cavity. If the distance is greater than the depth displayed, the sound cannot reach the transducer until after the next series of sound pulses have been sent. The computer interprets this as sound that has been reflected by an interface that is much closer to the transducer than it actually is (Figure 15-22).

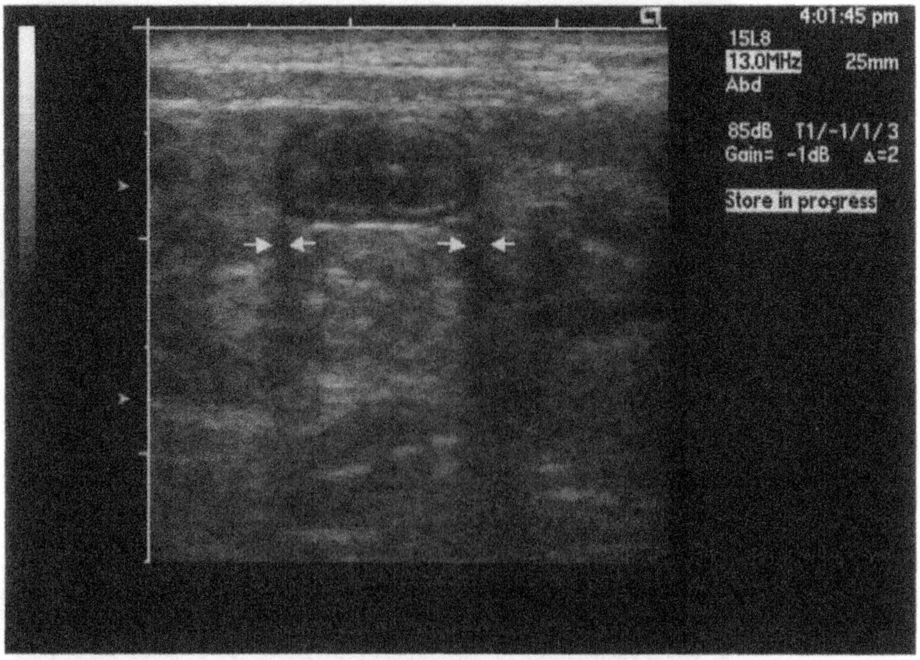

FIG. 15-21 Refraction artifact, *(arrows)*, coming off the curved surface of a transverse section of a small intestine.

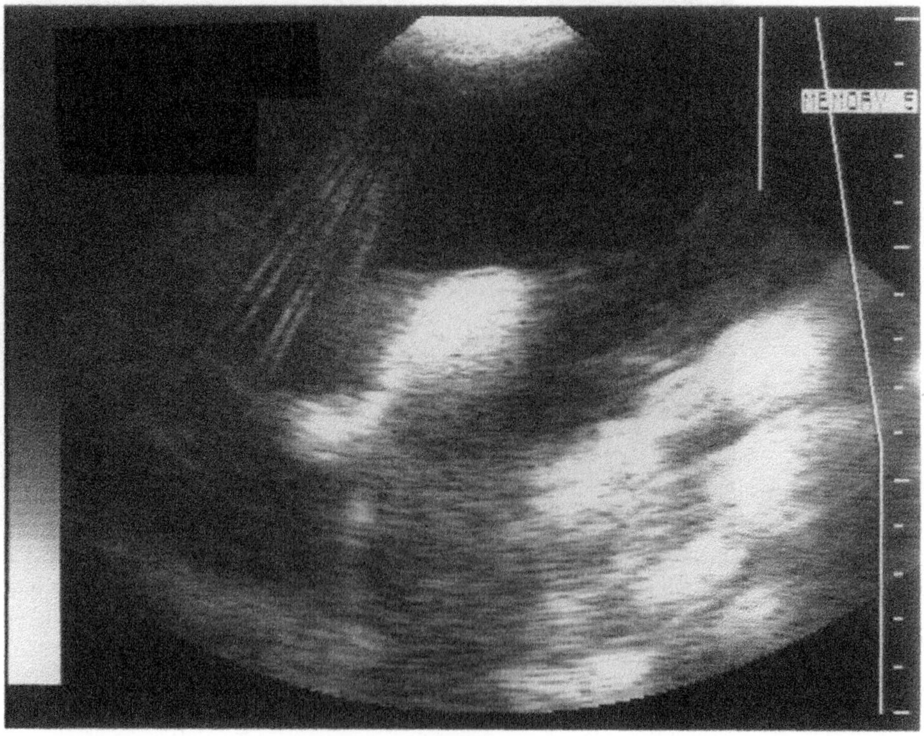

FIG. 15-22 Range ambiguity can be seen as poorly defined echoic lines within abdominal scan showing ascites.

Transducer Maneuvers

Ultrasound examination of the abdomen requires manipulation or maneuvering of the transducer to evaluate organs entirely and image them in different planes. The basic transducer maneuvers include slide, fan, roll, and rotate as well as using transducer pressure.

The *slide maneuver*, as the name implies, involves sliding the transducer along the abdomen ventrally, dorsally, cranially, caudally, or in any combination of these directions. This maneuver is used to progress from one area of the abdomen to another (Figure 15-23).

In the *fanning maneuver* the head of the transducer is held stationary on the patient and slowly rocked against the axis of the insonant sound beam. The transducer is "fanned" through the organ or tissue of interest, analogous to cooling oneself with a paper fan (Figure 15-24).

In the *roll maneuver* the head of the transducer is again held stationary on the patient, only this time it is rocked along the axis of the insonant sound beam. This maneuver is useful when an abdominal organ of interest is located at the edge of the image. By rolling the transducer, the organ can be brought to the center of the ultrasound image (Figure 15-25).

The *rotate maneuver* involves rotation of the transducer, typically to a location where the insonant sound beam is 90 degrees from the initial position. The head of the transducer is held stationary on the patient and rotated or twisted, usually clockwise, to obtain an image of an organ in an orthogonal plane (Figure 15-26).

The use of *transducer pressure* in an abdominal ultrasound examination can be either a benefit or a detriment. By increasing pressure, essentially pushing the transducer harder against the abdominal wall, organs in the far field can be brought up into the focal zone, improving resolution (Figure 15-27). In addition, organs such as gas-filled small intestinal loops that may interfere with visualization of deeper tissues can be displaced away from the central beam, allowing visualization of deeper structures or organs. Too much transducer pressure can be detrimental and interfere with evaluation of an organ. By decreasing pressure, tissues in the near field that may be less distinct because of near-field artifact are displayed deeper and closer to the focal zone and therefore are better visualized. Too much transducer pressure can also distort the normal shape of an organ (Figure 15-28). This is most evident when evaluating the urinary bladder, where too much pressure changes the shape of the urinary bladder, making it appear more ellipsoid and flattened. By simply lessening the pressure of the transducer, the urinary bladder becomes more spherical.

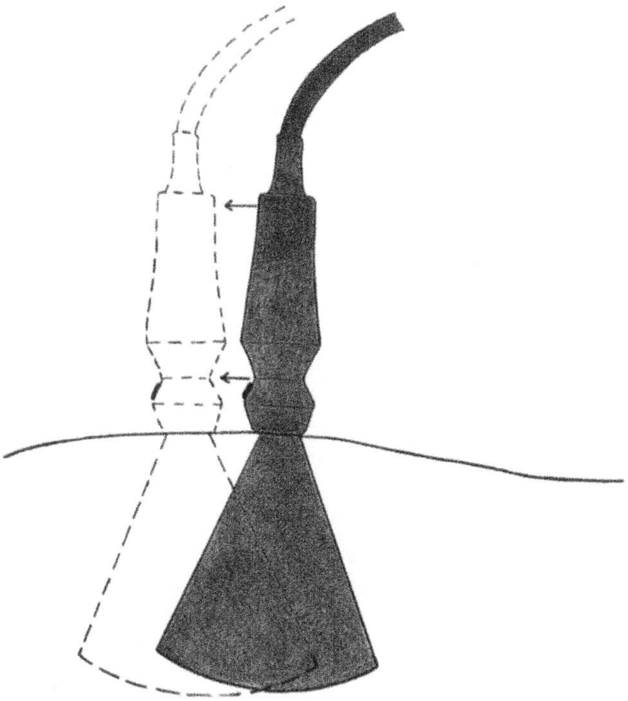

FIG. 15-23 Slide maneuver, used to cover large areas, as in following a loop of intestines or a vessel.

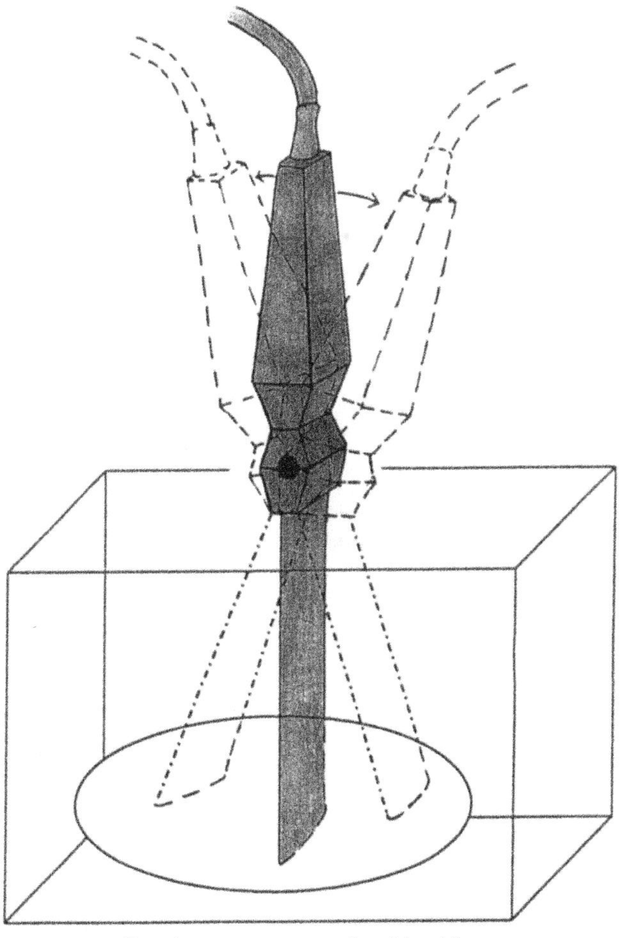

FIG. 15-24 Fanning maneuver, used to identify a structure as spherical or linear. When fanned, a spherical structure blinks in and out of the image on screen. A linear structure travels across the screen when fanned.

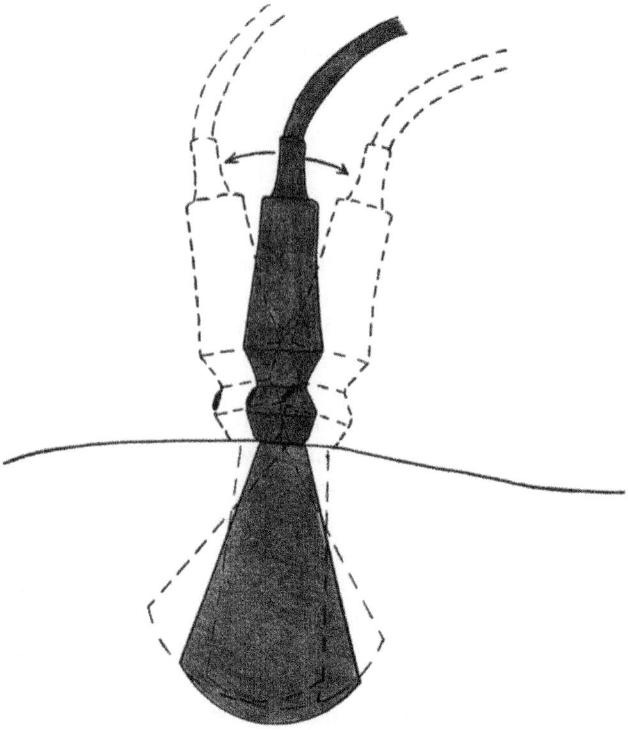

FIG. 15-25 Roll maneuver, used to bring an object that is at the edge of the image on the screen into the center of the screen.

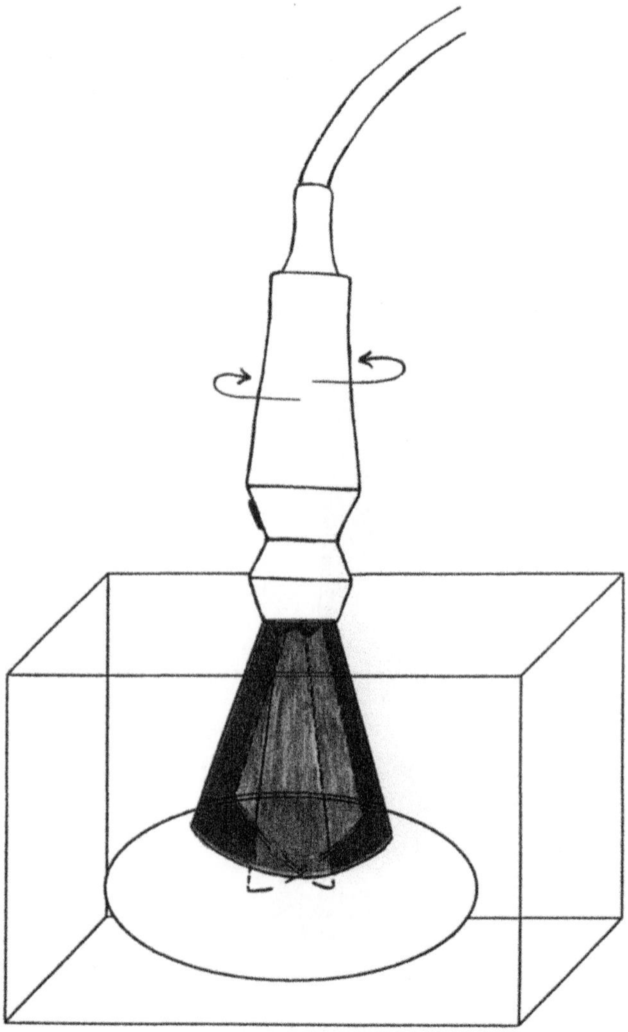

FIG. 15-26 Rotate maneuver, used to look at an object in two planes that are 90 degrees to one another.

A

B

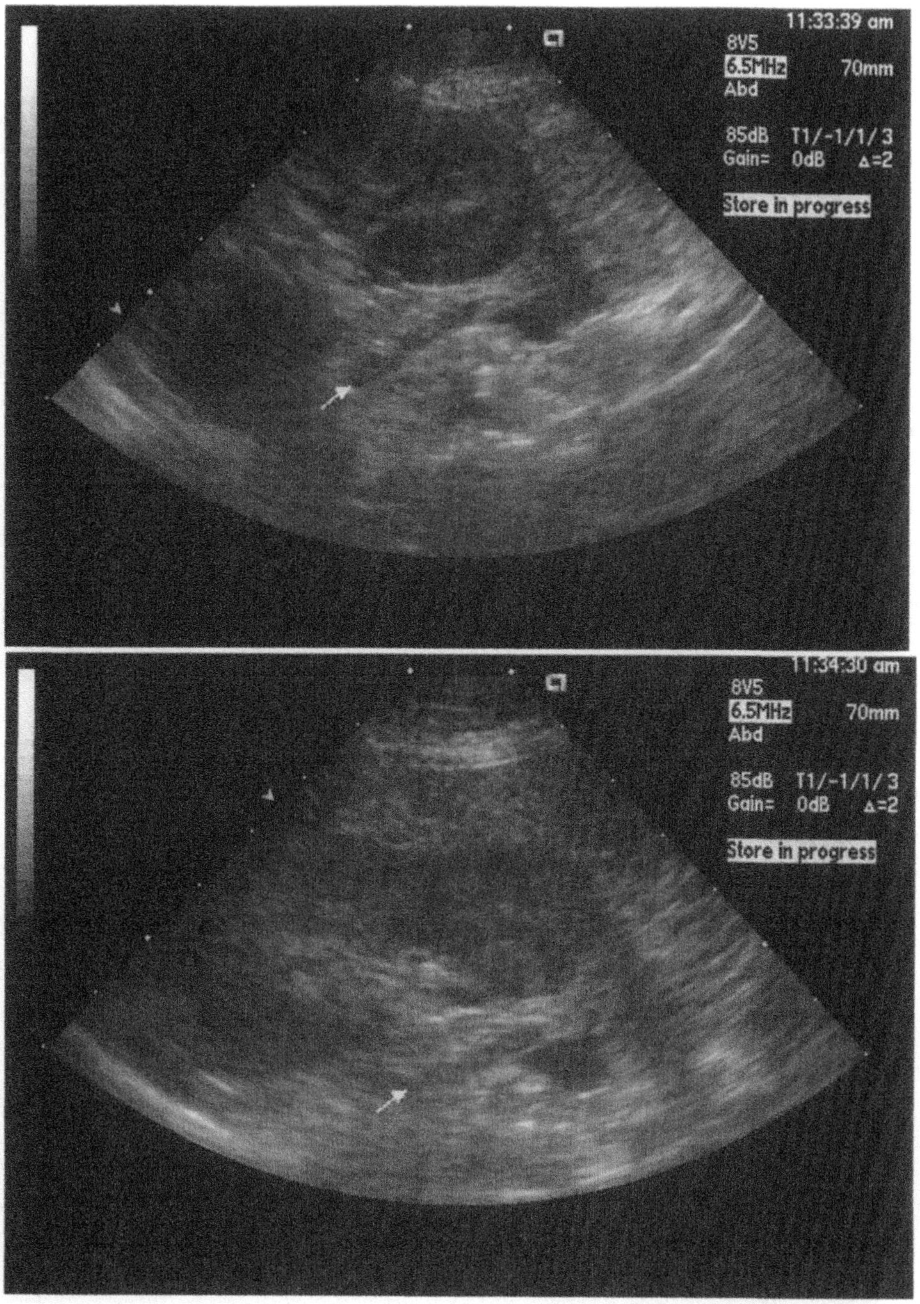

FIG. 15-27 Transducer pressure can be used to bring an object in the far field into the midfield focal zone, improving the resolution. **A,** Adrenal gland *(arrow).* **B,** Same adrenal gland *(arrow)* as in *A* with pressure to bring the gland closer to the focal zone. Note that the resolution is better in **B**.

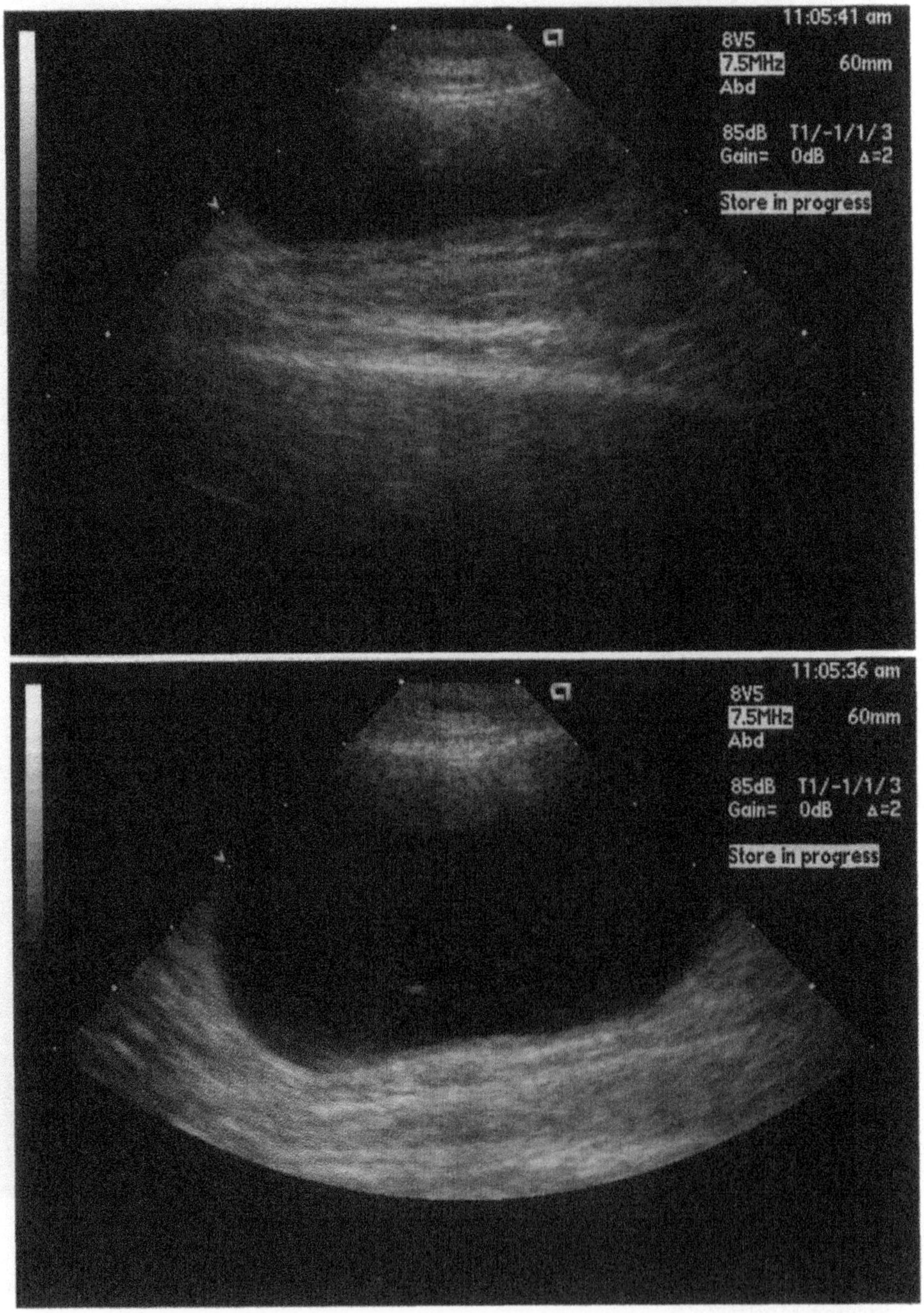

FIG. 15-28 Transducer pressure can impede the ability to image some organs. **A,** Urinary bladder. Too much pressure compresses the bladder, making visualization difficult. **B,** Same urinary bladder as in *A* after decreasing the amount of pressure applied.

Scanning Techniques for Normal Abdominal Anatomy

An ultrasound examination of the abdomen should be performed using a complete, systematic approach. Development of a systematic approach promotes thorough evaluation of abdominal organs and decreases the possibility of missing potential abnormalities.

Patient positioning for abdominal ultrasonography is important in that it affects the way abdominal organs lie within the peritoneal cavity, which ultimately affects how the different organs are imaged. Right and left lateral recumbent positioning and dorsal recumbent positioning are typically used. However, animals are more likely to lie quietly in lateral recumbency, and if patient restraint becomes necessary, this positioning requires less technical assistance.

A systematic approach begins with the patient in left lateral recumbency. The examination starts at the cranial aspect of the abdomen with evaluation of the liver. The examiner proceeds in a circular manner around the abdomen, evaluating the right kidney and then sliding caudally, following the aorta and caudal vena cava to the level of the bifurcation of the aorta into the external iliac arteries. Lymph nodes can be seen associated with the aorta and caudal vena cava. The examiner evaluates the urinary bladder and prostate gland and then slides cranially to image the small intestinal tract and stomach. Organs that are more difficult to image, such as the right limb of the pancreas and the right adrenal gland, can then be evaluated before imaging the opposite side of the abdomen.

The patient is then rolled over to right lateral recumbency, and the examination continues with imaging of the left kidney. Again in a circular fashion, the remainder of the abdomen is examined. Moving forward, the spleen is imaged, followed by the stomach and liver. By sliding caudally, the small intestinal tract can be reexamined. At the caudal extent of the abdomen, the urinary bladder and prostate can be evaluated again. The colon can then be followed cranially to the level of the transverse colon. The examination ends by evaluation of difficult organs to image, such as the left limb of the pancreas and the left adrenal gland.

When performing abdominal ultrasound examinations, knowledge of normal anatomy is essential. Successful recognition of disease processes requires a mental picture of normal ultrasonographic architecture, echotexture, and echogenicity of abdominal organs.

Liver

The liver is located in the cranial abdomen and is protected by the caudal rib cage. This feature necessitates subcostal and intercostal sonographic interrogation to image the entire liver effectively (Figure 15-29).

The liver is composed of five lobes: the caudate, right medial, quadrate, left medial, and left lateral. The borders between these lobes are almost imperceptible in the normal liver. Interlobar borders may be seen with real-time scanning, when the lobes can be observed sliding on one another during respiration. The internal echogenicity and echotexture of the liver are homogenous and coarse. In terms of relative echogenicity to other organs and structures, the liver is hypoechoic to the spleen, hypo- or isoechoic to falciform fat, and iso- or hyperechoic to the renal cortex.

Vascular structures that can be visualized within the liver include the portal and hepatic veins (Figure 15-30). Portal veins are anechoic tubular structures with echogenic walls and can be seen branching within the hepatic parenchyma. Hepatic veins are anechoic tubular structures similar in appearance to portal veins but lacking echogenic walls. Hepatic veins provide venous drainage of blood filtered by the hepatic lobules and can be seen communicating with the caudal vena cava deep in the liver near the caval hiatus of the diaphragm.

Deep in the liver, a curvilinear hyperechoic interface represents the interface between aerated lung and the parietal pleural surface of the diaphragm (Figure 15-31).

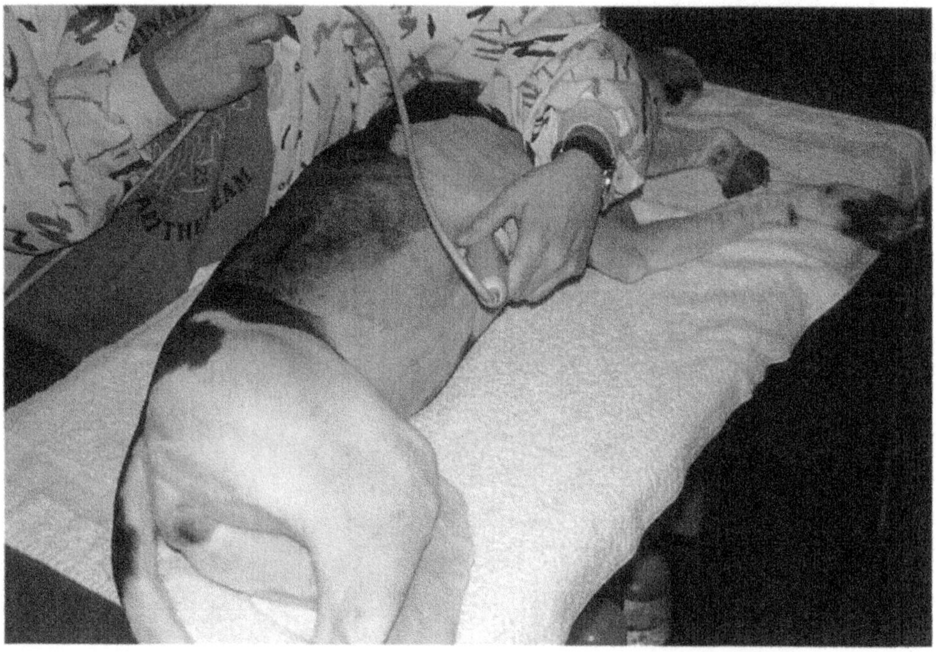

FIG. 15-29 Transducer positioning for ultrasound scan of the liver.

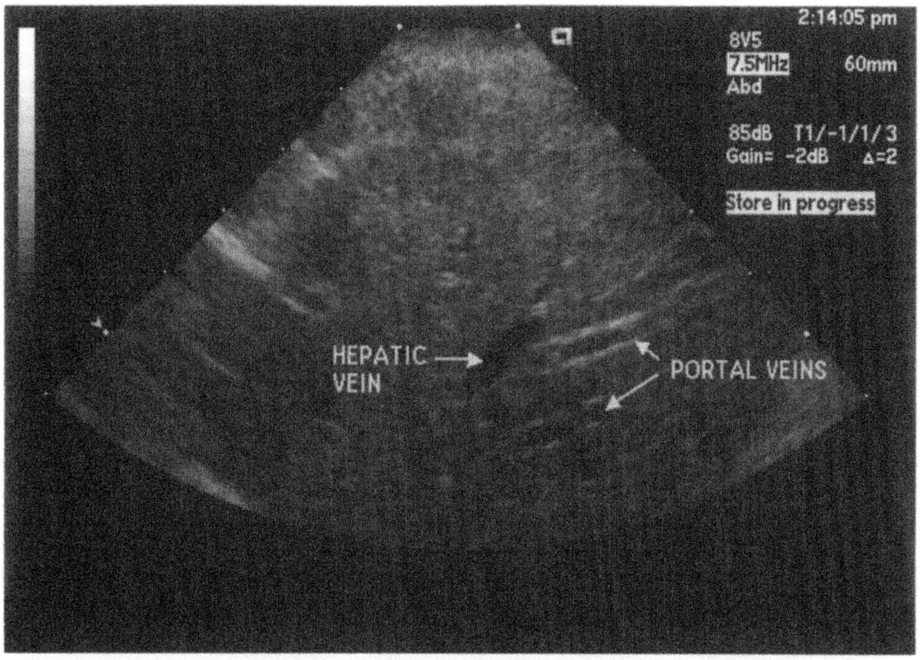

FIG. 15-30 Hepatic and portal veins can be visualized in the liver. Portal veins have echogenic walls; hepatic veins do not have echogenic walls.

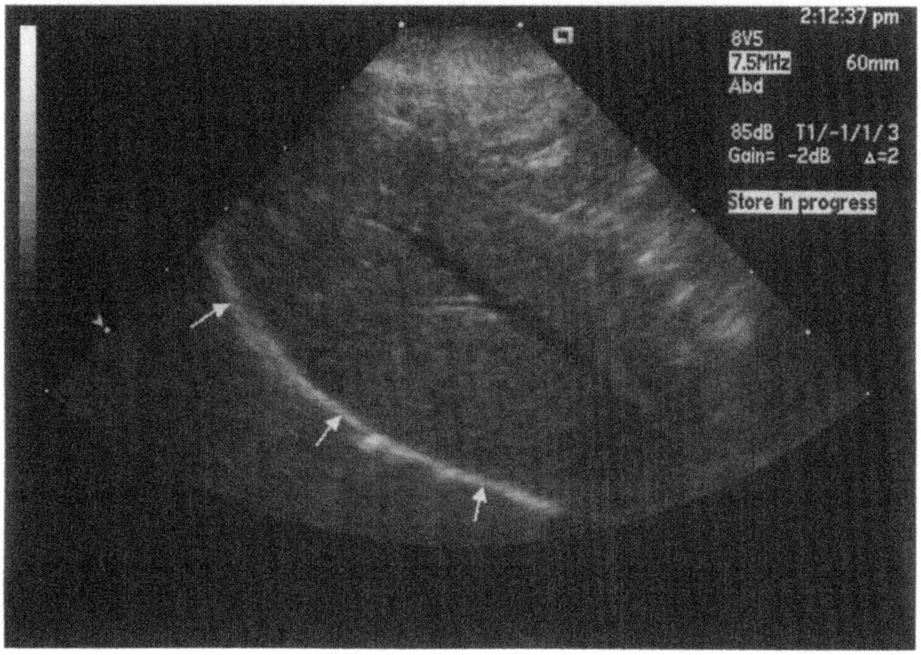

FIG. 15-31 Curvilinear echoic line deep in the liver *(arrows)* represents the interface between aerated lung and the diaphragm.

Gallbladder

The gallbladder is located between the right medial and quadrate lobes of the liver. The gallbladder can be imaged with a subcostal, midsagittal approach by fanning to the right of midline or from a right intercostal window immediately dorsal to the sternum.

The normal gallbladder appears as an anechoic, round or oval structure of variable size. Echogenic bile may be found and is visualized in a gravity-dependent location by fanning through the gallbladder. The wall of the gallbladder usually is not well visualized but may be seen as an echogenic line; visualization depends on transducer resolution, with normal thickness of the wall ranging from 1 to 2 mm. The cystic duct can normally be followed from the neck of the gallbladder to the porta hepatis. Acoustic enhancement of the liver parenchyma deep toward the gallbladder is evident to varying degrees, depending on the viscosity of the bile (Figure 15-32).

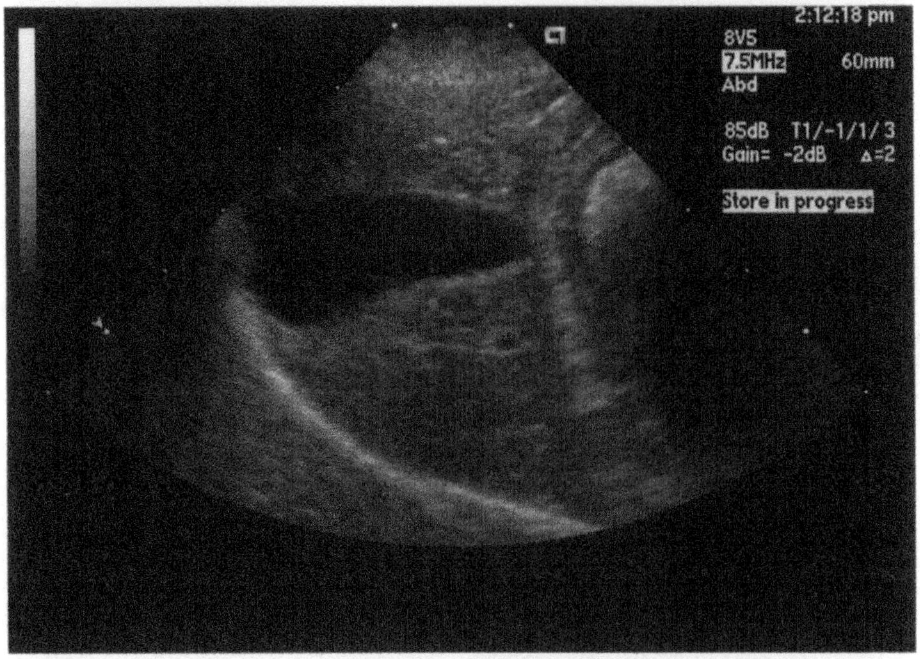

FIG. 15-32 Normal gallbladder.

Kidneys

The kidneys are located in the retroperitoneal space in the cranial to middorsal abdomen. The right kidney is positioned more cranially than the left, with the cranial pole extending to a fossa within the caudate lobe of the liver. The right kidney can be visualized using a subcostal or intercostal window (Figure 15-33). The intercostal window allows viewing of the kidney in a neutral anatomic position, whereas transducer pressure from a subcostal approach can alter the position of the kidney. The left kidney is typically best visualized immediately caudal to the last rib; however, in some cases an intercostal window is necessary to view the kidney in a neutral anatomic position.

Imaging of the kidneys is typically in two or more planes, including sagittal, transverse, and dorsal (Figure 15-34). The visible internal architecture of the kidney consists of the cortex, medulla, renal crest, peripelvic fat, and interlobar and arcuate arteries. The renal cortex has a homogenous echogenicity and a fine echotexture. The medulla is uniform in echogenicity and hypoechoic relative to the cortex. The demarcation between the cortex and the medulla is crisp. In the normal kidney the renal pelvis is not visible. Hyperechoic peripelvic fat surrounds the renal pelvis and envelops the renal crest in the transverse plane (Figure 15-35). The interlobar arteries are seen as hyperechoic lines radiating from the renal pelvis and extending to the corticomedullary junction in the sagittal plane. Arcuate arteries are seen as echogenic circular structures in the dorsal plane (Figure 15-36). In terms of relative echogenicity to other organs, the right kidney is hypoechoic or isoechoic to the caudate lobe of the liver, and the left kidney is hypoechoic to the spleen.

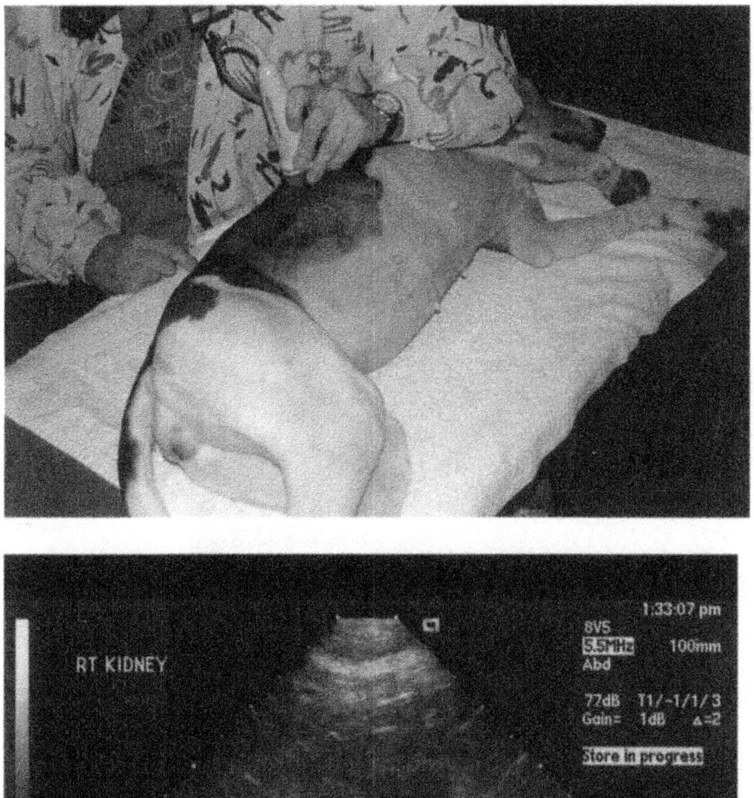

FIG. 15-33 Transducer positioning for ultrasound scan of the right kidney.

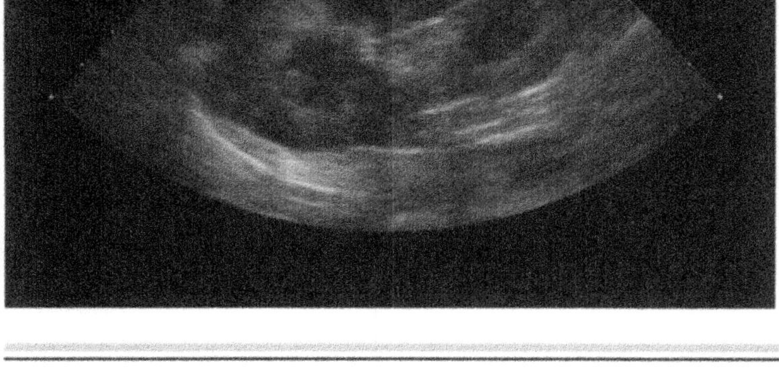

FIG. 15-34 Sagittal image of the right kidney.

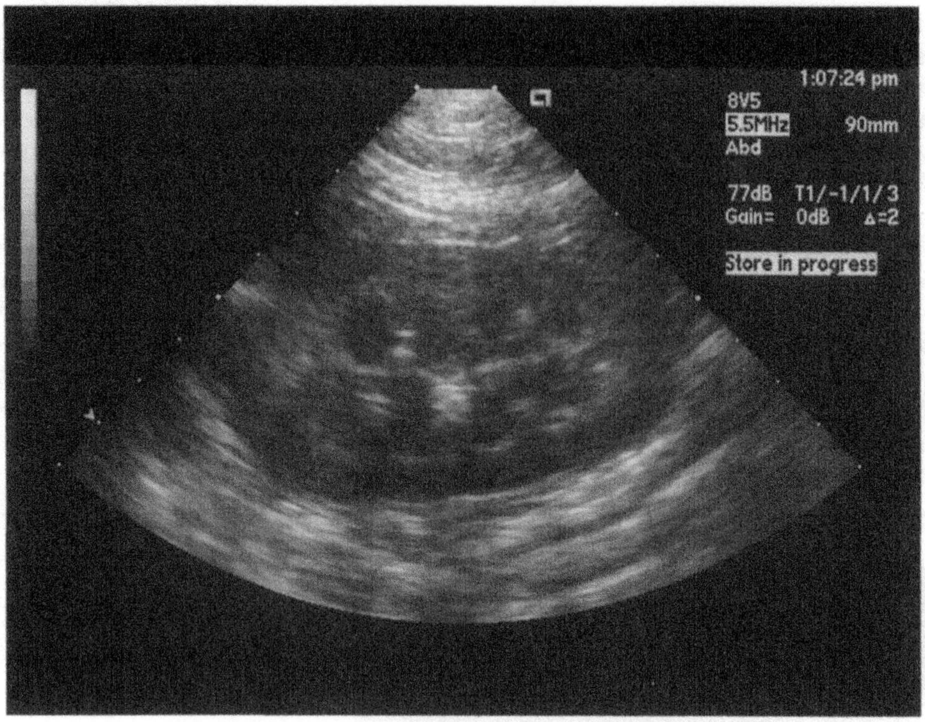

FIG. 15-35 Dorsal image of the right kidney.

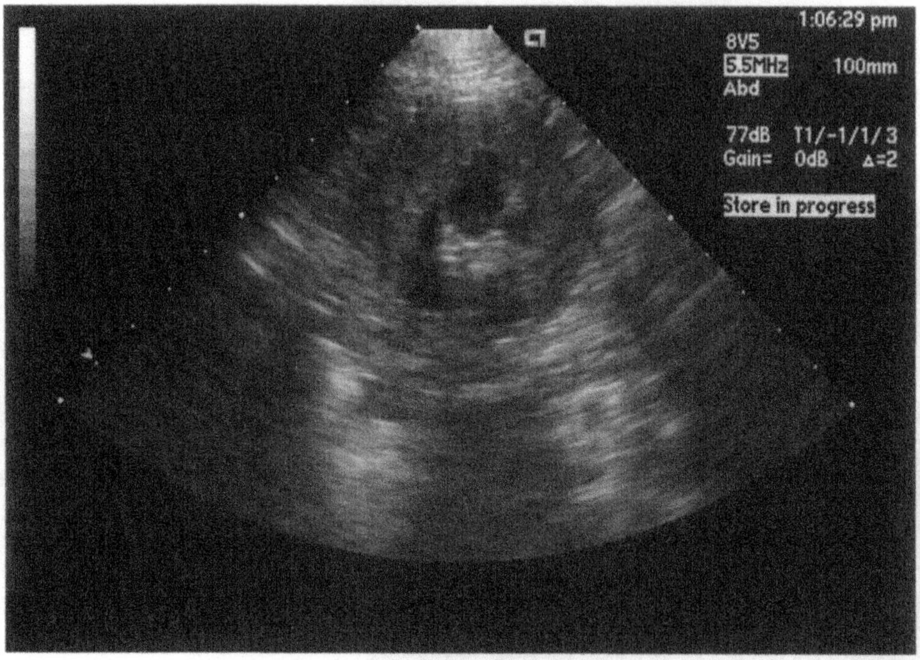

FIG. 15-36 Transverse image of the right kidney.

Urinary Bladder

The urinary bladder is located in the caudoventral abdomen and varies in size depending on distention (Figure 15-37). The normal urinary bladder contains anechoic urine. The urinary bladder is typically imaged in sagittal and transverse planes (Figure 15-38). In the transverse plane the colon is seen as a semicircular, highly echogenic structure that may deform the wall of the bladder. The colon must not be mistaken for a urolith. The wall of the urinary bladder is uniform in thickness and also varies in thickness, depending on degree of distention. Normal thickness of the bladder wall should not exceed 3 mm. The trigone region is located in the caudodorsal wall of the urinary bladder. The respective ureteral papillae are occasionally visualized.

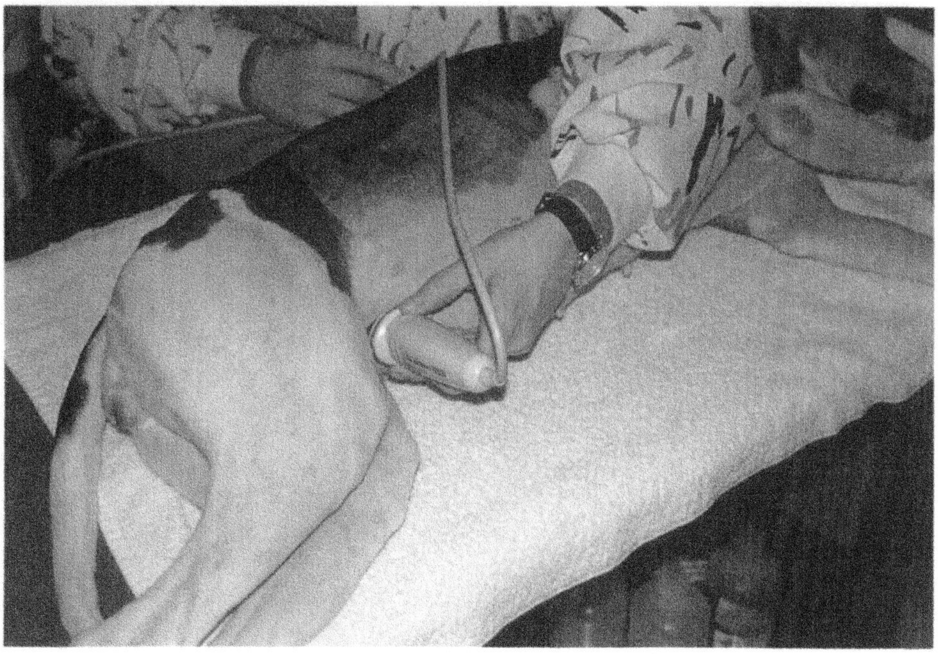

FIG. 15-37 Transducer positioning for ultrasound scan of the urinary bladder.

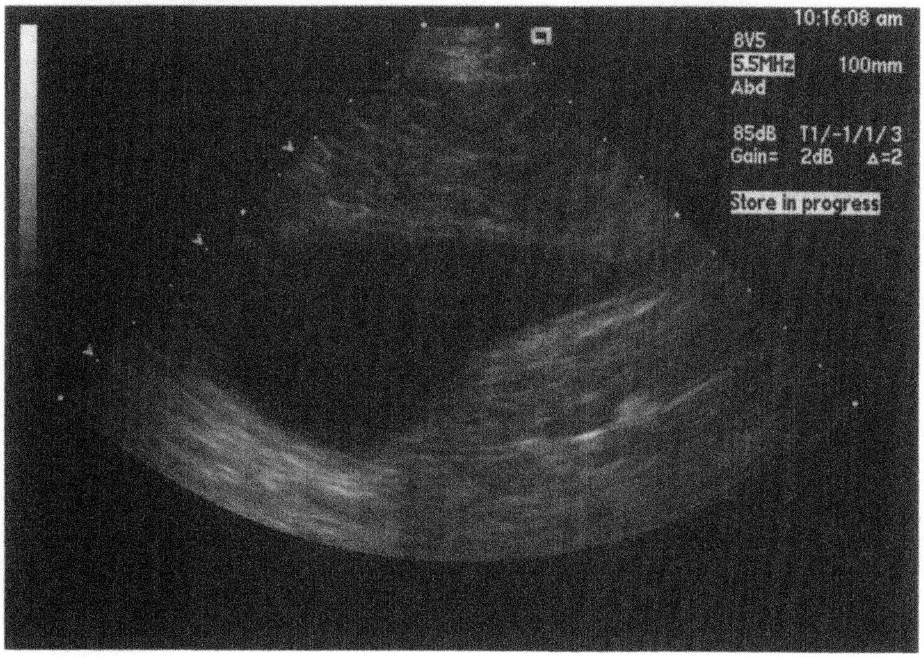

FIG. 15-38 Sagittal image of the urinary bladder.

Prostate

The prostate gland is a bilobed structure located caudal to the neck of the urinary bladder (Figures 15-39 and 15-40). The prostate can be visualized by imaging the urinary bladder in the transverse plane and sliding caudally through the neck of the urinary bladder to the urethra. Centrally within the gland the prostatic urethra is evident (Figure 15-41). The normal prostate of an intact male is homogenous in echogenicity and has a fine echotexture. The prostate is a relatively echogenic organ and is hyperechoic to the spleen, liver, and kidneys. The prostate of a neutered male is also homogenous in echogenicity and has a fine granular echotexture. However, the prostate of a neutered male is less echogenic than that of an intact male (Figures 15-42 and 15-43).

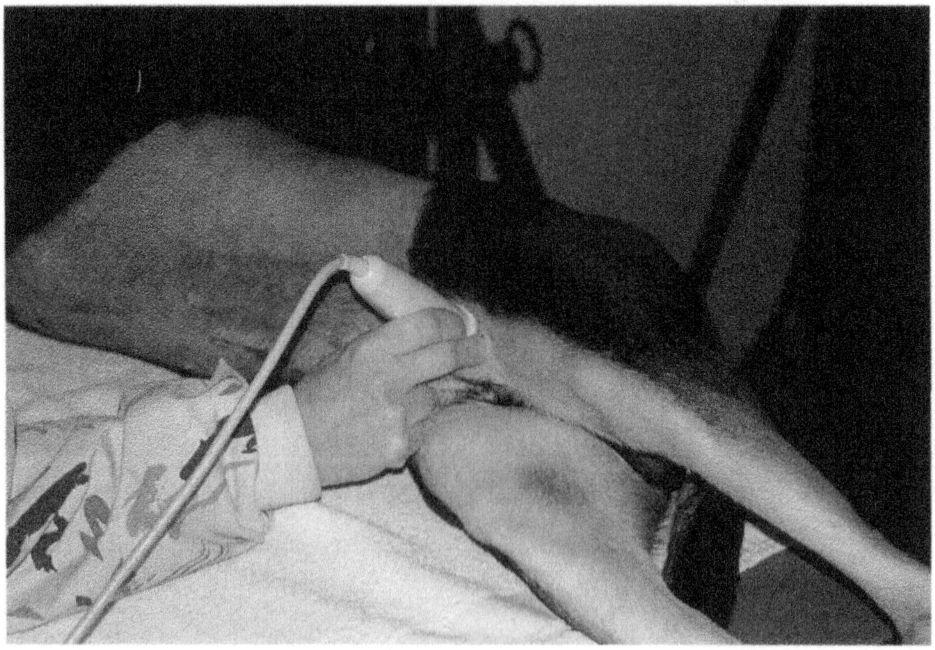

FIG. 15-39 Transducer positioning for ultrasound scan of the prostate.

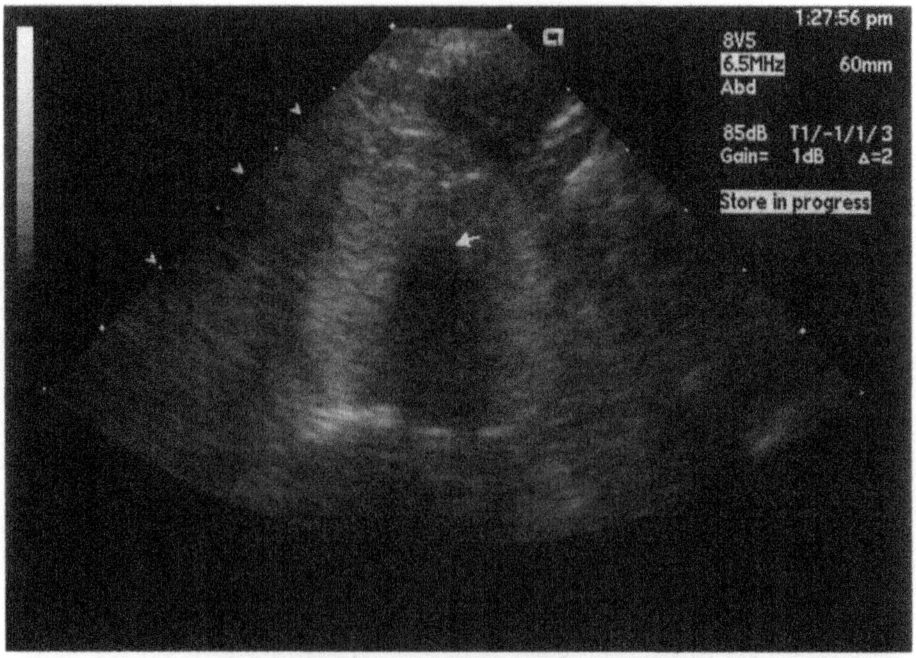

FIG. 15-40 Transverse image of an intact male prostate. The arrow indicates the prostatic urethra.

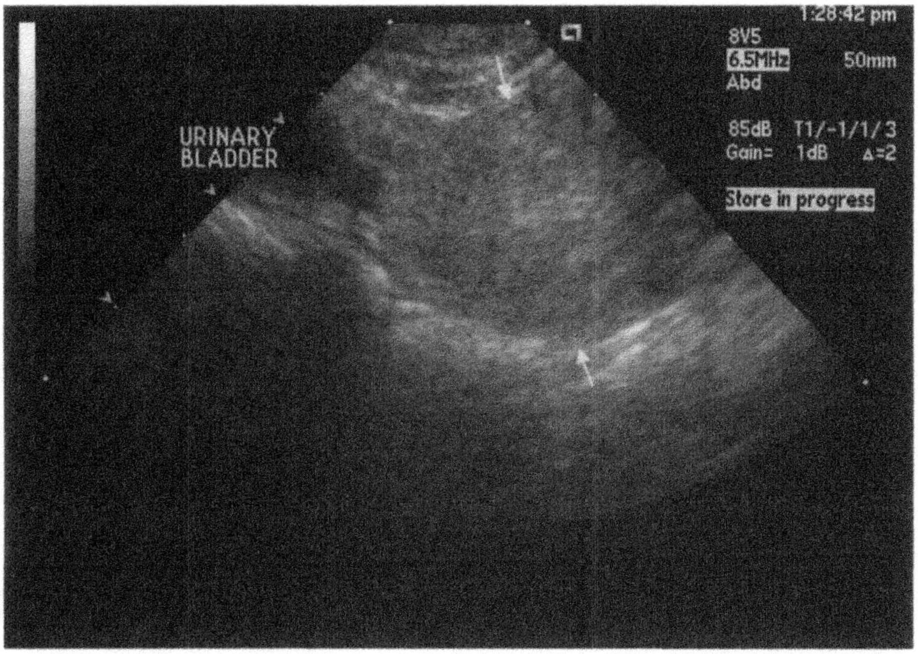

FIG. 15-41 Sagittal image of an intact male prostate *(arrows)*. A small amount of the urinary bladder can be visualized in the left near field of the image.

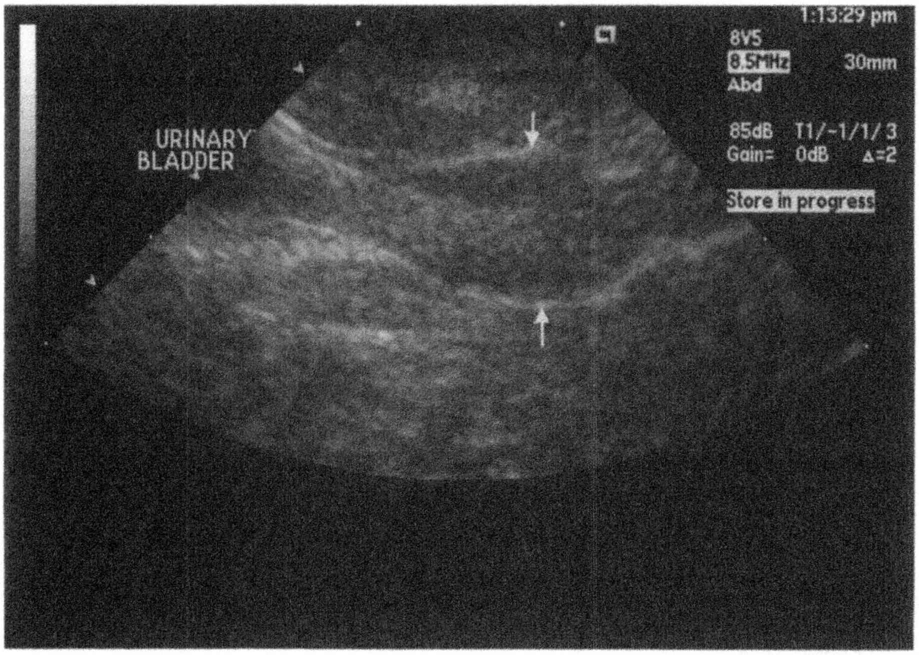

FIG. 15-42 Sagittal image of a neutered male prostate *(arrows)*. A small amount of the urinary bladder can be visualized in the left midfield of the image. Note that the image of the neutered male prostate is hypoechoic compared with that of the intact male prostate.

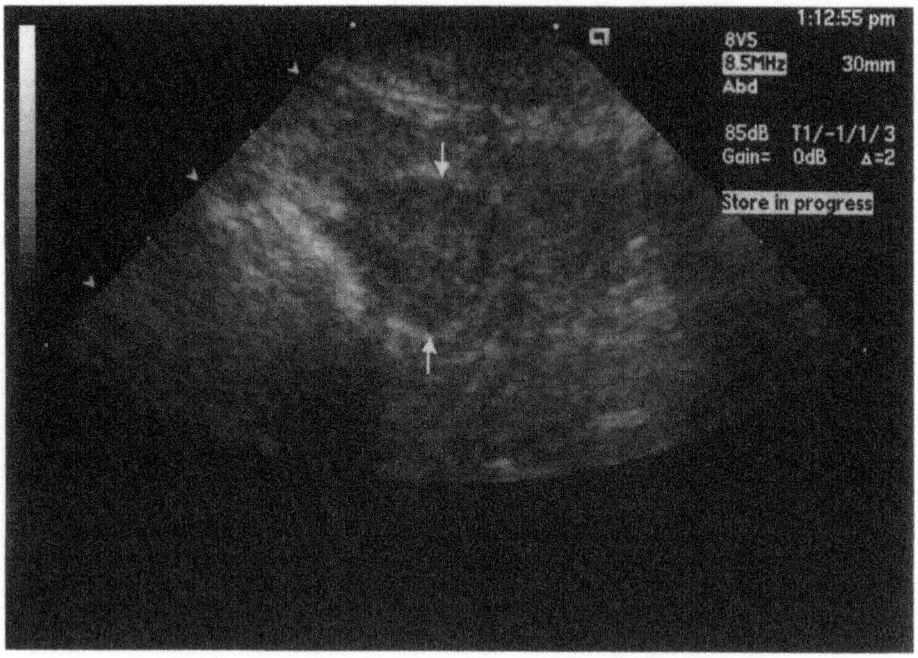

FIG. 15-43 Transverse image of a neutered male prostate *(arrows).*

Uterus and Ovaries

The body of the uterus is located in the caudal abdomen between the urinary bladder and the colon (Figure 15-44). To locate the uterus, scan the urinary bladder in the transverse plane and slide caudally; the colon is generally seen as a semicircular, highly echogenic line adjacent to or partially indenting the wall of the bladder. Interrogation of the tissue between the colon and the urinary bladder reveals the body of the uterus in short axis (Figure 15-45). Normally there is no distention of the uterine lumen; the lumen of the uterus is seen as an echogenic line where the endometrial mucosal surfaces come into contact. The wall of the uterus is homogenous with no characteristic layering. The uterine body can be followed cranially to the bifurcation of the uterine horns, generally near the apex of the urinary bladder (Figure 15-46). The uterine horns are difficult to follow cranially within the abdomen in the absence of pregnancy or pathologic condition.

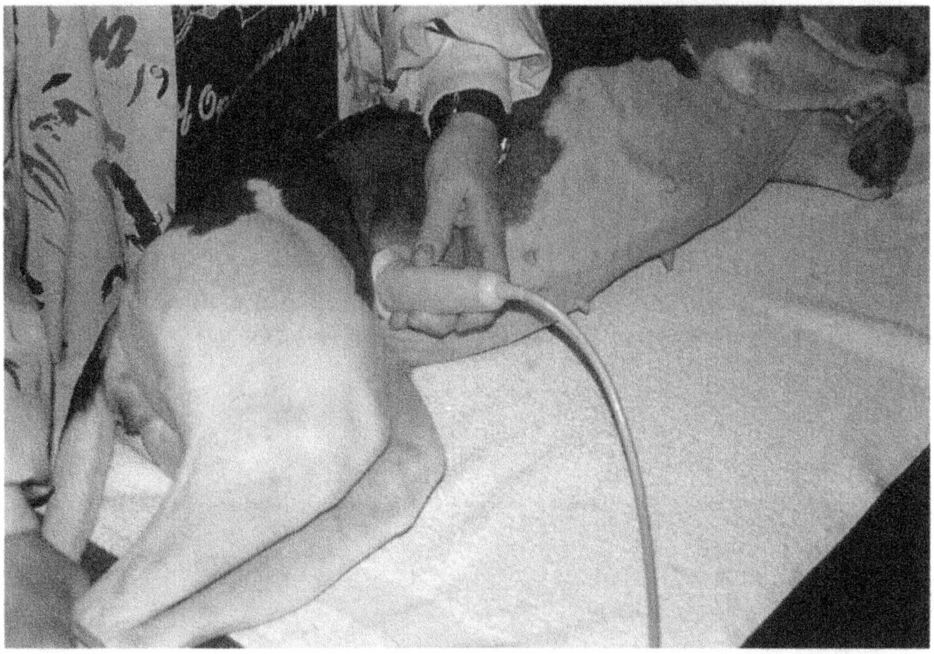

FIG. 15-44 Transducer positioning for transverse ultrasound image of the uterus.

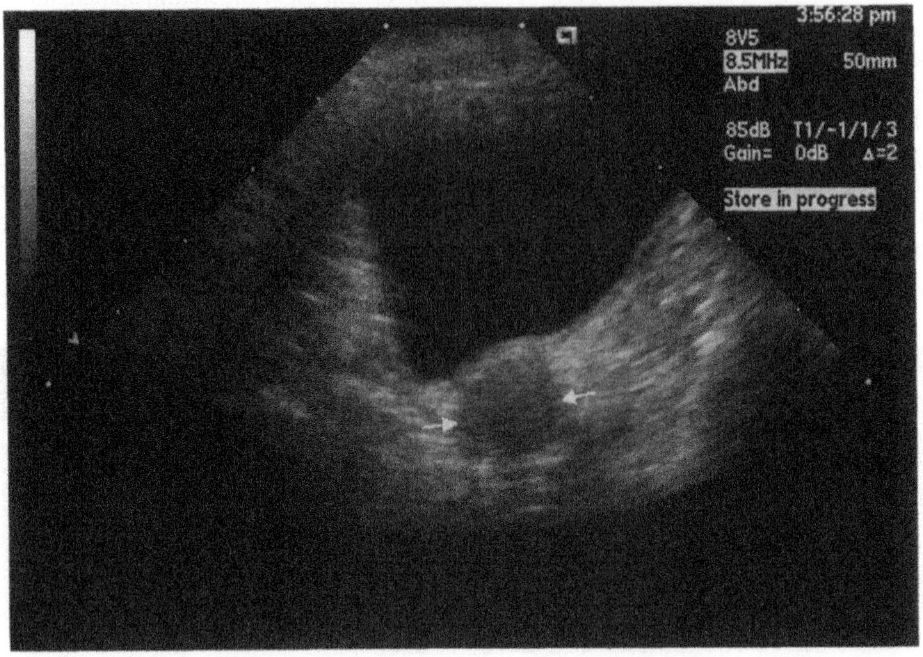

FIG. 15-45 Transverse image of the uterine body.

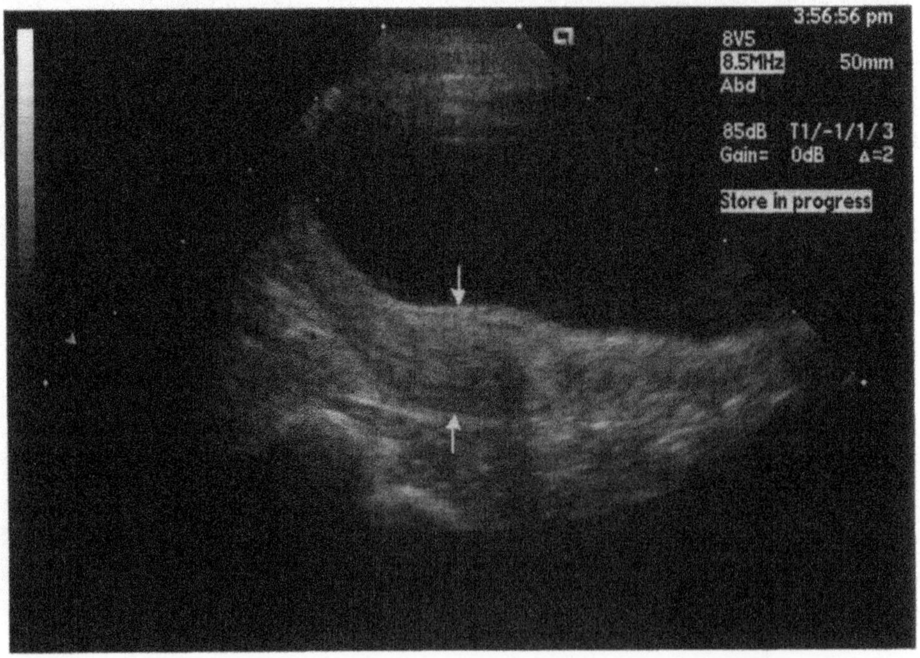

FIG. 15-46 Sagittal image of the uterine body *(arrows)*. The urinary bladder is in the near field.

The ovaries are located in the retroperitoneum immediately caudal to the respective kidneys (Figure 15-47). Optimal visualization of normal ovaries is enhanced with follicular activity. The ovaries may be visualized by imaging the caudal pole of the kidney, then sliding caudally and interrogating the retroperitoneal tissue with slow, meticulous fanning. Normal inactive ovarian tissue is echoic to the surrounding retroperitoneal fat (Figure 15-48). The ovary is circular to oval in shape. With follicular activity, anechoic cystic structures are seen within the ovary. Distal acoustic enhancement may be evident, depending on the size of the follicle(s) (Figure 15-49).

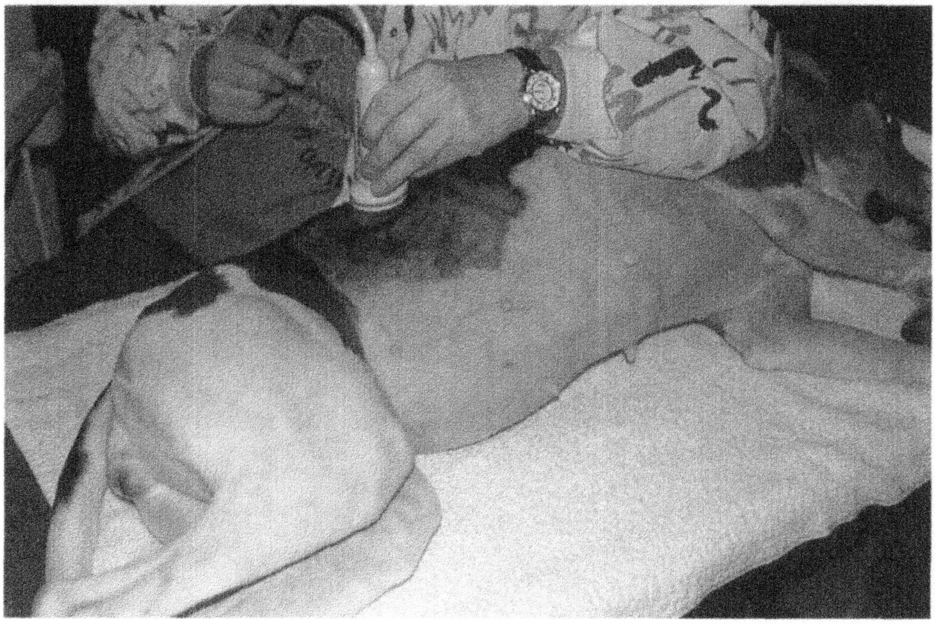

FIG. 15-47 Transducer positioning for ultrasound scan of the ovaries.

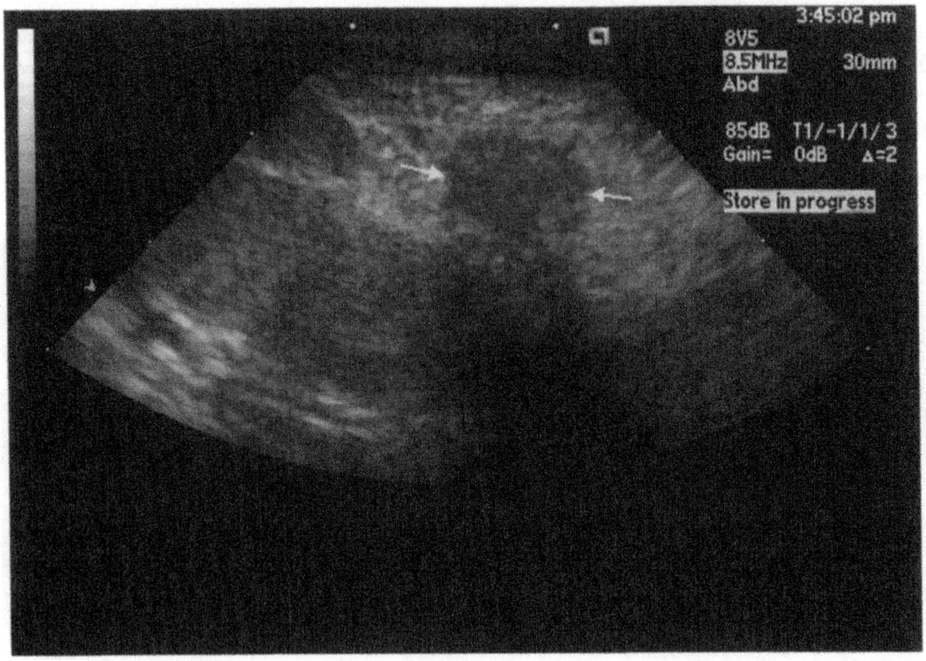

FIG. 15-48 Sagittal image of an inactive ovary *(arrows)*.

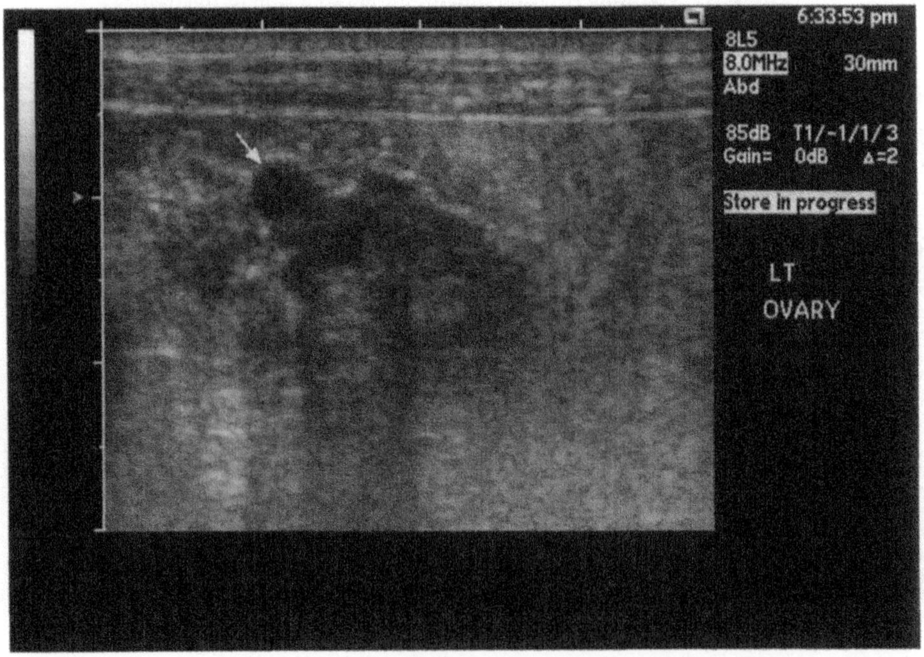

FIG. 15-49 Sagittal image of an ovary with follicular activity. The arrow indicates a follicle.

Spleen

The spleen is located predominantly on the left side of the abdominal cavity. Conventionally, the spleen is divided into the head, body, and tail regions. Complete imaging of the spleen requires visualization of each region.

The *head* of the spleen can be found by sliding one to two intercostal spaces cranial to the left kidney (Figure 15-50). With the transducer in a transverse orientation to the animal, gradual fanning through the intercostal space reveals the head of the spleen in a characteristic hook shape (Figure 15-51). Once the head of the spleen is imaged,

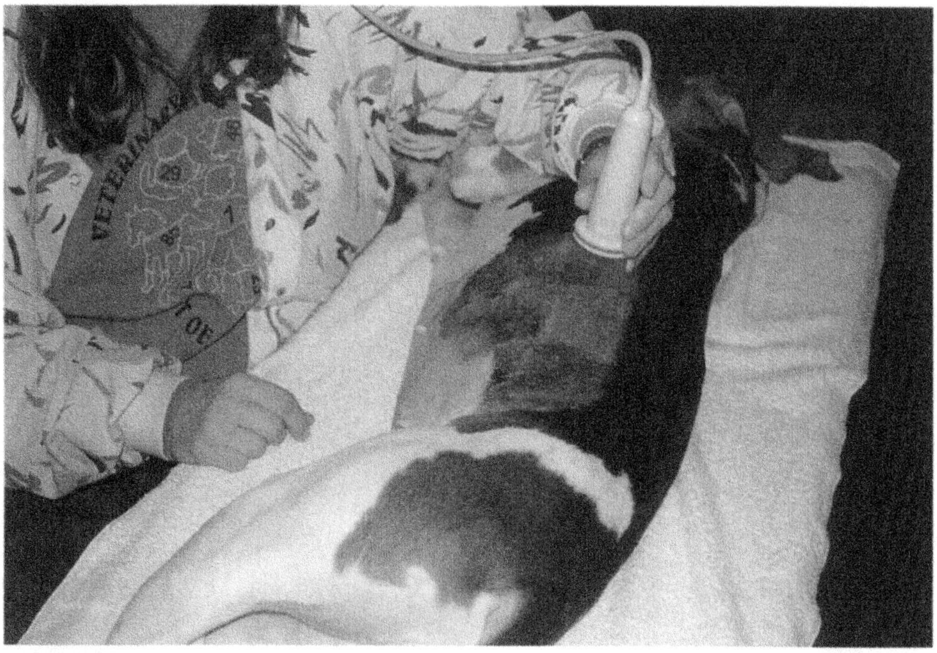

FIG. 15-50 Transducer positioning for ultrasound scan of the head of the spleen.

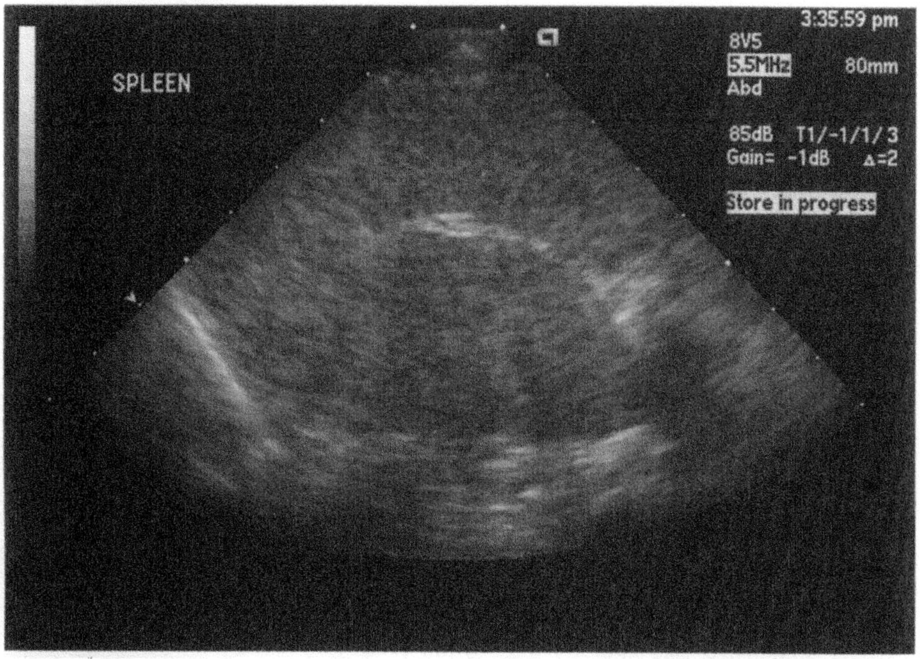

FIG. 15-51 Image of the head of the spleen. Note the characteristic hook shape of the spleen.

rotate the transducer 90 degrees and slide ventrally (Figure 15-52). The *body* of the spleen has a rounded triangular shape (Figure 15-53). To image the spleen completely, slide the transducer cranially and caudally to the respective edges of the spleen. Continue to slide ventrally, following the body of the spleen toward the tail region. Approximately one third to one half of the spleen is beneath the caudal rib cage, and visualization of the spleen around acoustic shadows from the ribs is necessary. The *tail* of the spleen may be seen as a gradual thinning of the rounded triangular shape of the body. In some cases the tail of the spleen may wrap around the ventral abdomen and extend to the right side.

The spleen normally has a homogenous echogenicity with fine echotexture. The spleen is hyperechoic to the liver and the cortex of the left kidney. Along the hilar surface of the spleen, anechoic tubular veins are visualized traveling from within the splenic parenchyma into the surrounding mesenteric fat. The population of these vessels is greater through the body of the spleen.

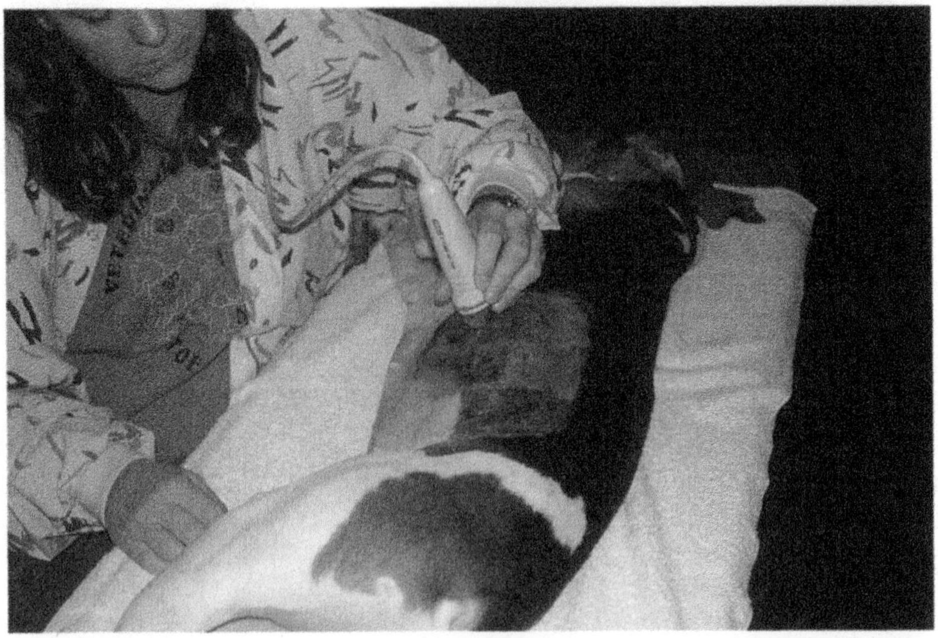

FIG. 15-52 Transducer positioning for ultrasound scan of the body of the spleen.

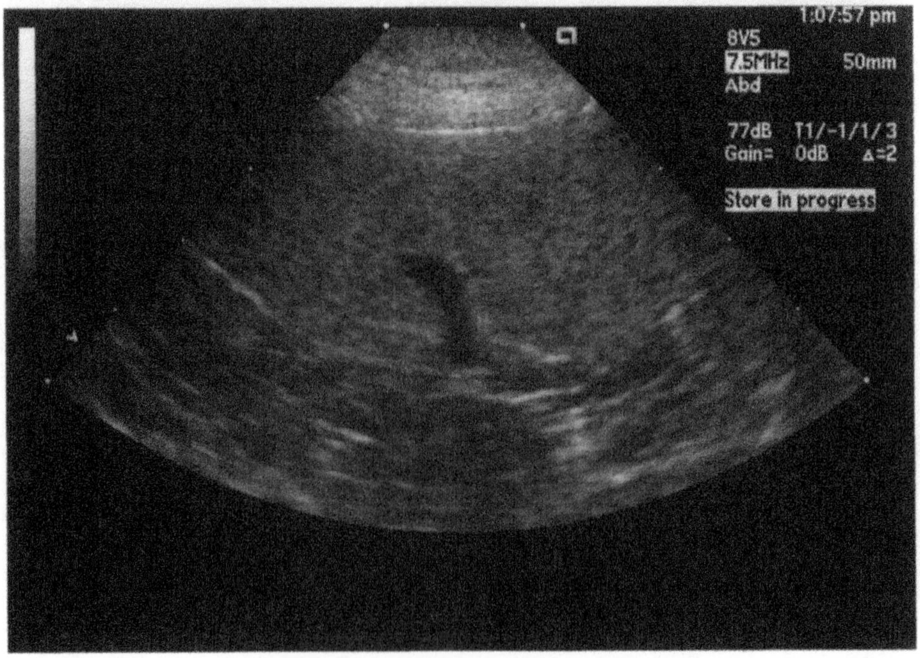

FIG. 15-53 Image of body of the spleen. Note anechoic tubular structure near the surface of the spleen. This is a splenic vein, which exits the spleen in the hilar region.

Gastrointestinal Tract

The stomach, small intestine, and colon make up the gastrointestinal (GI) tract. The *stomach* is located in the cranial abdomen, immediately behind the liver, and is divided into the fundus, body, and pyloric antrum (Figure 15-54).

Imaging of the stomach essentially involves visualization of the gastric wall (Figure 15-55). The normal stomach has a five-layer appearance consisting of the mucosal interface, mucosa, submucosa, muscularis, and serosa. The *mucosal interface* is typically seen as an echogenic line representing ingesta or gas within the stomach. The *mucosa*, the thickest of the layers, is homogenous and hypoechoic. The *submucosa* is seen as an echogenic thin band beneath the mucosa. The *muscularis* is an equally thin band of tissue that is hypoechoic similar to the mucosa. The *serosal surface* of the stomach is thin and is seen as the next echogenic interface beneath the muscularis. The normal thickness of the stomach should not exceed 7 mm (Figure 15-56).

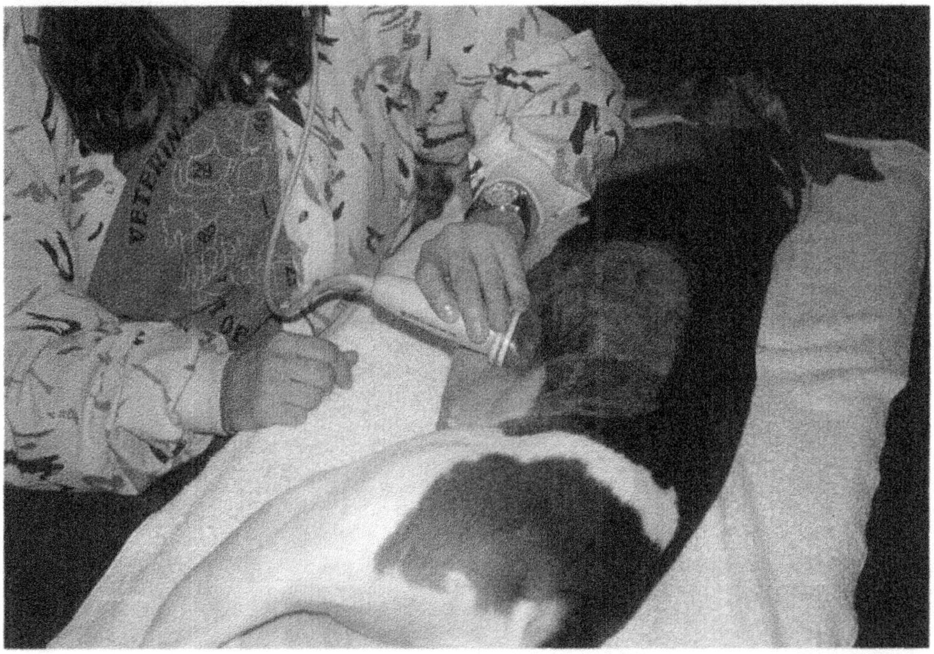

FIG. 15-54 Transducer positioning for ultrasound scan of the fundus and body of the stomach.

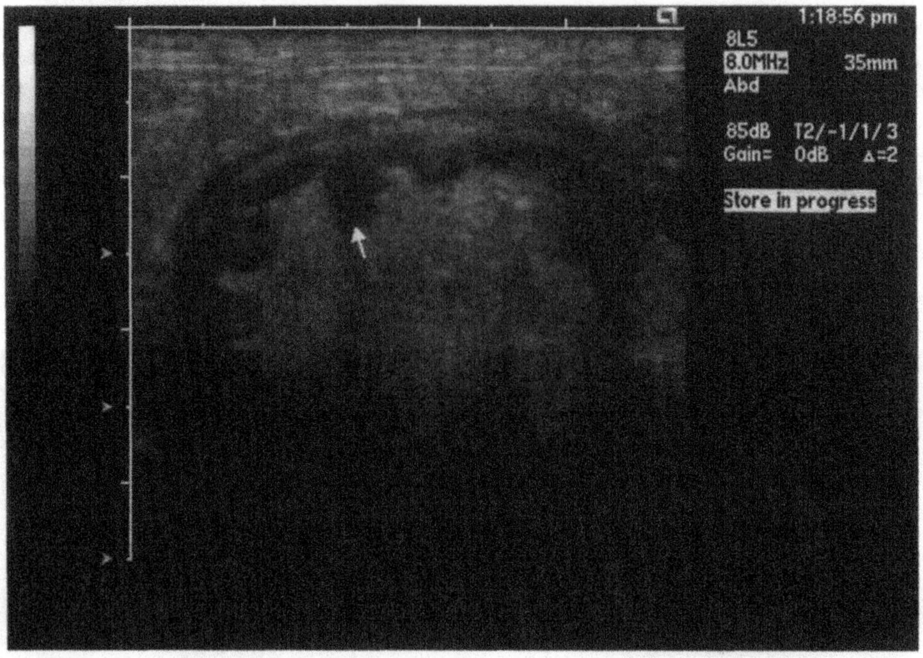

FIG. 15-55 Transverse image of the stomach. The arrow indicates a rugal fold in the stomach.

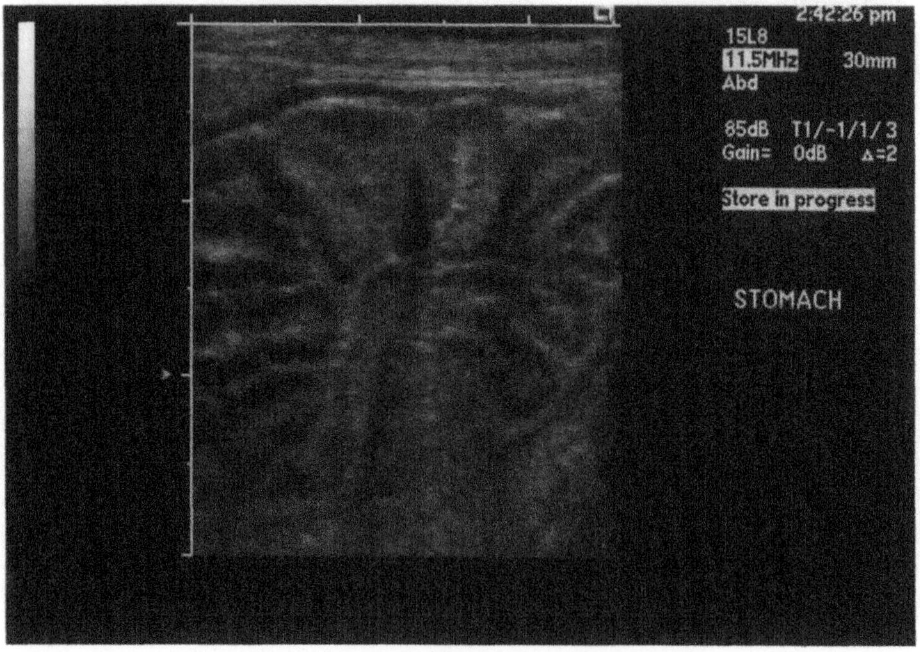

FIG. 15-56 Transverse image of an empty stomach.

The *small intestine* occupies the central ventral portion of the abdomen and is divided into the duodenum, jejunum, and ileum. The small intestine has a similar five-layer appearance as the stomach (Figure 15-57). Differentiation of the respective sections of the small intestine is difficult. The *duodenum* can be reliably imaged by following it from the pyloric antrum of the stomach along the right side of the abdomen to the caudal duodenal flexure (Figure 15-58). The duodenum is generally approximately 1 mm thicker than the remainder of the small intestine (Figure 15-59). The normal thickness of the small intestine is between 2 and 4 mm (Figure 15-60).

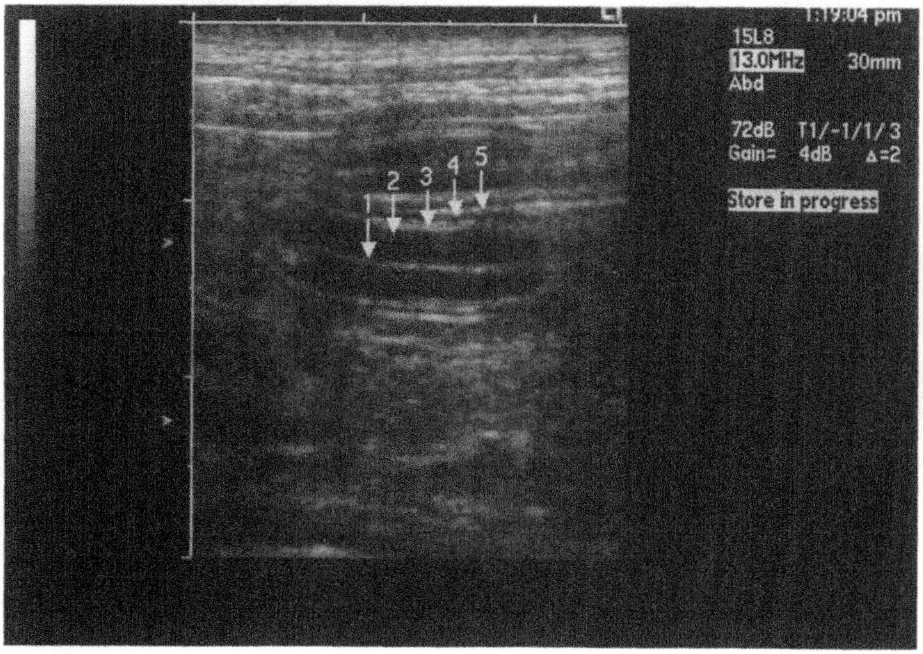

FIG. 15-57 Sagittal image of the small intestine. Note the different layers: *1,* lumen of the bowel; *2,* mucosa; *3,* submucosa; *4,* muscularis; *5,* serosa.

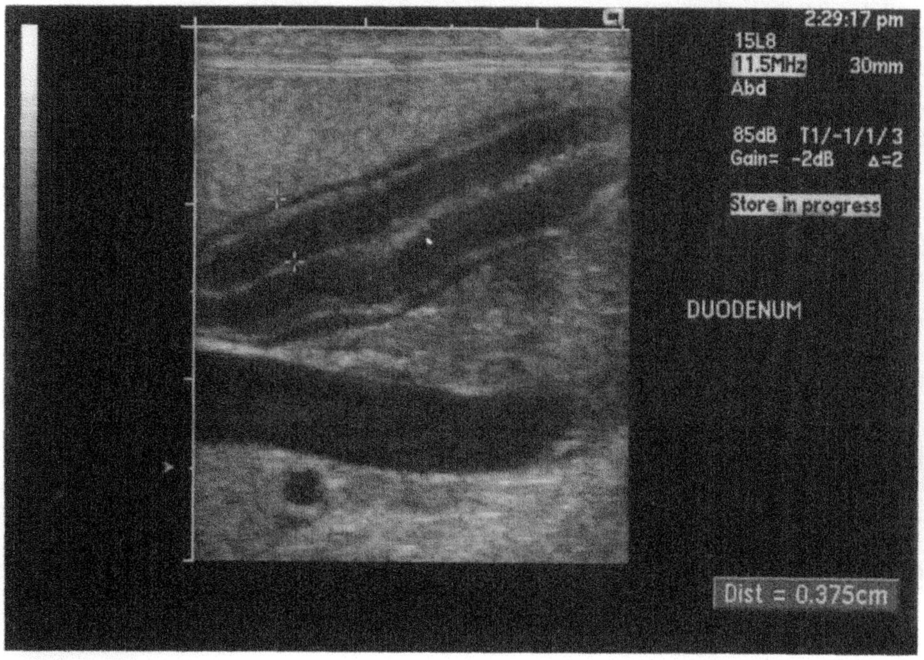

FIG. 15-58 Sagittal image of the duodenum.

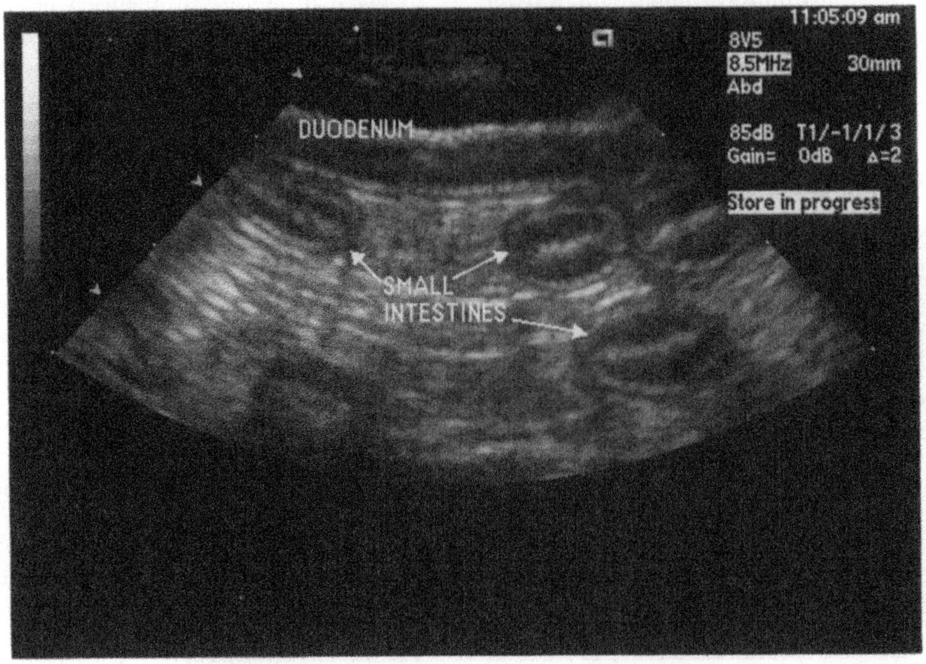

FIG. 15-59 Sagittal image of the duodenum and transverse image of the small intestine. Note the difference in thickness between the duodenum and the small intestines.

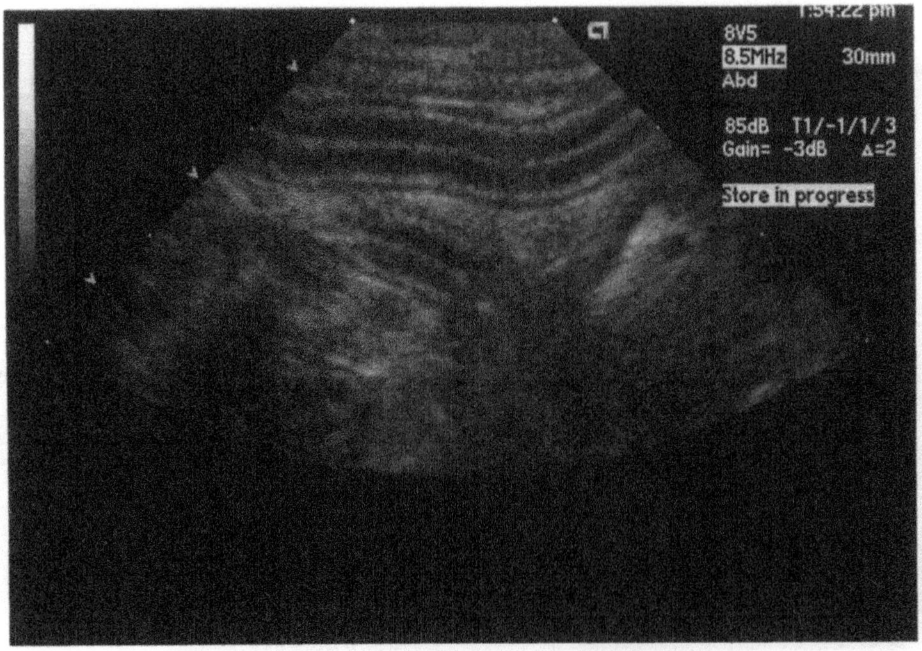

FIG. 15-60 Sagittal image of the small intestine.

The *colon* begins in the right cranial abdomen as the ascending colon, with the transverse portion coursing from the right to the left side of the abdomen immediately behind the stomach. The descending colon continues down the left side of the abdomen to the pelvic inlet. Wall layering within the colon is not evident. The wall of the colon is seen as a hypoechoic band of tissue. The thickness of the colonic wall is generally 1 to 2 mm. The colon is visualized as an echogenic interface with a distant acoustic shadow. This interface represents either gas or fecal material within the colon (Figure 15-61).

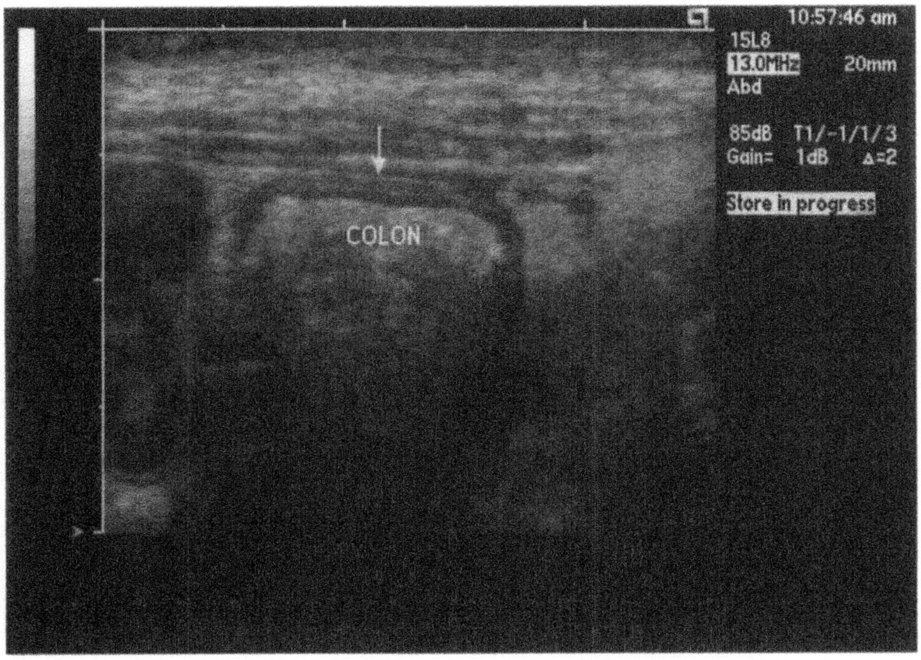

FIG. 15-61 Transverse image of the colon. The word "colon" is printed over the lumen, and the arrow points to the serosal surface.

Lymph Nodes

Lymph nodes that are reliably visualized within the abdomen are generally the cranial mesenteric and medial iliac lymph nodes. The *cranial mesenteric nodes* are found within the mesentery of small intestines generally associated with the celiac and cranial mesenteric arterial branches of the abdominal aorta (Figure 15-62). The nodes are generally seen in pairs with a vessel dissecting them. Mesenteric lymph nodes are homogenous in echotexture and slightly hypoechoic to the surrounding mesenteric fat. The nodes are oblong in shape and can measure as long as 7 cm (Figure 15-63).

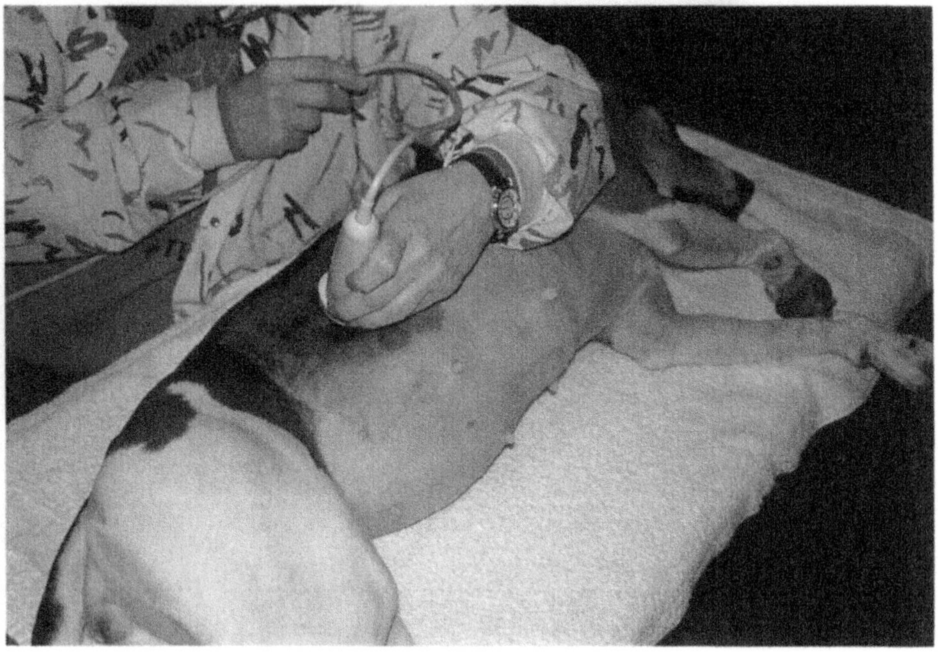

FIG. 15-62 Transducer positioning for ultrasound scan of the cranial mesenteric lymph nodes.

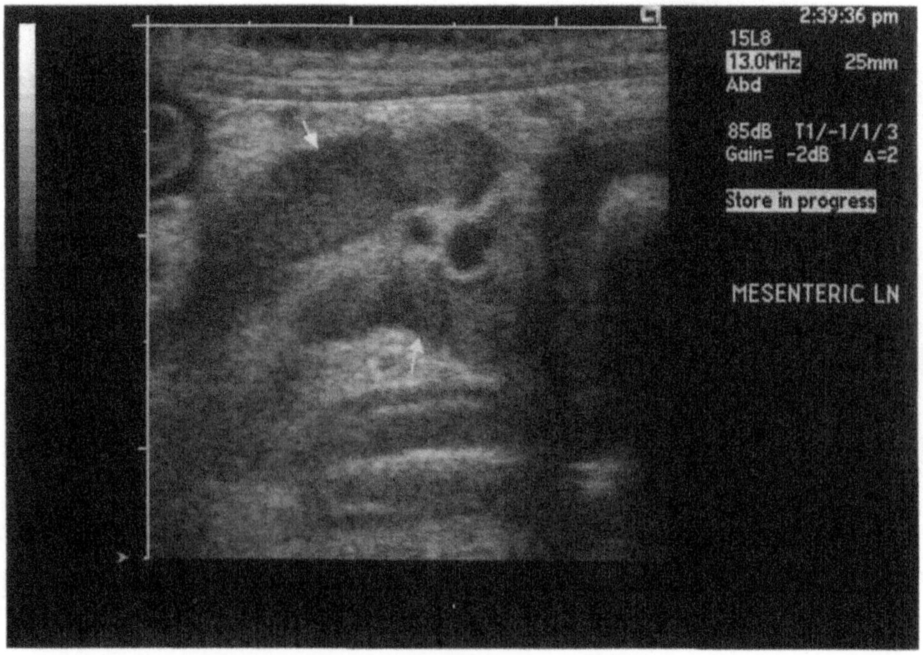

FIG. 15-63 Sagittal image of the cranial mesenteric lymph nodes *(arrows)*.

The *medial iliac lymph nodes* are located within the caudal retroperitoneum at the level of the bifurcation of the aorta to the external iliac arteries (Figure 15-64). Medial iliac lymph nodes are oblong in shape, have a homogenous echotexture, and are slightly hyperechoic or isoechoic to the retroperitoneal fat (Figure 15-65).

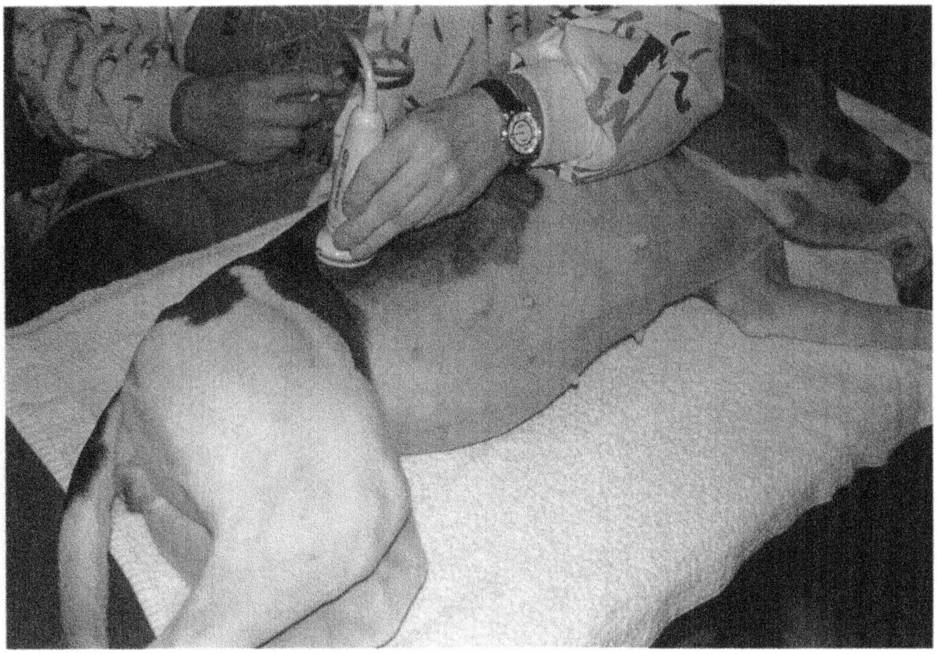

FIG. 15-64 Transducer positioning for ultrasound scan of the iliac lymph nodes.

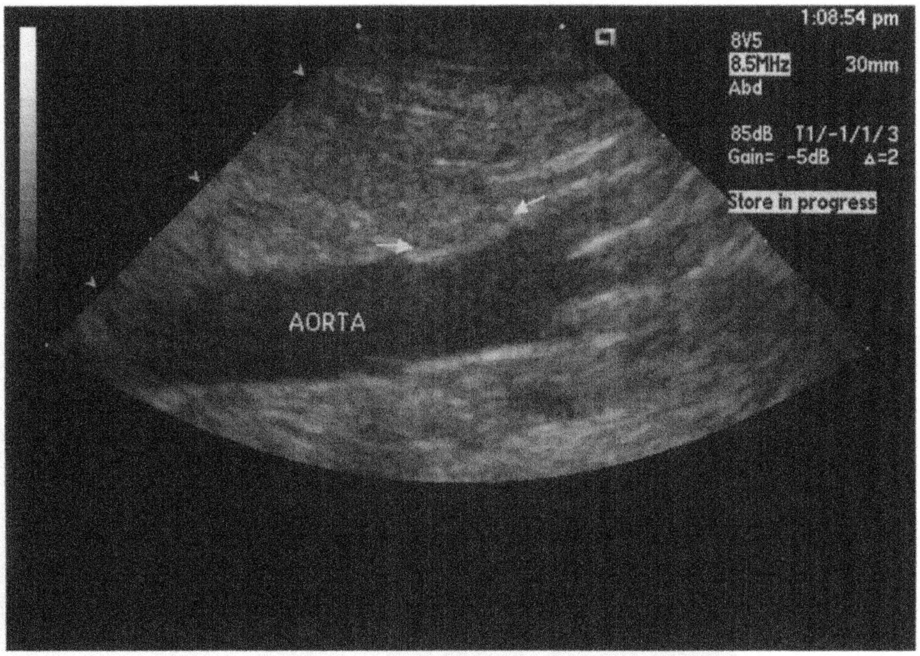

FIG. 15-65 Sagittal image of the iliac lymph node *(arrows)*.

Adrenal Glands

The adrenal glands are located within the retroperitoneal space in close association with the cranial poles of the respective kidneys (Figure 15-66). The vascular anatomy in the cranial abdomen provides a "roadmap" to aid in finding the adrenal glands. First, find the aorta in long axis immediately caudal to the respective kidney. Next, identify the renal artery, which has a characteristic "hook" from the aorta to the hilum of the kidney, and then slowly fan through the retroperitoneal tissue medial to the renal artery (Figure 15-67). The adrenal gland may or may not be within the same imaging plane as the renal artery. The characteristic shape of the adrenal gland is similar to a peanut, with the caudal pole generally slightly larger than the cranial pole. The phrenicoabdominal vein may be seen as an anechoic vessel traversing the midbody of the adrenal gland.

The adrenal gland is slightly hypoechoic to the surrounding retroperitoneal fat. With high-resolution transducers the internal architecture of the adrenal gland may be seen. The delineation between the adrenal cortex and medulla is seen as a fine echogenic line within the gland. The most significant normal dimension of the adrenal gland is the width, which should not exceed 7 mm.

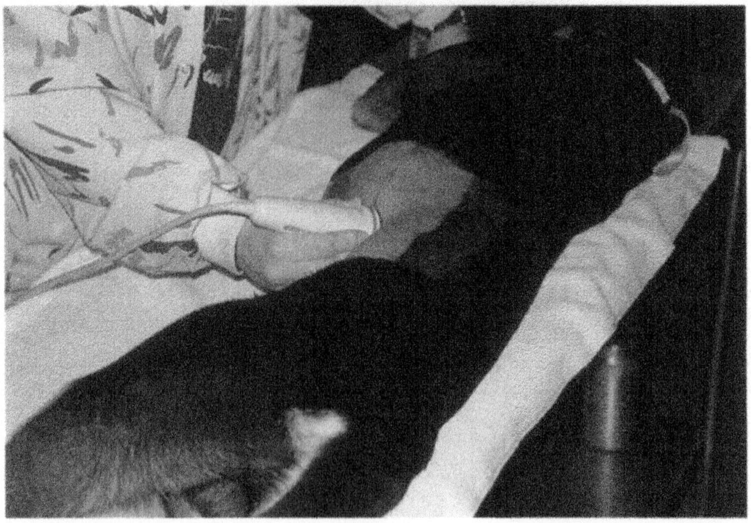

FIG. 15-66 Transducer positioning for the left adrenal gland.

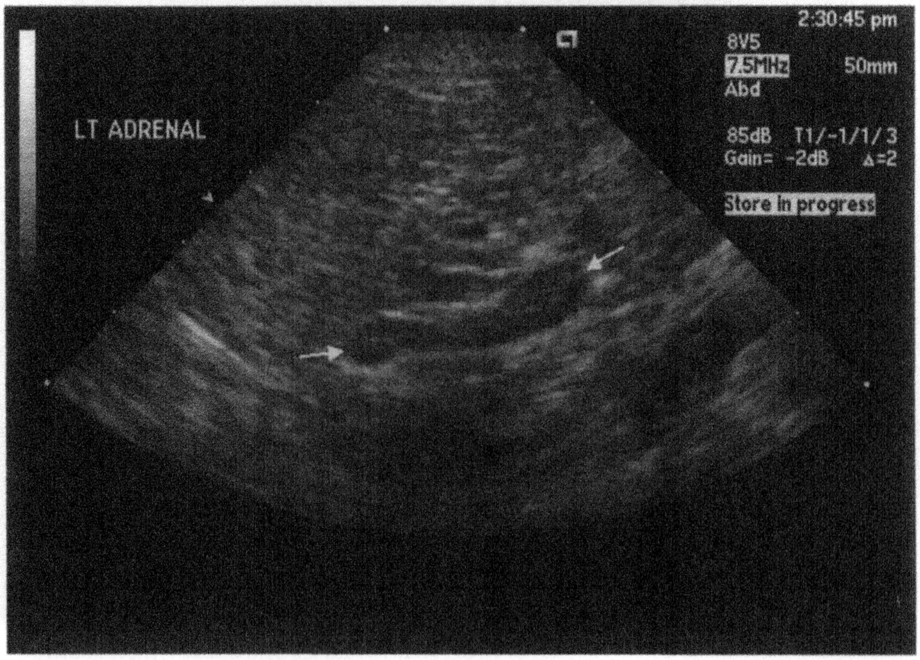

FIG. 15-67 Sagittal image of the left adrenal gland *(arrows)*.

Pancreas

The pancreas is located within the cranial abdomen in close association with the descending duodenum and greater curvature of the stomach and in close proximity to the colon and spleen. The pancreas is divided into three regions: the right limb, body, and left limb.

The *right limb* of the pancreas is located within the mesentery of the descending duodenum (Figure 15-68). To find the right limb of the pancreas, locate the descending duodenum in short axis. The pancreas is evident within the mesentery adjacent to the duodenum, generally at the level of the right kidney or cranial. The pancreas is homogenous in echotexture and slightly hypoechoic to the surrounding mesenteric fat (Figure 15-69). Centrally within the right limb of the pancreas, the accessory pancreatic duct can be seen. The duct appears as a tubular structure with echogenic walls, similar to the echogenicity of the intrahepatic portal veins. The *body* is the portion of the pancreas between the right and left limbs.

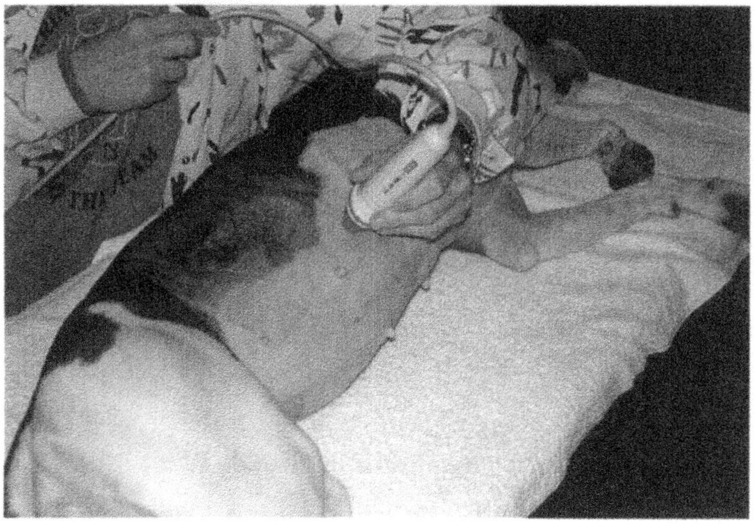

FIG. 15-68 Transducer positioning for ultrasound scan of the right limb of the pancreas.

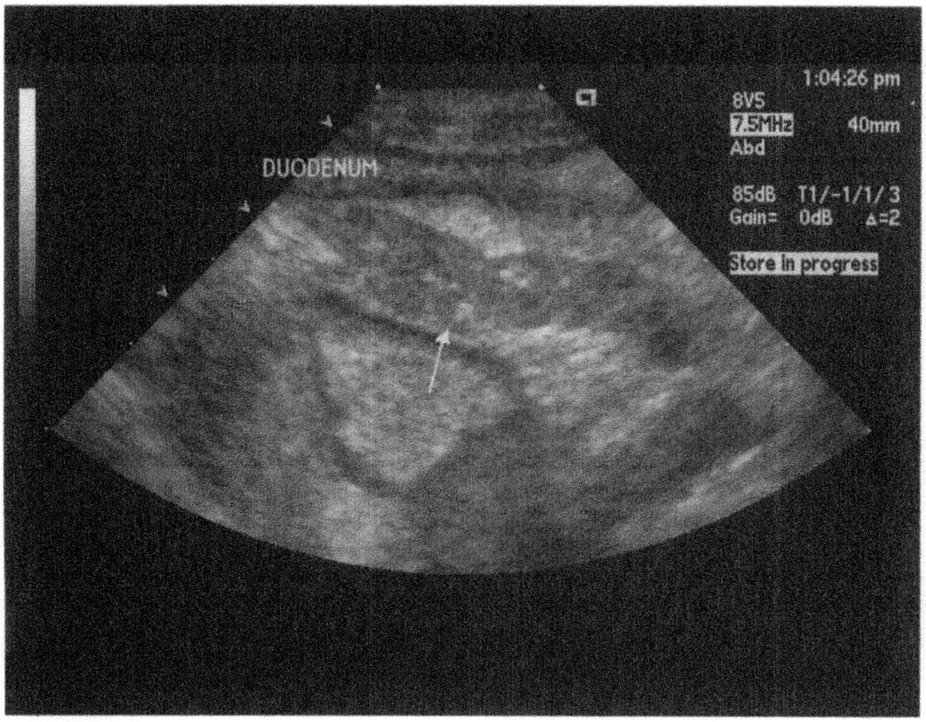

FIG. 15-69 Sagittal image of the right limb of the pancreas *(arrow)*.

The *left limb* of the pancreas can be imaged by following the splenic veins from the hilum of the spleen toward the portal vein (Figure 15-70). Within the mesentery, deep toward the spleen and caudal to the stomach and cranial to the colon, lies the left limb of the pancreas. In its normal state the pancreas is difficult to image reliably (Figure 15-71). Transducer resolution is important for successful imaging of the pancreas.

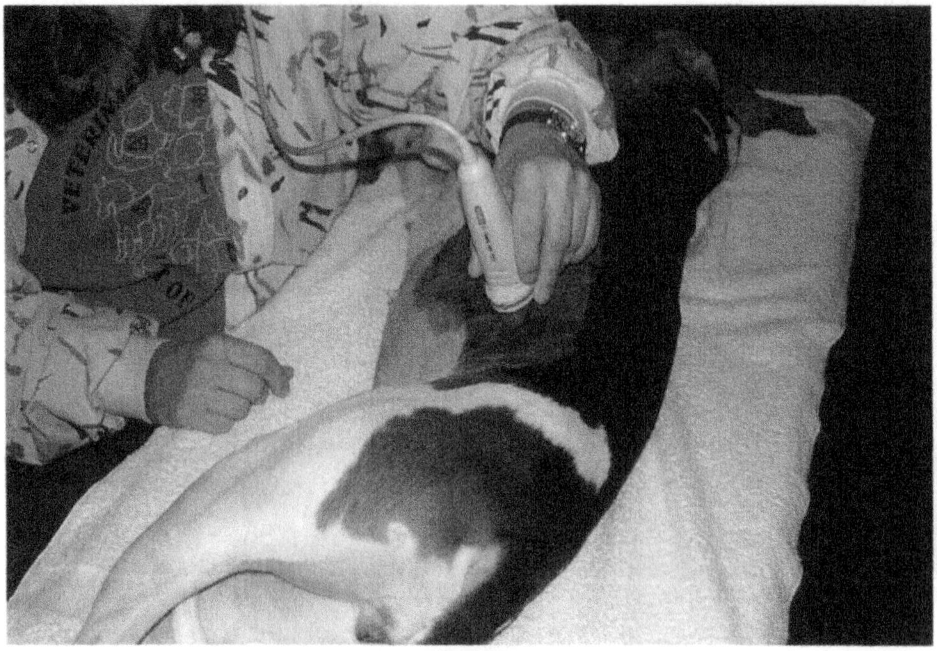

FIG. 15-70 Transducer positioning for ultrasound scan of the left limb of the pancreas.

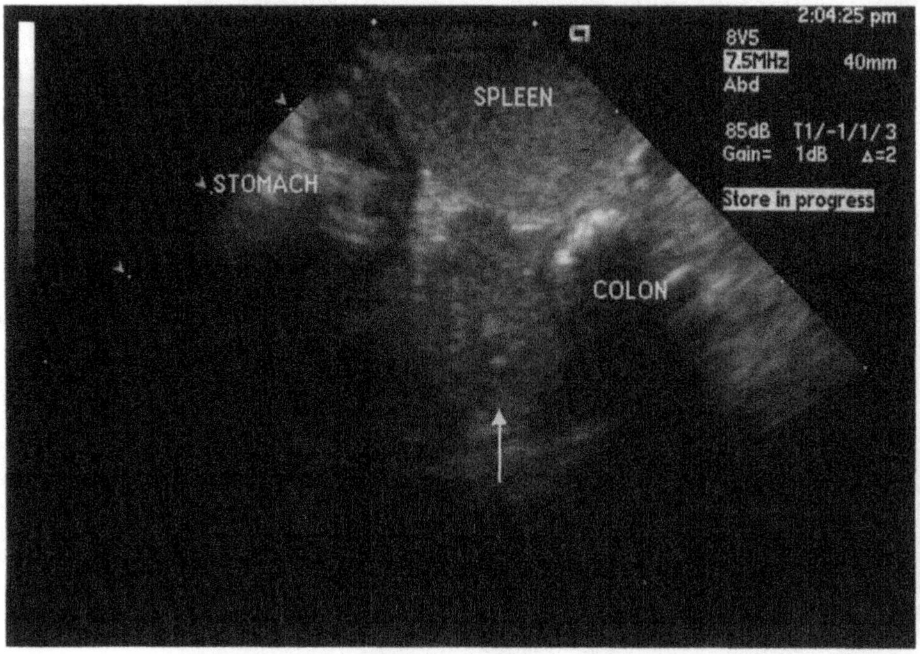

FIG. 15-71 Transverse image of the left limb of the pancreas *(arrow)*.

Scanning Techniques for Normal Cardiac Anatomy

Similar to abdominal ultrasonography, *echocardiography* should be performed using a systematic approach. A series of standard views should be obtained as well as routine measurements. The bulk of a routine study is performed through a right parasternal window. Specialized views, primarily for better Doppler angles, are obtained from the left side of the thorax from cranial and caudal parasternal locations.

Patient Preparation

A small area of fur is clipped on the right side of the thorax, where the precordium of the heart is the strongest (Figure 15-72). Some animals have thin fur in this area, and clipping may not be necessary. The patient is positioned in right lateral recumbency on a cardiac table. Many varieties of cardiac tables are available, as well as some homemade versions (Figure 15-73). A *cardiac table* allows the heart to be imaged from the dependent side of the thorax. Lateral recumbency takes advantage of the animal's weight forcing air out of the dependent lung, thereby providing a larger acoustic window. The patient can also be imaged in a standing position with the front leg held forward (Figure 15-74). The standing position can be more difficult because of restraint issues but may be necessary in some giant breed dogs.

A series of two-dimensional views (two long-axis views, five short-axis views) are obtained in a routine cardiac examination. M-mode tracings are also obtained at three different positions along the heart in a basic cardiac ultrasound examination.

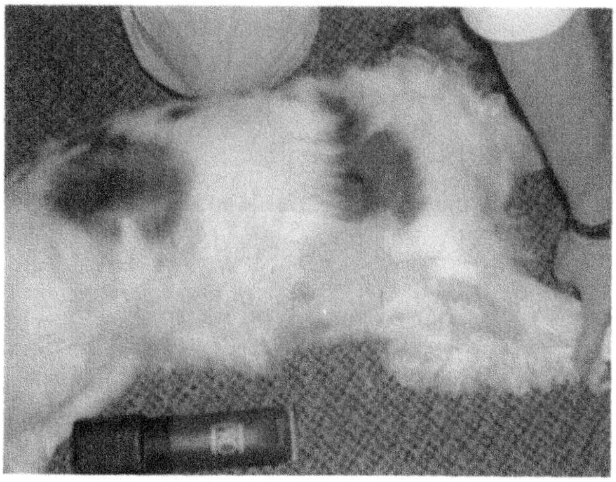

FIG. 15-72 Proper patient preparation is important to achieve a good-quality echocardiographic image.

Two-Dimensional Imaging (Right Parasternal Location)

Long-axis four-chamber view

The long-axis four-chamber view displays the right and left atria as well as both ventricles (Figure 15-75, *A*). The overall size of the heart chambers can be evaluated, with a subjective initial impression of myocardial function. The motion of the mitral valve and tricuspid valve can be observed. The patient is placed in right lateral recumbency, and the transducer is positioned perpendicular to the body wall. The image of the heart should have the ventricles displayed on the left and the atria to the right (Figure 15-75, *B*). This image shows the length of the heart as it lies in the thorax. Slight fanning of the transducer caudally can be used to maximize the size of the atria.

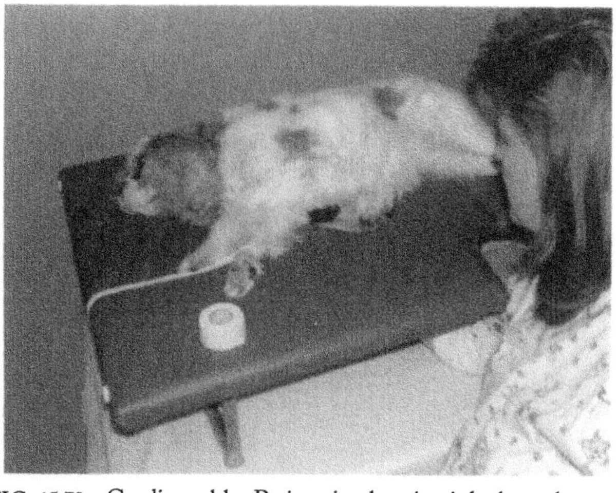

FIG. 15 73 Cardiac table. Patient is place in right lateral recumbency and is imaged from the recumbent side.

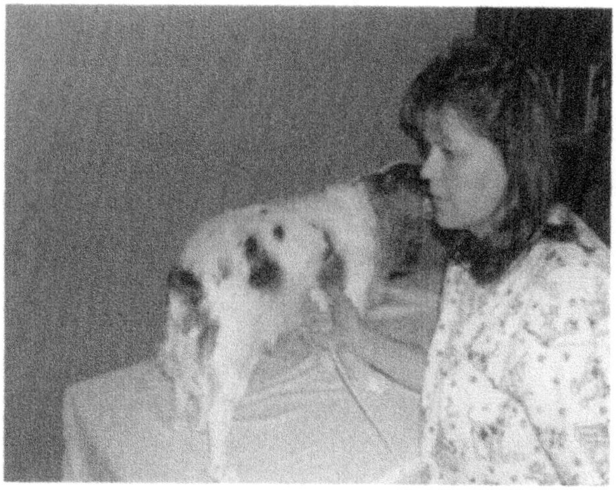

FIG. 15-74 Standing echocardiogram.

A

B

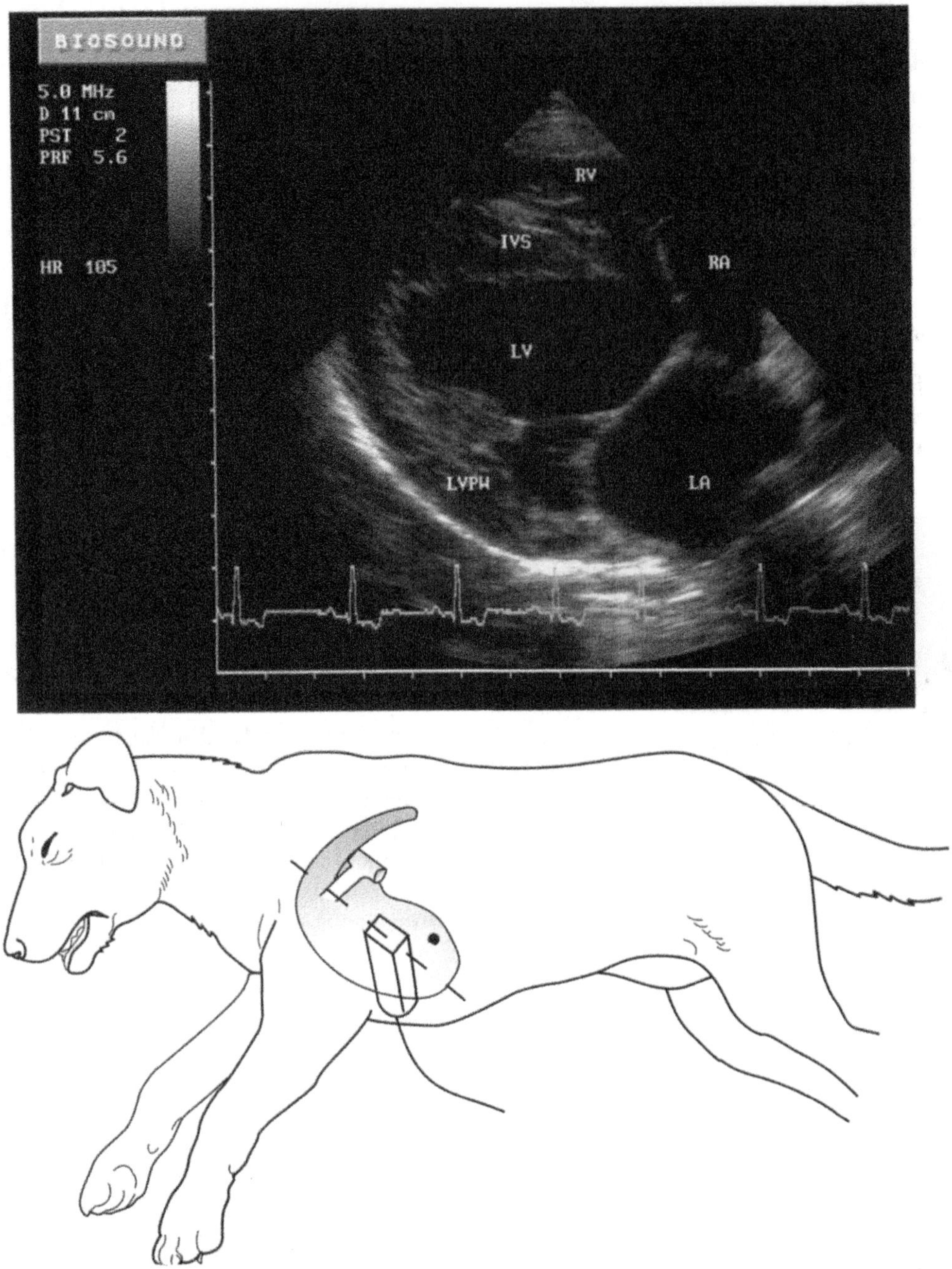

FIG. 15-75 **A,** Long-axis four-chamber view. *RA,* Right atrium; *RV,* right ventricle; *IVS,* interventricular septum; *LV,* left ventricle; *LA,* left atrium; *LVPW,* left ventricular posterior wall. **B,** Transducer positioning for long-axis four-chamber view.

Long-axis left ventricular outflow view

The long-axis left ventricular (LV) outflow view displays the left ventricle, the left ventricular outflow tract (LVOT) area, the aortic valve, and the aorta (Figure 15-76, *A*). The right atrium and ventricle can also be imaged from this view. From the long-axis four-chamber view, a very slight counterclockwise rotation of the transducer is made to bring the LVOT and aorta into view. To optimize the image, it may be necessary to fan cranially ever so slightly. The movements of the transducer are miniscule to achieve this image (Figure 15-76, *B*).

A

B

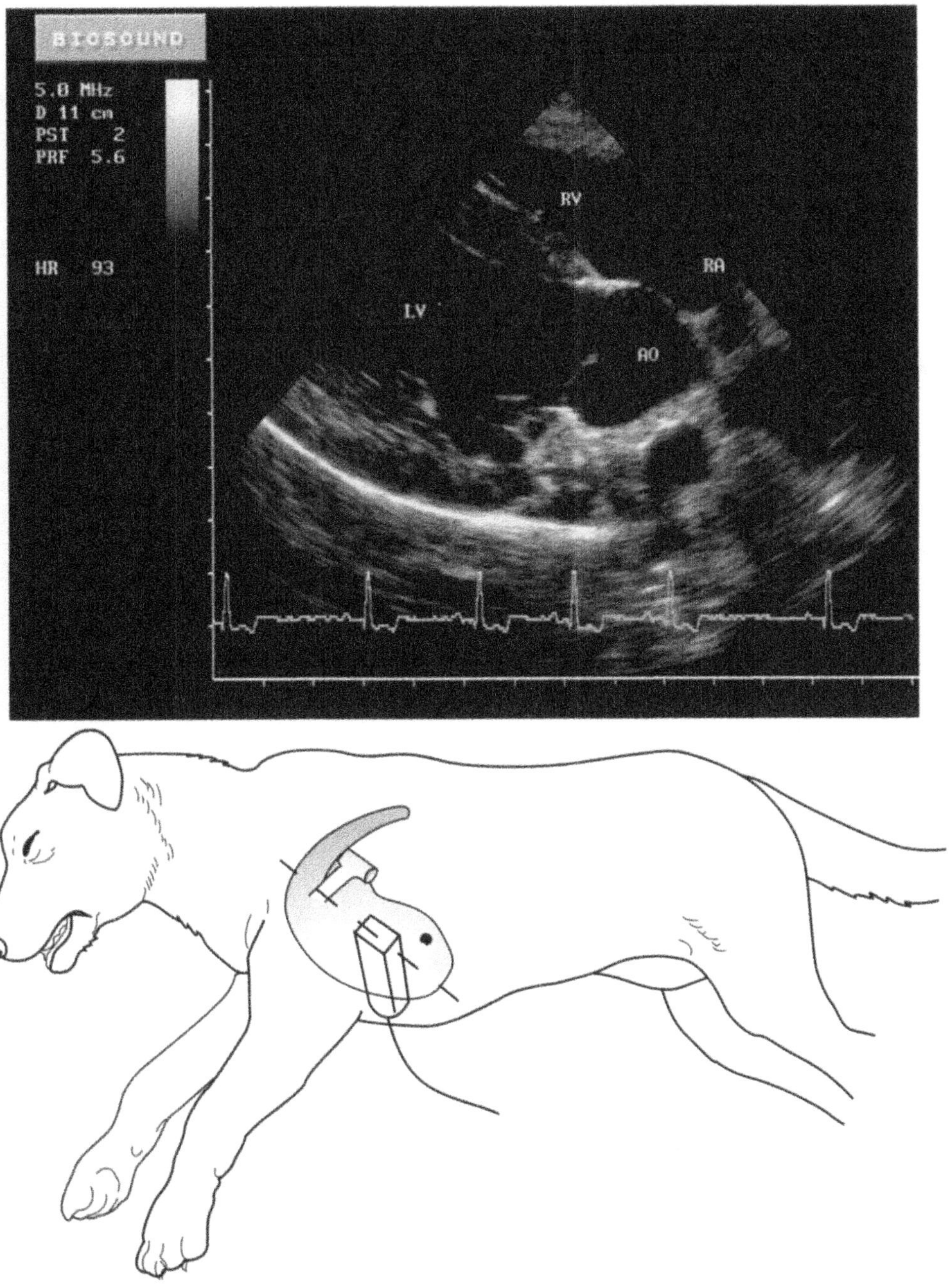

FIG. 15-76 **A,** Long-axis left ventricular outflow view. *AO,* Aorta. **B,** Transducer positioning for long-axis left ventricular outflow view.

Short-axis papillary muscle view

The short-axis papillary muscle view displays a cross-sectional image of the left ventricle at the level of the papillary muscles and the right ventricle (Figure 15-77, *A*). From the long-axis LV outflow view, an approximate 90-degree counterclockwise rotation of the transducer is made. The direction indicator on the transducer is in the cranioventral position (Figure 15-77, *B*). Fanning the transducer either craniodorsal toward the base of the heart or caudoventral toward the apex of the heart allows for optimized imaging of the papillary muscles.

A

B

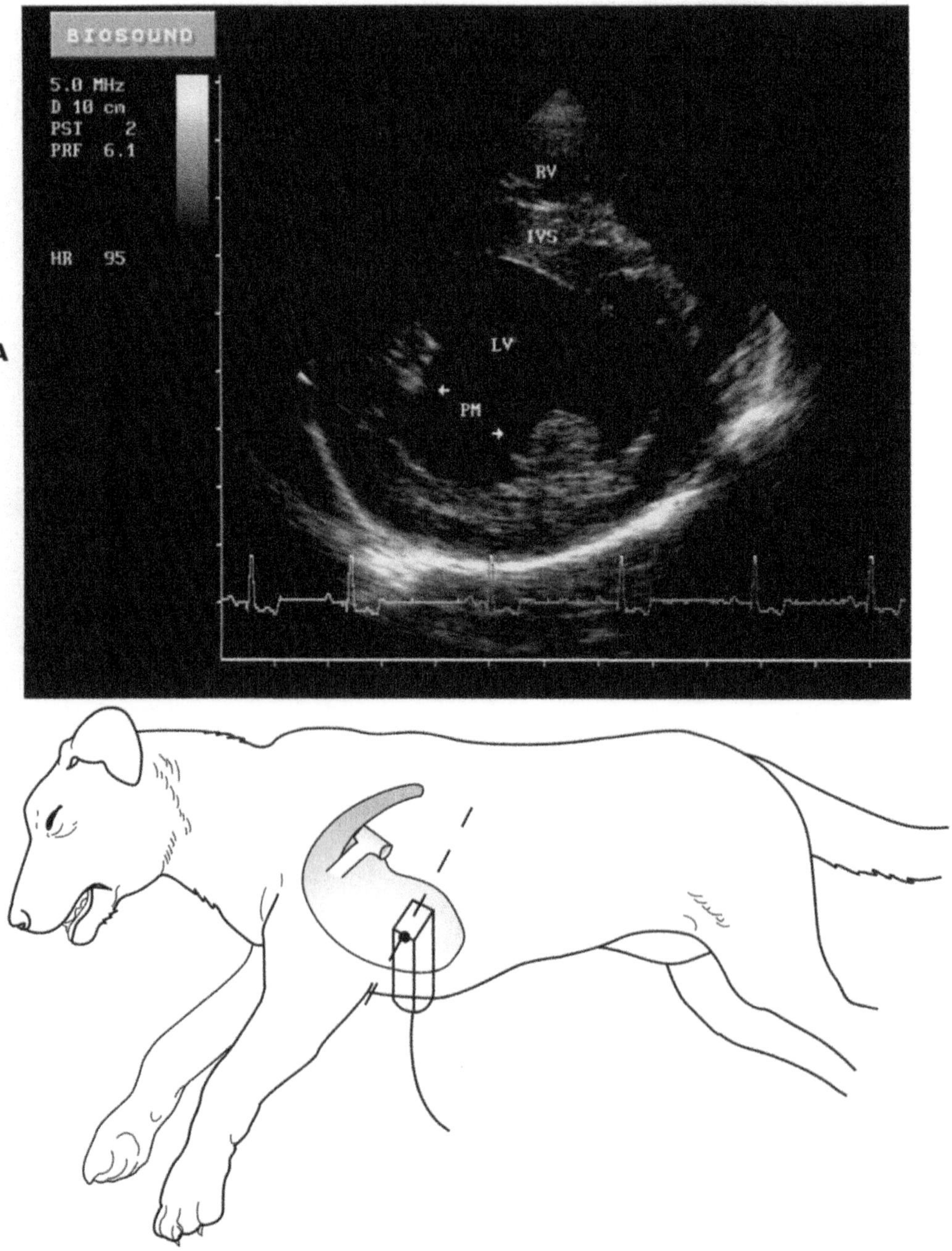

FIG. 15-77 **A,** Short-axis papillary muscle view. *PM,* Papillary muscle. **B,** Transducer positioning for short-axis papillary muscle view.

Short-axis mitral valve view

The short-axis mitral valve view ("fish lips" view) displays a cross-sectional image of the LVOT at the level of the mitral valve, the mitral valve, the right ventricle, and papillary muscles in the right ventricle (Figure 15-78, *A*). From the short-axis papillary view, slightly slide or fan the transducer craniodorsally until the mitral valve leaflets come into view (Figure 15-78, *B*). Slight fanning of the transducer either craniodorsal to the base of the heart or caudoventral to the apex of the heart allows for optimal visualization of the mitral valve.

A

B

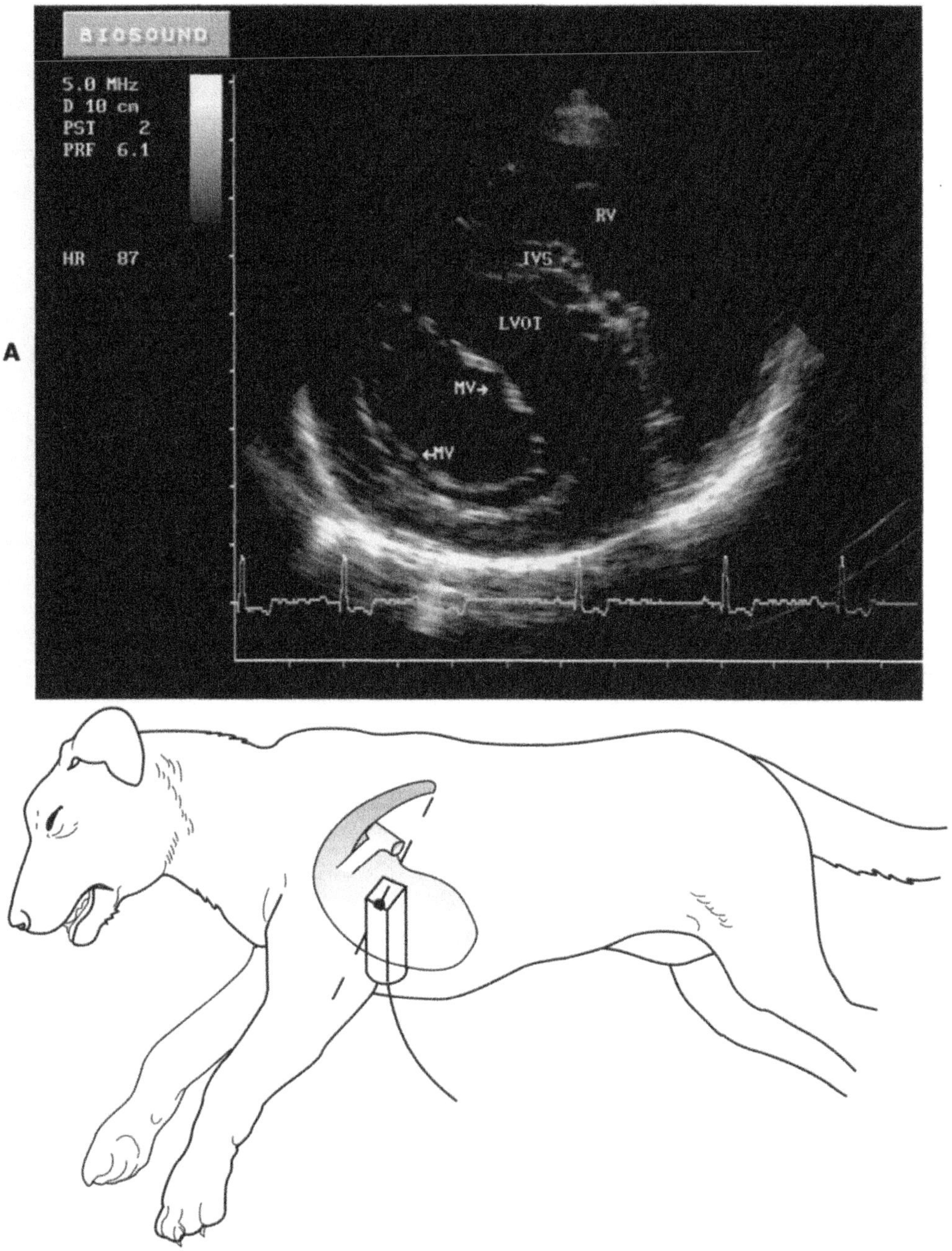

FIG. 15-78 **A,** Short-axis mitral valve view ("fish lips" view). *LVOT,* Left ventricular outflow tract; *MV,* mitral valve. **B,** Transducer positioning for short-axis mitral valve view.

Short-axis aorta/left atrium view

The short-axis aorta/left atrium view displays a cross-sectional image of the left atrium at the level of the aortic valve (Figure 15-79, *A*). From the short-axis mitral valve view, slightly fan the transducer craniodorsally until the left atrium is maximized and the cross section of the aortic valve cusps comes into view. Fan the transducer either craniodorsal to the base of the heart or caudoventral to the apex of the heart until the left atrium appears as a rounded triangle and the aortic valve is visualized (Figure 15-79, *B*). This view is used to compare the aortic diameter to the width of the left atrium. Normal values have been established for both canine

A

B

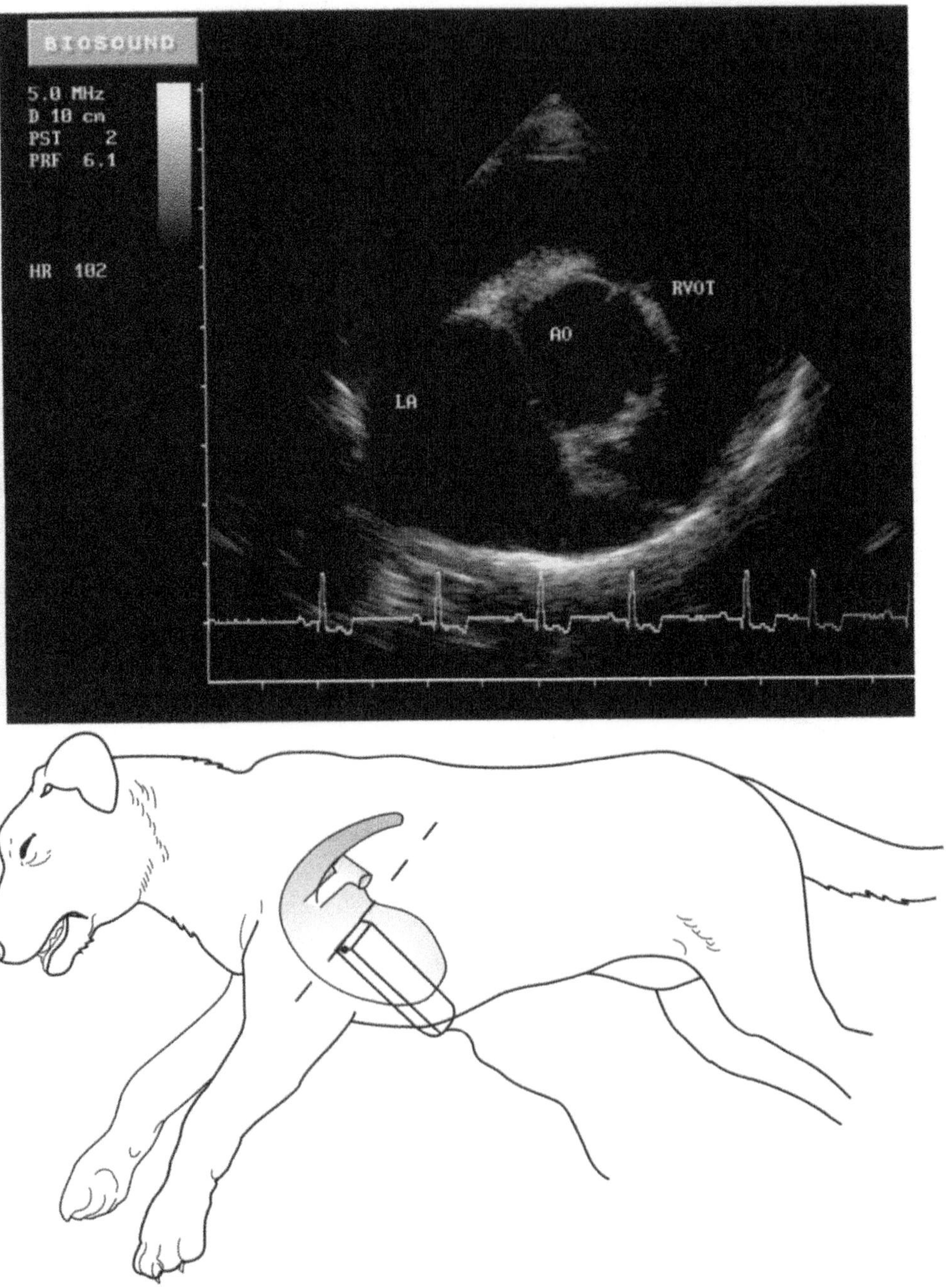

FIG. 15-79 A, Short-axis aorta/left atrium view. *RVOT,* Right ventricular outflow tract. **B,** Transducer positioning for short-axis aorta/left atrium view.

and feline patients. The aortic diameter measurement is made from the origin of the noncoronary cusp across the aorta to a point approximately midway between the right coronary and left coronary cusps. The width of the left atrium is measured through the body of the left atrium at the widest point in an orientation nearly paralleling the aortic diameter measurement (Figure 15-80).

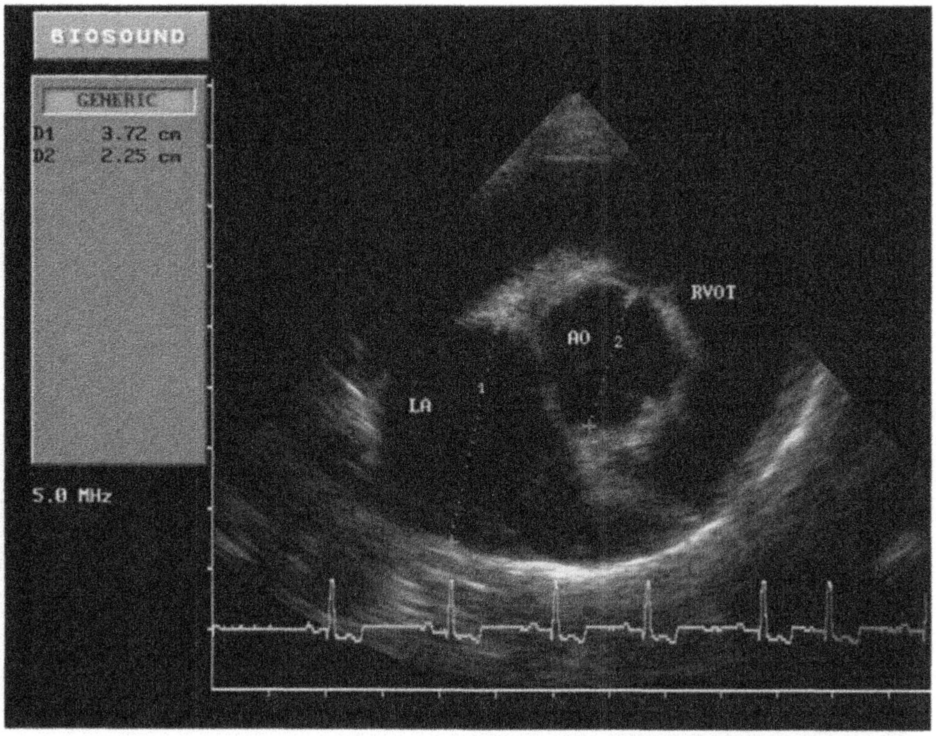

FIG. 15-80 One method of measuring the aorta *(AO)* and the left atrium *(LA)* to derive an Ao:LA ratio.

Short-axis pulmonic valve view

The short-axis pulmonic valve view displays a long-axis image of the right ventricular outflow tract, the pulmonic valve, and a cross-sectional view of the aorta (Figure 15-81, *A*). The short-axis aorta/left atrium view may allow visualization of the pulmonic valve. If the pulmonic valve is not seen, slightly fanning the transducer craniodorsally or sliding the transducer cranially one rib space may be necessary to visualize the valve (Figure 15-81, *B*).

A

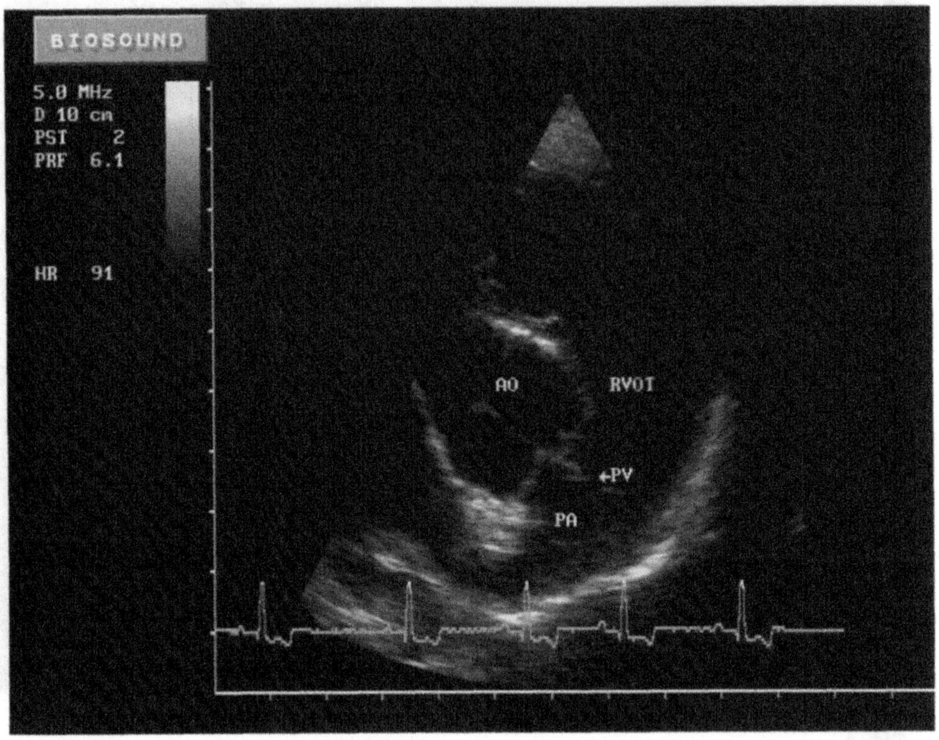

B

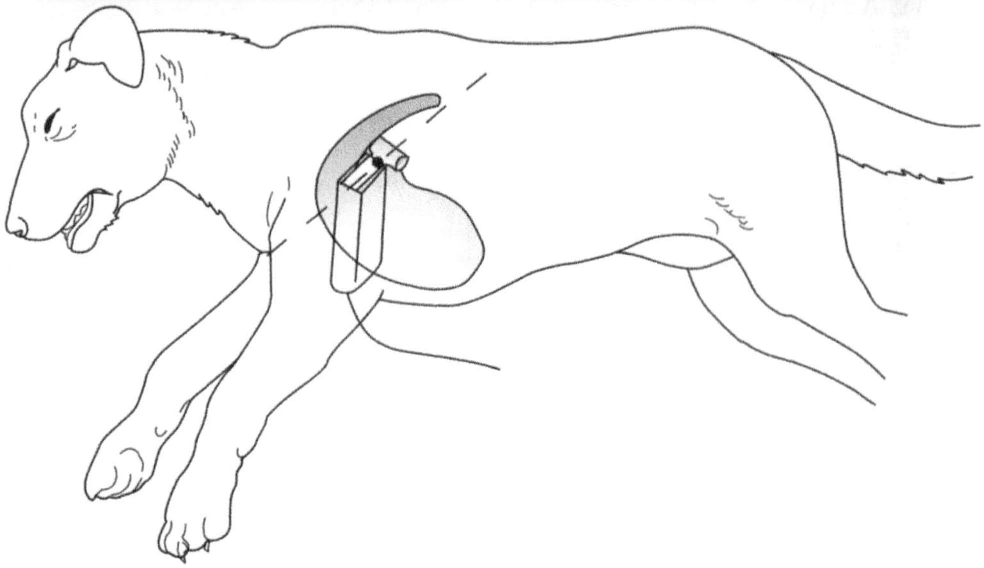

FIG. 15-81 A, Short-axis pulmonic valve view. **B,** Transducer positioning for short-axis pulmonic valve

M-Mode Imaging

M-mode is a useful method to document the motion of the left ventricle and the mitral and aortic valves toward or away from the transducer. M-mode echocardiography uses an extremely thin ultrasound beam across different positions of the heart to detect the motion of ventricular walls and valve leaflets in relation to the transducer. With M-mode echocardiography the motion of the heart along this thin ultrasound beam is recorded over a time-oriented baseline (horizontal axis). Three common positions are used to evaluate valve motion and measure chamber size and ventricular wall thickness.

The *first position* places the M-line across the left ventricle at a level between the papillary muscles and chordae tendineae. The M-line can be placed with the cardiac image in either a short axis or a long axis. With either view, care must be taken to maintain the M-line perpendicular to the interventricular septum and the LV free wall. Misalignment of the M-line can result in a false LV free wall and interventricular septum thickening. Paradoxical motion of the interventricular septum and LV free wall could also be seen with improper placement of the M-line. Once a clean M-mode run is obtained, measurements of the interventricular septum, LV lumen, and LV free wall in diastole and systole can be made (Figure 15-82). Most ultrasound machines have a cardiac package that run through these measurements step by step.

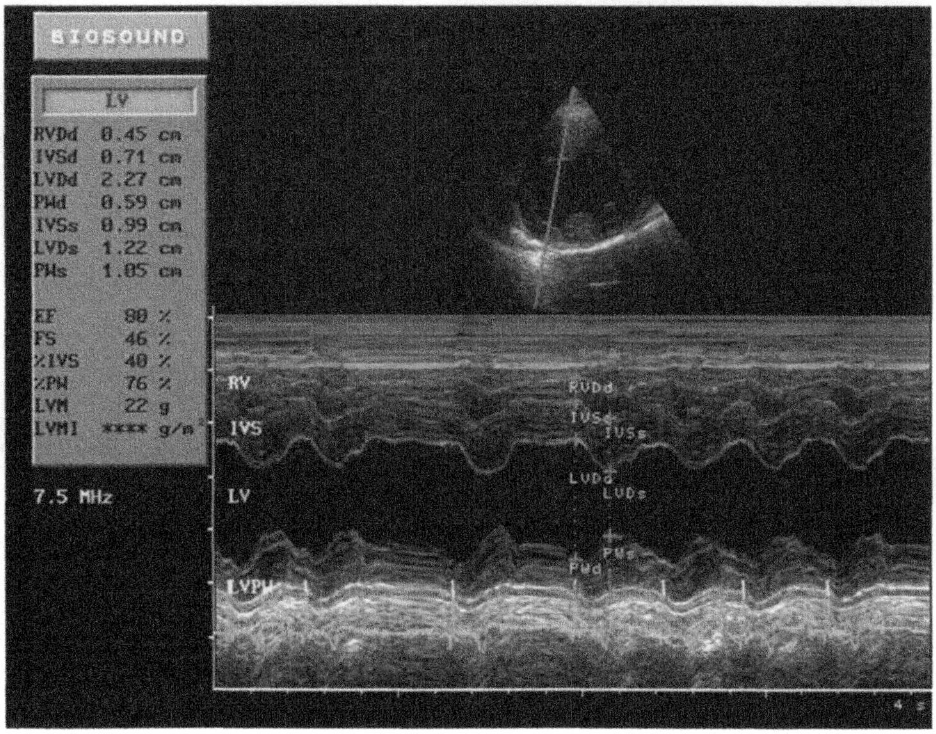

FIG. 15-82 Standard M-mode tracing through the left ventricle.

The *second position* places the M-line at the tip of the mitral valve. Again, this can be obtained in either the long-axis four-chamber view or the short-axis mitral valve view. This M-mode position is used to evaluate the motion of the mitral valve. The anterior leaflet of the mitral valve produces a double-peaked line during ventricular diastole. The first (and largest) peak is called the *E peak*, which represents the passive filling of the left ventricle following ventricular systole. The second peak is called the *A peak*, which represents movement of the mitral valve following atrial contraction to further fill the left ventricle with blood before systole (Figure 15-83).

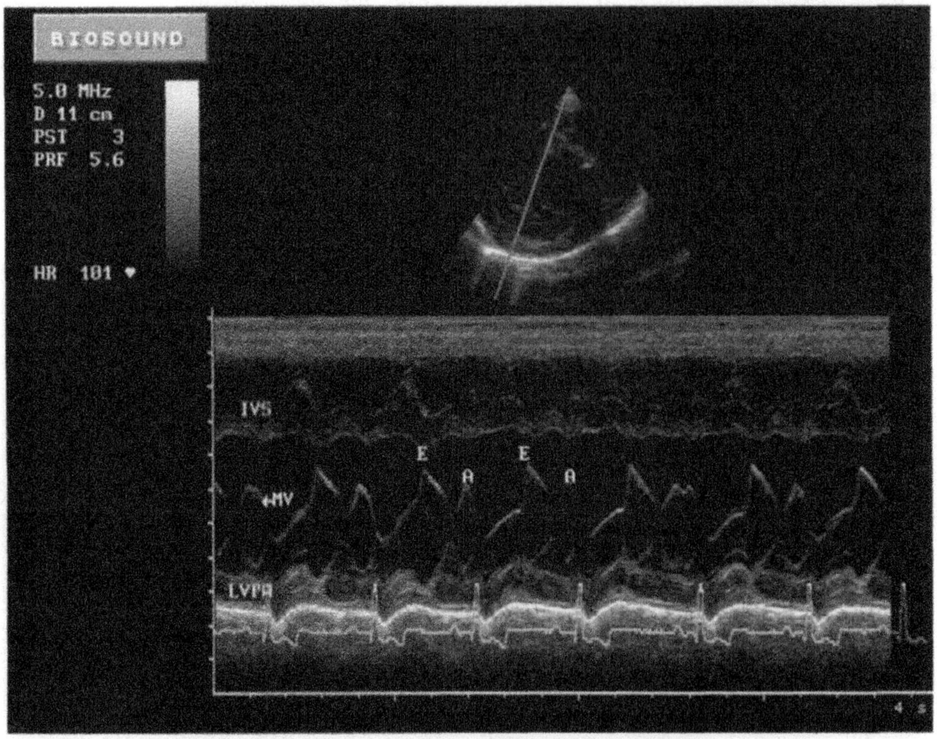

FIG. 15-83 Standard M-mode tracing across the mitral valve.

The *third position* places the M-line across the aortic valve. Again, this M-mode tracing can be obtained in either the long-axis LV outflow view or the short-axis aorta/left atrium view. This M-mode position is used to evaluate the motion of the aortic valve during opening and closing (Figure 15-84).

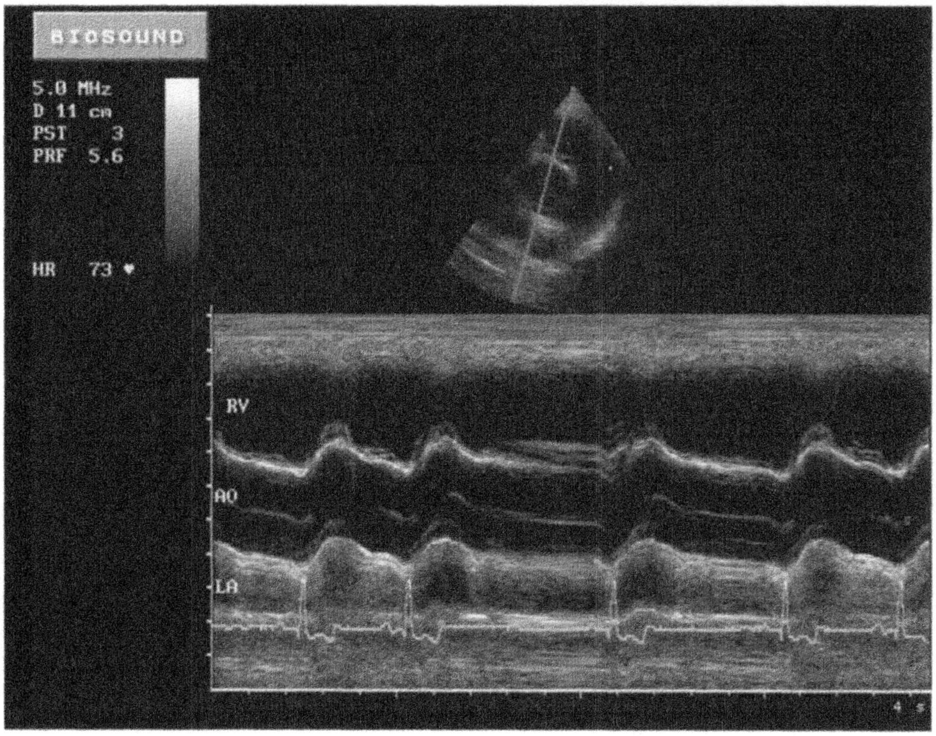

FIG. 15-84 Standard M-mode tracing across the aortic valve.

Recommended Reading

Curry TS III et al: *Christensen's physics of diagnostic radiology*, ed 4, Philadelphia, 1990, Lea & Febiger.

Miles KG: Basic principles and clinic applications of diagnostic ultrasonography, *Compendium* 11(5):609, 1989.

Nyland TG, Mattoon JS: *Veterinary diagnostic ultrasound*, ed 2, Philadelphia, 2002, Saunders.

Park RD et al: B-mode gray-scale ultrasound: imaging artifacts and interpretation principles, *Vet Radiol* 22(5):204, 1981.

Powis RL, Powis WJ: *A thinker's guide to ultrasonic imaging*, Baltimore, 1984, Urban and Schwarzenberg.

Rantanen NW, Ewing RL: Principles of ultrasound applications in animals, *Vet Radiol* 22(5):196, 1981.

Toal RL: *Ultrasound for the practitioner*, 1992, Wallingford, Conn, Corometrics Medical Systems.

Glossary

A-mode Amplitude mode; displays the returning echoes as a series of peaks on a graph. The greater the intensity of the returning echo, the higher the peak on the graph.

Absorbed dose Quantity of energy imparted by ionizing radiation to matter per unit mass of the matter.

Acoustic impedance Ability of living tissue to resist or impede transmission of sound. Acoustic impedance varies slightly among most tissue, depending on the density and elasticity of the tissue.

Air-gap technique Method used to decrease scatter radiation when a grid is not available. The technique uses a 6-foot focal-film distance (FFD) and a 6-inch object-film distance (OFD). The increased OFD decreases the amount of scatter that reaches the film, and the increased FFD decreases the amount of penumbra and magnification created by increasing the OFD.

Anechoic Describes tissue that transmits sound through to deeper tissues, reflecting none back to the transducer. Anechoic areas appear black on the monitor.

Anode Site of x-ray generation in x-ray tube; contains a tungsten metal plate on which electrons are focused.

Arthrography Radiographic study in which contrast medium is injected into the synovial fluid to contrast the articular surface and joint capsule.

Attenuation Process in which ultrasound waves traveling through tissues lose their intensity, or *attenuate*, as a result of scatter or absorption.

Axial resolution Ability to differentiate between two reflecting interfaces that lie along the axis of the transmitted sound beam.

B-mode Brightness mode; uses bright pixels on the monitor to represent the intensity of the returning echoes. The brighter the pixel, the greater its intensity. The image generated is a two-dimensional slice that is continually being updated.

Barium enema Contrast study used to evaluate the cecum and rectum by administering contrast medium directly into the colon.

Cathode Site of electron generation in x-ray tube; contains a filament consisting of a tightly coiled tungsten wire. As current is applied to the filament, electrons are "boiled off" and become available to be accelerated toward the anode.

Caudal Pertaining to structures or areas situated toward the tail.

Celiography Contrast study used to evaluate the abdominal cavity and the integrity of the diaphragm.

Collimator Device used to restrict the size of the x-ray beam.

Contralateral Pertaining to the opposite side.

Contrast media Substances used to opacify or delineate an organ system against the surrounding organs.

Cranial Pertaining to structures or areas situated toward the head.

Cystography Contrast study used to evaluate the urinary bladder.

Developer Processing chemical that changes the sensitized silver halide crystals into black metallic silver.

Distal Pertaining to structures or areas situated away from the point of attachment.

Dorsal Pertaining to body areas situated toward the back or topline of quadrupeds.

Dose equivalent Quantity obtained by multiplying the absorbed dose in tissue by the quality factor.

Dosimetry Method used to measure ionizing radiation exposure to personnel.

Double contrast Contrast procedure that uses both positive-contrast and negative-contrast media.

Echoic Describes tissue that reflects most of the sound back to the transducer. Echoic tissue appears white on the monitor; also referred to as *echogenic*.

Electron cloud When current is applied to the cathode filament, electrons are "boiled off." These electrons make up the electron cloud.

Esophography Contrast study used to evaluate the esophagus.

Excitation Process by which an electron is moved to a higher energy level within the atom.

Excretory urography Contrast study used to evaluate the kidneys, ureters, and urinary bladder; provides information relative to renal function.

Exposure latitude Range of exposures that produce a film density of diagnostic quality.

Filament Tightly coiled tungsten wire that is placed in the focusing cup of the cathode.

Fistulography Contrast study that delineates the extent and possible origin of fistulous tracts.

Fixer Processing chemical responsible for removing the remaining silver halide crystals from the film emulsion.

Focal-film distance (FFD) Distance from the focal spot to the recording surface (film or cassette).

Focal spot Site on the anode where the electrons are focused. The focal spot is oriented at an 11- to 20-degree angle.

Focal zone Method of improving the resolution of the returning echoes. The sound beam can be focused either by electronic means or by an acoustic lens.

Focusing cup Part of the cathode that restricts the diameter of accelerating electrons to the focal spot on the anode.

Fog Decrease in the differences in tissue densities between two adjacent shadows. Fog can be caused by a low-grade light leak in the darkroom, scatter radiation, high temperatures, and improper processing techniques.

Foreshortening Radiographic effect occurring when the object is not parallel to the recording surface. This causes a distortion of the size and length of the object.

Frequency Number of complete waveforms (cycles) per unit of time.

Gastrography Contrast study used to evaluate the stomach.

Grid Series of thin linear strips made of alternating radiodense and radiolucent interspacers. Grids are used to decrease the amount of scatter radiation and increase the contrast on the radiograph.

Grid cutoff Absorption of excessive amounts of x-rays caused by improper alignment of the grid to the center of the primary beam or placement of the primary beam at an angle other than perpendicular to the grid.

Heel effect Uneven distribution of the x-ray beam intensity emitted from the x-ray tube.

High frequency Referring to x-ray generators that use a series of conversions and manipulations in the current to produce a more constant radiation output.

Hyperechoic Describes tissues that reflect more sound back to the transducer. Hyperechoic tissues appear brighter than surrounding tissues.

Hypoechoic Describes tissues that reflect less sound back to the transducer. Hypoechoic tissues appear darker than surrounding tissues.

Inverse square law Intensity of the x-ray beam is inversely proportional to the square of the distance from the source of the x-rays.

Ionization Process in which an outer electron is completely removed from the atom so that the atom is left positively charged.

Isoechoic Describes tissues that have the same echotexture as surrounding tissues.

kVp Kilovoltage peak; voltage applied between the cathode and anode. Increasing the kVp results in a shorter-wavelength x-ray beam that is more penetrating.

Latent image Silver halide crystals in the film emulsion that have been exposed to a radiant energy become sensitized and susceptible to chemical change. These susceptible crystals make up the latent image.

Lateral Pertaining to structures or body areas situated away from the median plane or midline.

Lateral resolution Ability to differentiate between two reflecting interfaces that lie in a plane perpendicular to the transmitted sound beam.

Linear scanner Device that produces a rectangle-shaped image; useful when imaging areas with an unrestricted acoustic window (e.g., equine tendons).

M-mode Motion mode; continuous display of a thin slice of an organ over a time-oriented baseline.

mA Milliamperage; controls the number of electrons generated at the filament of the cathode, increasing the number of x-rays produced.

mAs Product of milliamperage and exposure time.

Medial Pertaining to structures or body areas situated toward the median plane or midline.

Myelography Contrast study used to evaluate the spinal cord for the site and nature of lesions not seen on survey radiographs.

Negative contrast Contrast media low in atomic number, appearing radiolucent on the radiograph.

Nonselective angiography Contrast study used to obtain specific information about cardiac abnormalities.

Object-film distance (OFD) Distance from the object being imaged to the recording surface (film or cassette).

Oblique Radiographic projection used to set off an area that would normally be superimposed over another area.

Palmar Pertaining to structures or body areas situated on the caudal aspect of the front limb, distal to the antebrachiocarpal joint.

Penumbra Blurring at the tissue interfaces.

Photons Small packets of energy; also referred to as *quanta.*

Plantar Pertaining to structures or body areas situated on the caudal aspect of the rear limb, distal to the tarsocrural joint.

Pneumoperitoneography Contrast study used to evaluate the abdominal organs better when subject contrast in the animal is decreased.

Positive contrast Contrast medium high in atomic number, appearing radiodense on the radiograph.

Potter-bucky diaphragm Device that sets the grid in motion, blurring the white lines on the finished radiograph that are produced by the grid.

Proximal Pertaining to structures or body areas situated closer to the point of attachment.

Radiodense Describes an area that absorbs x-rays, appearing white on the finished radiograph.

Radiographic contrast Differences in radiographic density between adjacent areas on the radiographic image.

Radiographic density Degree of blackness on a finished radiograph.

Radiographic detail When the tissue interfaces are sharp and possess good contrast.

Radiolucent Describes an area that absorbs fewer x-rays than other areas, appearing darker on the finished radiograph.

rem (roentgen-equivalent-man) Unit of measurement of the absorbed dose of ionizing radiation.

Rostral Pertaining to structures or body areas on the head situated toward the nose.

Rotating anode Disc-shaped piece of metal (usually molybdenum alloy) containing a tungsten insert around the periphery.

Scatter radiation Longer-wavelength x-ray that has no usefulness to the formation of the image; results in a great decrease in the contrast on the finished radiograph.

Sector scanner Device that produces a pie-shaped image with a narrow near field and a wide far field; useful when imaging areas with a restricted acoustic window (e.g., intercostal).

Sialography Contrast study used to evaluate salivary ducts and glands.

Sonolucent Describes the tissue that transmits most of the sound to deeper tissues, with only a few waves being reflected back to the transducer; appears dark on the monitor.

Stationary anode Part of x-ray tube that consists of a block of tungsten embedded into a block of copper on the anode side of the tube.

Subject density Ability of different tissue densities to absorb x-rays. These differences depend on the average atomic number and thickness of the area.

Time gain compensation (TGC) Series of controls on an ultrasound machine that are used to make like tissues look the same.

Transducer Instrument used to conduct an ultrasound of tissues; emits a series of pulses and then receives the returning echoes.

Tube overload Combined kVp and mA are too high for the machine. Too much heat is created, causing the anode to crack.

Tube rating chart Measurements that help to determine the maximum exposure characteristics that allow safe operation of the machine, prolonging the life of the x-ray tube.

Tube saturation Situation in which the positive potential (voltage) between the cathode and the anode is insufficient to pull all the electrons across the tube. Extra electrons build up on the glass envelope, causing it to crack.

Ultrasound Noninvasive method of imaging soft tissues by sending low-intensity, high-frequency sound waves into tissues and then listening for the returning echoes that have been reflected.

Upper gastrointestinal series Contrast study used to evaluate the stomach and small intestine.

Urethrography Contrast study used to evaluate the urethra.

Vaginography Contrast study used to evaluate the vagina and urethra.

Velocity Speed at which sound travels through a medium.

Ventral Pertaining to structures or body areas situated toward the underside of the quadrupeds.

Wavelength Distance of one complete waveform. With ultrasound, it is the distance from one band of compression or rarefaction to the next.

X-rays Form of electromagnetic radiation; similar to visible light, with shorter wavelengths.

Index

Page numbers followed by f indicate figures; t tables.

Q

R

S

CPI Antony Rowe
Eastbourne, UK
January 04, 2023